Color Atlas of
Infectious and Inflammatory Diseases
of the External Eye

Color Atlas of Infectious and Inflammatory Diseases of the External Eye

H. Bruce Ostler, M.D.

Clinical Professor of Ophthalmology and
Research Ophthalmologist
Francis I. Proctor Foundation
and Department of Ophthalmology
University of California
San Francisco

Chandler R. Dawson, M.D.

Professor of Ophthalmology
and Director
Francis I. Proctor Foundation
University of California
San Francisco

Masao Okumoto, M.A.

Specialist in Ocular Microbiology
Francis I. Proctor Foundation
University of California
San Francisco

Urban & Schwarzenberg · Baltimore–Munich 1987

Urban & Schwarzenberg, Inc.
7 E. Redwood Street
Baltimore, Maryland 21202
USA

Urban & Schwarzenberg
Pettenkoferstrasse 18
D-8000 München 2
West Germany

Printed in Germany

NOTICES

The Editors (or Author(s)) and the Publisher of this work have made every effort to ensure that the drug dosage schedules herein are accurate and in accord with the standards accepted at the time of publication. The reader is strongly advised, however, to check the product information sheet included in the package of each drug he or she plans to administer to be certain that changes have not been made in the recommended dose or in the contraindications for administration.

The Publishers have made an extensive effort to trace original copyright holders for permission to use borrowed material. If any has been overlooked, it will be corrected at the first reprint.

Library of Congress Cataloging in Publication Data

Ostler, H. Bruce.
Color atlas of infectious and inflammatory diseases of the external eye.

Includes index.
1. Eye–Diseases and defects–Diagnosis–Atlases.
2. Eye–Infections–Diagnosis–Atlases.
3. Inflammation–Diagnosis–Atlases. I. Dawson, Chandler R., 1930– . II. Okumoto, Masao.
III. Title. [DNLM: 1. Eye Diseases–diagnosis–atlases. WW 17 085c]
RE71.088 1986 617.7'15 86-15941
ISBN 0-8067-1411-5

Sponsoring Editor: Charles W. Mitchell
Manuscript Editor: Linda Hansford
Proofreader: Linda Powell

ISBN 0-8067-1411-5 Baltimore
ISBN 3-541-71411-5 Munich

Foreword

It is a pleasure to write a foreword to this long-awaited *Atlas of Infectious and Inflammatory Diseases of the External Eye,* prepared by three distinguished senior members of the Francis I. Proctor Foundation for Research in Ophthalmology. In accordance with the express wishes of its founder, Mrs. Francis I. Proctor, the Foundation's special mission is research devoted to infectious and immunological ocular disease, to be accompanied by the training of fellows in external ocular disease and uveitis. This mission has provided the authors of the Atlas — Dr. H. Bruce Ostler, in charge of fellowship training; Dr. Chandler R. Dawson, Director of the Foundation; and Mr. Masao Okumoto, principal microbiologist — with the ammunition they needed to produce an outstanding volume.

Dr. Ostler is a highly esteemed consultant on external eye disease, and his experience has been worldwide. He has examined ocular infections in patients of all races and nationalities in the line of duty as a consultant and by virtue of his great and growing interest in ocular leprosy. Dr. Dawson is an authority on chlamydial and viral diseases of the eye. His work as consultant to the World Health Organization and his many years of research on trachoma in Egypt, Tunisia, and other countries have given him worldwide knowledge of and experience with the whole field of infectious ocular disease. And Mr. Okumoto, who has developed at Proctor a highly sophisticated ocular microbiology laboratory, has to his credit a notable record of studies of ocular infections and many years of teaching advanced ocular microbiology to the Proctor fellows. Over the years he has acquired a very special ability to solve difficult diagnostic problems on the basis of his microbiological and cytological observations. He has spent his entire career at Proctor, and his contributions to the Atlas will be of special interest and value to the lesser microbiologists among us.

The Proctor Foundation is a memorial to the late Dr. Francis I. Proctor, whose primary interests in his latter days were the diagnosis, treatment, and prevention of trachoma and other infectious ocular diseases. In September 1987, the Proctor Foundation, established in 1947 by his widow in Dr. Proctor's memory, will celebrate 40 years of teaching and research. The publication of this fine Atlas is a most fitting event at this time in the Foundation's 40-year history. It will be a most valuable addition to every ophthalmologist's library, but it will also be, I have no doubt, a very special delight to the Foundation's worldwide roster of former fellows.

Phillips Thygeson
April 24, 1986

Preface

In this book, we describe with both text and photographs the major infectious and inflammatory diseases of the external eye. Despite the proliferation of therapeutic modalities, we have deliberately not discussed treatment, but have emphasized identification of specific diseases and syndromes. Because appropriate treatment must be based on the identification of the specific disease process, we have focused on the diagnostic entities. A second volume will be devoted to the management of the various infections and inflammatory diseases.

In writing this text, we have become increasingly conscious of the limitations in the present knowledge of medicine, but we hope that errors in this volume will be brought to our attention for correction in the future.

In ophthalmology, the disease processes are perceived by direct visual observation or measurement of functional change (e.g., loss of vision). This characteristic has led to the description of disease processes in the eye by their appearance as syndromes that incorporate separate disease processes; for example, in describing disease of the peripheral cornea, the syndromes described as Mooren's ulcer, Fuchs' superficial marginal keratitis, and Terrien's degeneration have very different outcomes and need radically different treatments.

While infections and inflammatory eye diseases occupied a major part of 19th century ophthalmology texts, they have been relatively neglected in training programs for ophthalmologists in the last 20 years. Treatment of these diseases is making rapid strides, however, and we hope this Atlas will provide a basis for the identification of these disease processes.

Acknowledgments

We wish to acknowledge the help of Nancy Thomas and Kathie Strack, who typed the manuscript, and Dr. Devron Char, who supplied many of the slides used in the chapter on orbital infections and inflammations.

We also wish to acknowledge and thank our publishers for their patience and advice, and to especially thank Mr. Charles Mitchell, who was so patient with us and willing to help.

Contents

Chapter 1

Introduction

Throughout the world, infectious and inflammatory diseases of the eye constitute a major portion of the problems encountered in ophthalmology. Trachoma, hypovitaminosis A (often becoming manifest during a measles infection), and onchocerciasis are major causes of blindness, especially in developing countries. Other infections that play major roles in loss of sight include herpes simplex keratitis, Hansen's disease, various bacterial corneal ulcers, and endophthalmitis. Iritis, iridocyclitis, and many of the chorioretinitities are major causes of blindness in both emerging and developed countries.

Because the eye and the ocular adnexa serve as a meeting place for the skin and mucous membranes, they also serve as a common ground for many disciplines of medicine. Furthermore, the structures of the external eye are accessible to direct observation with a variety of instruments, and there is an increasing base of specialized information about the external eye and adnexa in both sickness and health. In addition, the etiologies of different inflammatory reactions of the eye are becoming better understood, allowing clinical differentiation between viral, bacterial, and chlamydial infections and their pathogenesis.

Laboratory Tests

Identification of potential pathogenic organisms can be made using cultures of an infected lid, conjunctiva, or cornea, of the ocular fluids of the eye, and of exudates from draining sinuses or fluctuant areas in the orbit, lacrimal sac, or lacrimal gland. The identification of these organisms is essential for the adequate treatment and management of the infectious process of the eye.

Bacterial Cultures

For routine cultures of the external eye, cultures from the lid margin and conjunctiva of both eyes are placed on the same bacteriological culture plate. This procedure provides detailed information on the etiology of conjunctival and lid margin infections and is efficient in terms of cost and time.

For cultures of the lid margin and conjunctiva, the cotton tip of a sterile applicator stick premoistened with sterile broth, sterile saline, or sterile water without inhibitors is used; this increases the detection of bacterial organisms by at least 50% when compared with the use of a dry cotton-tipped applicator stick. To sample bacterial flora of the right conjunctiva, the swab is rubbed or rolled gently across the tarsal conjunctiva of the right eye and is then used to streak a blood agar plate and a mannitol salt agar plate. (The letters "RC" are made on the culture media to represent the right conjunctiva.) The same swab is rubbed across the base of the eyelashes and the inner canthal region of the skin and is then streaked on the blood agar and mannitol salt agar plates in the form of the letters "RL" (right lids) (Fig. 1–1 A). For the left conjunctiva and left eyelids, a new swab is used in a similar fashion and the letters "LC" and "LL" are used (Figs. 1–1 A, 1–1 B). The highest yields are obtained if the swabs are immediately streaked onto the culture media rather than placed in a sterile tube or in transport media for plating in the laboratory. A substantial overgrowth of commensals and failure of detection of pathogenic organisms occurs when transport media are used or when there is a delay in plating. The recovery of pathogenic organisms, and especially the more fastidious organisms, is also reduced by the use of a topical anesthetic prior to making the cultures.

When cultures are made of the cornea, separate bacteriological plates are used, and several C-shaped smears are made (Fig. 1–1 C) on the medium so that there is no mistake about where the culture has originated. To obtain adequate specimens from the cornea, anesthesia is usually required and is readily achieved by dropping a topical anesthetic into the conjunctival sac. Scrapings are then made of the cornea with a platinum spatula, Bard-Parker knife, or any instrument that is sufficiently rigid. The scrapings are transferred to the appropriate culture media.

If cultures are made of ocular fluids or fluids from fluctuant areas, the specimens should be transported to the laboratory, where one or two drops of the material can be placed on the medium and spread evenly over the surface with a bacteriological loop.

Once the specimens have been transferred to culture media, the plates or tubes should be quickly transported to the laboratory for incubation. The mannitol salt agar is placed in a standard incubator (without CO_2) at 35° C. The sheep's blood agar and all other media except for Sabouraud's medium and media for anaerobic cultures are placed in a CO_2 incubator at 35° C. The Sabouraud's medium is sealed and placed in a 30° C incubator or kept at room temperature.

Although we routinely use sheep's blood agar and mannitol salt agar (Fig. 1–2), other culture media, such as chocolate blood agar, cooked meat, thioglycolate, and Lowenstein-Jensen media, may be used, as clinically indicated (Table 1–1).

Table 1–1 Media Recommended for Culturing of Various Infectious Agents from the Eye

Clinical Impression	Organism	Culture Media
Bacterial blepharitis	*Staphylococcus aureus*	Blood and mannitol agar
	Staphylococcus epidermidis	Blood and mannitol agar
	Moraxella lacunata	Blood agar or Loeffler's medium
	Streptococcus spp. (including *S. pneumoniae*)	Blood agar
	Acinetobacter calcoaceticus	Blood agar
	Corynebacterium diphtheriae	Blood agar
	Mycobacterium tuberculosis	Lowenstein-Jensen medium
Fungal blepharitis	*Candida* spp.	Sabouraud's agar
	Trichophyton mentagrophytes	Sabouraud's agar
	Coccidioides immitis	Sabouraud's agar
Bacterial conjunctivitis	*Staphylococcus aureus*	Blood and mannitol agar
	Streptococcus spp. (including *S. pneumoniae*)	Blood agar
	Haemophilus spp.	Chocolate blood agar; sheep's blood agar inoculated with *Staphylococcus*
	Moraxella spp.	Blood agar
	Actinomyces spp.	Thioglycolate medium fluid; blood agar in anaerobic jar
	Neisseria gonorrhoeae and *meningitidis*	Chocolate blood agar
	Francisella tularensis	Chocolate blood agar supplemented with cystine or cysteine
	Mycobacterium tuberculosis	Lowenstein-Jensen medium
	Corynebacterium diphtheriae	Blood agar
	Proteus spp.	Blood agar
Chlamydial conjunctivitis	*Chlamydia trachomatis* and *psittaci*	Yolk sac, tissue culture (McCoy cells or a heteroploid mouse line require centrifugation to facilitate growth)
Bacterial keratitis	*Pseudomonas aeruginosa*	Blood agar
	Streptococcus spp. (including *S. pneumoniae*)	Blood agar
	Moraxella spp.	Blood agar or Loeffler's medium
	Staphylococcus aureus	Blood and mannitol agar
	Serratia marcescens	Blood agar

Clinical Impression	Organism	Culture Media
	Proteus spp.	Blood agar
	Klebsiella spp.	Blood agar
	Branhamella catarrhalis	Blood agar
	Peptostreptococcus spp.	Thioglycolate medium (fluid); cooked meat; or blood agar in anaerobic jar
Fungal keratitis	*Candida* spp.	Sabouraud's agar
	Fusarium spp.	Sabouraud's agar
	Aspergillus spp.	Sabouraud's agar
	Penicillium spp.	Sabouraud's agar
	Acremonium spp. *(Cephalosporium)*	Sabouraud's agar
	Alternaria spp.	Sabouraud's agar
Bacterial endophthalmitis	*Staphylococcus epidermidis*	Blood agar
	Staphylococcus aureus	Blood agar
	Streptococcus spp. (including *S. pneumoniae*)	Blood agar
	Pseudomonas aeruginosa	Blood agar
	Serratia marcescens	Blood agar
	Proteus spp.	Blood agar
	Escherichia coli	Blood agar
	Klebsiella pneumoniae	Blood agar
	Enterobacter aerogenes	Blood agar
	Propionibacterium acnes	Thioglycolate medium, cooked meat medium; blood agar in anaerobic jar
	Clostridium perfringens	Blood agar in anaerobic jar or cooked meat
	Nocardia asteroides	Blood agar or Sabouraud's agar
	Bacillus cereus	Blood agar

Cytological Study

To obtain cytological specimens from the lid margin, conjunctiva, or cornea, a platinum (Kimura or Lindner) spatula or any sterile instrument that is moderately thin and sharp can be used (Fig. 1–3). It is critical to obtain sufficient material for cytological examination if the laboratory work is expected to be of any value.

Scrapings of the lid margin can be taken without anesthetic by pulling the lid margin away from the surface of the eye and scraping only the margin of the eyelid. On the other hand, a topical anesthetic is necessary to obtain scrapings of the conjunctiva and cornea.

To obtain maximum information, the area of greatest inflammation should be scraped with the edge of the spatula, exerting sufficient pressure to cause blanching but not bleeding of the conjunctiva (if the conjunctiva is being scraped). The material is transferred to a microscope slide, and should be spread evenly over a few centimeters of the slide (Yoneda et al., 1975). If the slide is observed under bright light, the unstained specimen should be clearly visible on the slide (Sanderson et al., 1980; Motyl et al., 1984).

To obtain a scraping from the cornea, a topical anesthetic should be instilled into the conjunctival sac and the area of infiltration or ulceration scraped; the material should then be transferred to a microscope slide. In many instances, the scraping is more readily performed under magnification at the slit lamp.

For most cytological specimens, the smears should be air dried and treated with fixative within a few hours. For Giemsa staining, the fixative, absolute methanol, is applied to the slide at room temperature for five minutes. If wet fixation is desired, smears must be fixed immediately, before they dry.

Diagnosis of Chlamydial Infections

In suspected cases of trachoma, inclusion conjunctivitis, or other chlamydial infections, conjunctival smears can be made and stained with Giemsa or fluorescein-conjugated monoclonal antibodies (FMAB) (Taylor et al., 1984), or conjunctival cultures for *Chlamydia* can be made. The presence of Giemsa-stained inclusions or FMAB elementary bodies is diagnostic of active chlamydial infection. If the procedure is available, specimens for chlamydial culture can be obtained by vigorously rubbing the anesthetized conjunctiva with a dry swab; the swab is then placed immediately into the medium and transported to the laboratory so that tissue cultures can be inoculated the same day (Mahony and Chernesky, 1985).

Antibody to *C. trachomatis* in blood or tears is detected by a micro-titer indirect immunofluorescent test (micro IF). In adults this test is of little value for detecting current infection because any prior infection (commonly, genital infection) will induce a long-lasting antibody response. In infants with conjunctivitis or pneumonitis during the first six months of life, the presence of serum IgM antibody is diagnostic, but the presence of IgG antibody is *not* diagnostic because it can be passively acquired during the gestation period.

Aspiration of Aqueous and Vitreous Humors

For patients with suspected endophthalmitis, aqueous and vitreous specimens should be obtained without delay. Satisfactory specimens from cooperative patients can be obtained at the bedside or in the examining room of the office or emergency room, although vitrectomy under sterile conditions is a preferred procedure.

The conjunctiva and cornea must be adequately anesthetized before obtaining aqueous or vitreous specimens. To accomplish this, a topical anesthetic is instilled into the eye, and a subconjunctival injection of 1% or 2% xylocaine (or other suitable anesthetic) is then made into the quadrant where the keratocentesis is to be performed. Materials required to perform a keratocentesis or vitreous aspiration include a topical and injectable anesthetic, two 27-gauge disposable needles and two tuberculin syringes, one 18- or 20-gauge disposable needle and one 1- or 2-ml syringe, a lid speculum, a small toothed forceps (e.g., Bishop-Harmon), microscope slides, and culture media (Fig. 1–4).

To perform a keratocentesis, a lid speculum is inserted into the eye and the limbal conjunctiva is grasped with a Bishop-Harmon or similar small toothed forceps in the area where the cornea is to be entered. A 27-gauge disposable needle attached to a 1- or 2-ml syringe is then used to penetrate the cornea at an oblique angle, 1–2 mm from the limbus. Penetration of the cornea is facilitated if the needle is rotated as pressure on the syringe is directed toward the eye. Once the needle enters the anterior chamber, aqueous is gently aspirated. A sample of 0.1–0.2 ml of fluid can be easily obtained in this fashion for cultures and cytology. When the corneal wound is beveled, it quickly seals following removal of the needle because of swelling of the corneal stroma, and no sutures are required.

In an aphakic eye, vitreous can be aspirated in a similar fashion, except that an 18- or 20-gauge disposable needle is used and the needle, once the anterior chamber is entered, is directed through the vitreous face. In some instances, the tip of the needle may have to be repositioned within the vitreous several times to locate a pocket of liquid vitreous.

When the lens-iris diaphragm is intact, the vitreous cavity should be approached through the pars plana region (4 mm behind the limbus), and between the insertion of the recti muscles. The limbus is grasped with a fine-toothed forceps, and the conjunctiva and sclera are entered with an 18- or 20-gauge disposable needle attached to a hypodermic syringe. The clinician must be aware of the location of the needle in relationship to the lens and retina at all times, and frequently the needle must be repositioned several times to find a pocket of fluid vitreous. A sample of 0.2–0.5 ml of fluid vitreous can be removed in this fashion. The area of penetration need not be closed, for it seals rapidly from swelling of the sclera. If an operating room and suitable vitrectomy instruments are readily available, a surgical approach to obtain vitreous is preferable.

References

Mahony, JB, and Chernesky, MA: Effect of swab type and storage temperature on the isolation of *Chlamydia trachomatis* from clinical specimens. *J. Clin. Microbiol.* 22: 865–867, 1985.

Motyl, MR, Bottone, EJ, and Janda, JM: Diagnosis of herpesvirus infections: Correlation of Tzanck preparations with viral isolation. *Diagn. Microbiol. Infect. Dis.* 2: 157–160, 1984.

Sanderson, TL, Pustai, W, Shelly, L, Gelender, H, and Ng, AB: Cytologic evaluation of ocular lesions. *Acta Cytol. J.* 24: 391–400, 1980.

Taylor, HR, Agarwala, N, and Johnson, SL: Detection of experimental *Chlamydia trachomatis* eye infection in conjunctival smears and in tissue culture by use of fluorescein-conjugated monoclonal antibody. *J. Clin. Microbiol.* 20: 391–395, 1984.

Yoneda, C, Dawson, CR, Daghfous, T, Hoshiwara, I, Jones, P, Messadi, M, and Schachter, J: Cytology as a guide to the presence of chlamydial inclusions in Giemsa-stained conjunctival smears in severe endemic trachoma. *Br. J. Ophthalmol.* 59: 116–124, 1975.

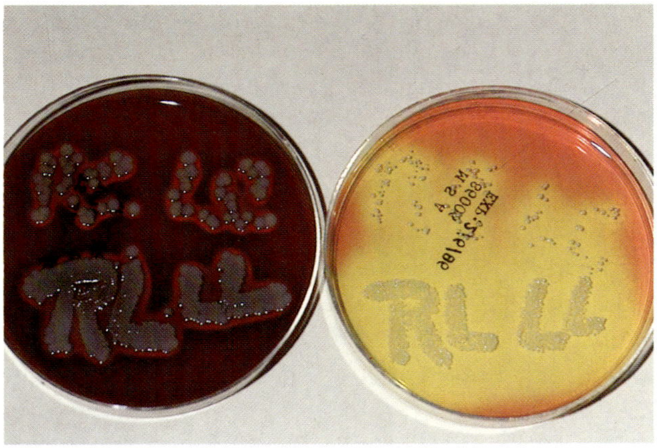

1–1A Method for streaking bacteriological plates after cultures are taken from the lid and conjunctiva; *Staphylococcus aureus* growing on blood and mannitol salt agar. A swab is moistened with sterile broth, gently rubbed over the tarsal conjunctiva, then streaked on the bacteriological plate as the letters RC (right conjunctiva); the same swab is then rubbed on the right lid margins and streaked on the media as the letters RL (right lid). A second sterile moistened swab is used to repeat the procedure in the left eye, with the conjunctival specimen streaked as the letters LC (left conjunctiva) and the lid as LL (left lid).

Because of the high (7.5%) salt concentration in mannitol salt agar, most organisms, except staphylococci, fail to grow on mannitol salt agar; this medium is thus selective for staphylococcal organisms. Furthermore, staphylococci that use mannitol (as manifested by a change in the color of the medium to yellow because of the indicator present in the medium) are more likely to be pathogenic. The bacteriologist can then select these colonies for antibiotic sensitivity testing. The change to a yellow color in the mannitol salt *(right)* suggests that the staphylococcus isolated in this instance is probably pathogenic. (See Fig. 1–1B.)

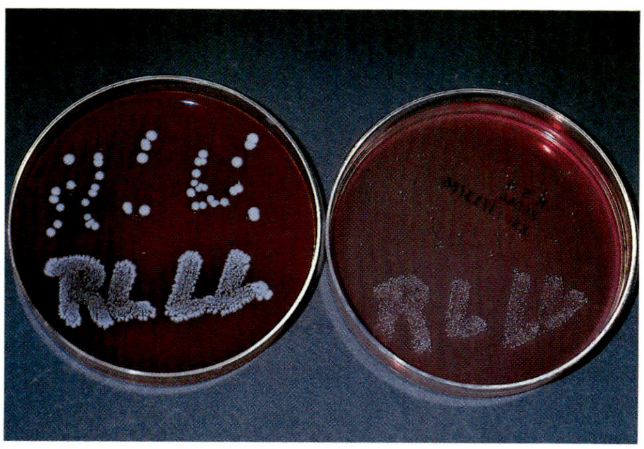

1–1B *Staphylococcus epidermidis* growing on blood agar and mannitol salt agar. Staphylococci such as *S. epidermidis* are less pathogenic than *S. aureus* and usually do not use mannitol; the mannitol plate remains pink in color. (See Fig. 1–1A.)

1–1C Method for streaking bacteriological plates after cultures are taken from the cornea. The streaks are made as the letter C at multiple sites in the medium. If colonies of bacteria grow in areas other than those where the streaks have been placed, the colonies should be regarded as contaminants.

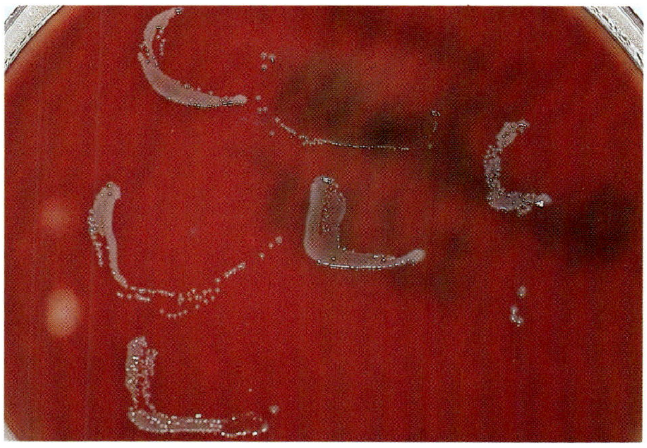

1–2 Routine culture media used for cultures of the conjunctiva and lid margin. The materials preferred by the authors include: blood agar, mannitol salt agar, cotton-tipped applicator sticks, and cooked meat broth.

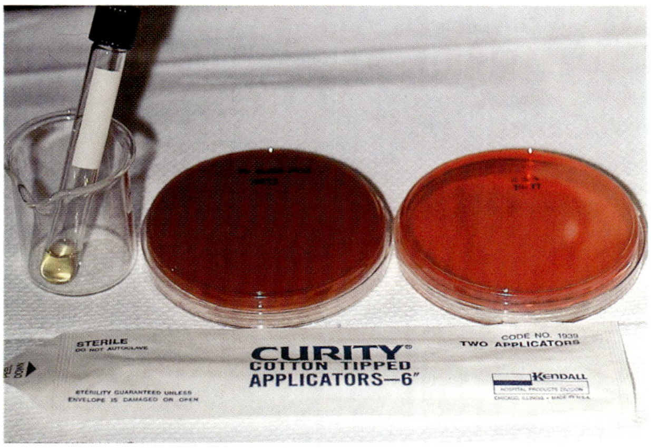

1–3 Materials recommended for obtaining cytological specimens of the lid, conjunctiva, and cornea. Although a Kimura or Lindner spatula is preferable for scraping of the lid, conjunctiva, and cornea, almost any small bladed instrument that can be easily sterilized can be used. The authors prefer the firm blade of the Kimura or Lindner spatula, which provides an adequate specimen when scraped over the conjunctiva or cornea. It is also readily sterilized by heating in the alcohol lamp, cools rapidly, and does not char even after repeated use.

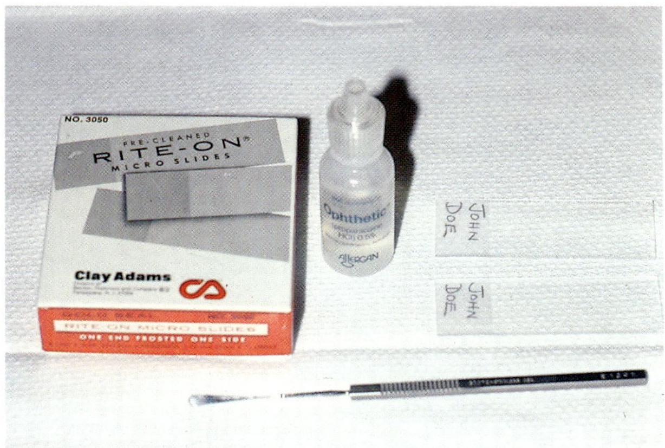

1–4 Materials for performing a keratocentesis and/or a vitreous aspiration as an office or outpatient procedure: two 27-gauge disposable needles, two or three tuberculin syringes, one 18- and one 20-gauge disposable needle, a topical anesthetic such as proparacaine, 1% or 2% xylocaine, Bishop Harmon forceps, a lid speculum, blood agar, Sabouraud's agar without inhibitors, cooked meat broth, and microscope slides. For vitreous aspiration, vitrectomy is preferred when appropriate instruments and an operating room are immediately available and there is no delay in obtaining specimens.

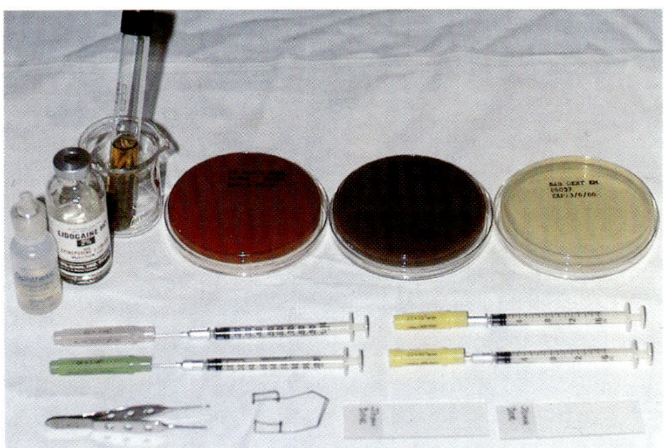

Chapter 2

Infections and Inflammations of the Eyelid and Lid Margin

With only a few exceptions (for example, the lack of subcutaneous fat and the presence of the tarsus), the skin of the eyelid and the lid margin is similar to the skin of other parts of the body and is therefore readily infected by most organisms capable of infecting the skin in general. Several factors, however, such as the spacing of the eyelashes and the presence of secretions (tears, mucus, and meibomian oil), encourage the development and/or persistence of infections that are uncommon in other areas of the body.

Infections and inflammations of the eyelid and lid margin are commonly referred to as blepharitis, with no distinction being made about location or whether the condition is an infection or inflammation. Infections and inflammations of the eyelid are associated with erythema and crusting or discharge.

Staphylococcal Infections

The staphylococci commonly infect the lid margin (Dougherty and McCulley, 1984). They are extremely resistant to treatment, and the recurrent symptoms of pain, photophobia, redness, and conjunctivitis are often severe.

Staphylococcal organisms characteristically infect the lash follicles (folliculitis) (Fig. 2–1), leading to a localized abscess which then ulcerates with exudation of fibrin (Valenton and Okumoto, 1973). Upon healing, the fibrin remains attached to the skin and eyelashes, and, as the eyelashes grow, the fibrin is carried away from the lid margin and resembles a thin sheet of paper impaled on a stick. This finding is termed a collarette (Figs. 2–2A, 2–2B) and is highly suggestive of staphylococcal infection.

In the more severe staphylococcal infections, a frank ulcerative blepharitis occurs (Fig. 2–3) (Smolin and Okumoto, 1977). Pain is commonly noted in staphylococcal blepharitis and arises from an external hordeolum (stye), which is an acute infection of a gland of Zeis or gland of Moll (Fig. 2–4), or from corneal involvement in the form of blotchy epithelial keratitis, marginal (catarrhal) corneal infiltrate (Fig. 2–5A), or marginal corneal ulcer. A fascicular form of keratitis may also occur (Fig. 2–5B).

The epithelial keratitis that occurs with a staphylococcal blepharitis is located in the inferior part of the cornea and is produced by the action of the staphylococcal exotoxins on the corneal epithelium. The marginal corneal infiltrates and marginal corneal ulcers develop from an antigen-antibody reaction in the cornea, which fixates complement and attracts neutrophils. (The antigen arises from the staphylococcus or staphylococcal products that are absorbed into the cornea; the antibody is brought to the area by way of the limbal circulation.) Subsequently the infiltrate regresses and heals with little or no scarring, or it progresses to epithelial breakdown and formation of a marginal corneal ulcer. Both the marginal infiltrate and marginal corneal ulcer remain confined to the corneal periphery and bear a distinct relationship to the limbal vasculature. They are typically located at the 2:00, 4:00, 8:00, and 10:00 positions (Fig. 2–5A), and a lucid interval usually separates the infiltrate or ulcer from the limbal vasculature. When there is corneal involvement due to a staphylococcal blepharitis, the patient characteristically wakes up with a feeling of pain and photophobia.

The signs of staphylococcal blepharitis are listed in Table 2–1. The premature loss of eyelashes and the misdirected, broken, and white eyelashes (Fig. 2–6) result from damage inflicted on the lash follicle by the staphylococcal infection. The infectious eczematoid dermatitis (Fig. 2–7) that may occur in staphylococcal blepharitis is the result of an antigen-antibody reaction in which the staphylococcal products act either as an antigen or a hapten.

Cultures of the lid margin in staphylococcal blepharitis generally reveal colonies of mannitol-positive staphylococci, which are usually but not always coagulase-positive. Scrapings of the lid margin sometimes reveal Gram-positive cocci, which if present in large numbers are probably causing disease (Fig. 2–8). (A few Gram-positive cocci may not be significant.)

Table 2–1 Signs of Staphylococcal Infection of the Eyelid

Absent, broken, and misdirected eyelashes (Fig. 2–2A)
Poliosis (Fig. 2–6)
Folliculitis of lash follicle (Fig. 2–1)
Ulceration of lid margin (Figs. 2–3, 2–5B)
Collarettes (fibrin impaled upon an eyelash) (Figs. 2–2A, 2–2B)
Stye or external hordeolum (Fig. 2–4)
Multiple or recurrent chalazia (Figs. 2–38A, 2–38B, 2–38C, 2–38D, 2–39)
Chronic conjunctivitis
Angular blepharitis or conjunctivitis (Fig. 2–16)
Blotchy epithelial keratitis (lower part of cornea)
Marginal catarrhal infiltrates or ulcers (Fig. 2–5A)
Impetigo contagiosum (Fig. 2–13)
Infectious eczematoid dermatitis (Fig. 2–7).

Seborrhea

Seborrhea (excessive oiliness of the skin) affects the scalp, face, chest, and intertriginous areas of the body. The lid and lid margin, eyebrows, and glabellar region are commonly involved (Fig. 2–9); seborrhea is the most common cause of blepharitis. A seborrheic blepharitis is often associated with staphylococcal infection (mixed blepharitis).

Seborrhea of the eyelids is characterized by erythema of the lid margin and greasy yellow crusts on the eyelashes and lid margin (Fig. 2–10), or by dry bran-like flakes (scurf) of the eyelashes and lid margin without evidence of erythema.

Scrapings of the lid margin in seborrhea reveal *Pityrosporum ovale* and/or *Pityrosporum orbiculare* (Fig. 2–11), which are saprophytic yeast-like organisms.

Mixed Blepharitis

A mixed blepharitis is very common and is composed of a staphylococcal infection superimposed upon seborrhea. The findings in mixed blepharitis include the erythema and greasy scales of seborrhea along with the findings of staphylococcal blepharitis (Fig. 2–12). Scrapings of the lid margin reveal *P. ovale* and/or *P. orbiculare* together with Gram-positive cocci.

Other Bacterial Infections of the Lid Margin

Non-staphylococcal bacterial infections of the lid margin are uncommon. Streptococcal infections of the eyelid are usually associated with streptococcal infections of the face, such as impetigo contagiosum (Fig. 2–13) and erysipelas. Although streptococcal impetigo is characteristically associated with regional adenopathy and cellulitis, it can be differentiated from staphylococcal impetigo only by laboratory means.

Blepharitis caused by *Moraxella* is uncommon except in the southwestern region of the United States. Manifestations of the infection include erythema, crusting and fissuring of the medial or lateral canthal region (angular blepharitis) (Fig. 2–14), and angular conjunctivitis. Scraping of the lid margin reveals large square-ended diplobacilli (Fig. 2–15). A staphylococcal infection of the lid margin may also cause an angular blepharitis (Fig. 2–16), and the two may be confused unless cultures or scrapings are taken of the infected area. *Moraxella* and *Staphylococcus* may also occur concurrently (Fig. 2–17).

Other Gram-negative infections of the lid margin are unusual and are associated with minimal or no signs unless the patient is immunosuppressed. In the presence of immunoincompetence, necrosis and ulceration of the eyelid or lid margin may occur, as is demonstrated in Fig. 2–18: a woman who developed a necrotizing cellulitis of the eyelid due to *Pseudomonas aeruginosa* was found to have an agranulocytosis from an idiosyncratic reaction to methimazole.

Acid-fast infections of the lid and lid margin in the form of lupus vulgaris due to tuberculosis and Hansen's disease are unusual. However, the most frequent ocular manifestations of Hansen's disease are thinning and loss of the eyebrow and/or loss of the eyelashes (Fig. 2–19); nodules or thickening of the eyelid and eyebrows may also be seen.

Fungal Infections

Although the yeast-like organisms, *Pityrosporum ovale* and *P. orbiculare* (discussed in the section on seborrhea) are common inhabitants of the lid margin, true fungal infections of the eyelid are uncommon.

Candidal infections of the lid margin may develop following the prolonged use of topical glucocorticoids and/or broad-spectrum antibiotics. In many instances, the infections simulate staphylococcal infections by the erythema, ulceration, and crusting produced, but small granulomas often serve as a clue to the presence of *Candida* (Figs. 2–20A, 2–20B). A candidal infection may also simulate a ringworm infection (see below).

The dermatophytes infect the eyelid primarily, or secondarily by spreading to the eyelid from the glabrous regions of the face (Ostler et al., 1971). The infection usually resembles a ringworm infection in other areas of the body, which is characterized by circumferentially spreading circles of erythema, edema, and crusting as central healing takes place (Fig. 2–21A). Rarely, the infection may simulate a pyoderma at onset (Fig. 2–21B). In many instances, the infection causes temporary loss of the eyebrows and eyelashes in the affected area. Scrapings of the lesion usually demonstrate one of the various causes of ringworm: *Trichophyton* spp. (Fig. 2–21C), *Epidermophyton* spp., or *Microsporum* spp.

Ocular rhinosporidial infections involve the medial aspect of the lid margin or conjunctiva or involve the lacrimal system. They begin as papillomatous growths which later become pedunculated or verrucous in nature (Prevost et al., 1980). Biopsy of the lesion reveals thick-walled cysts (sporangia) containing endospores (Fig. 2–22).

Viral Infections

Viral infections of the eyelid occur in the form of verruca, herpes simplex, primary and secondary varicella, orf, and molluscum contagiosum, as well as in others forms.

Verruca of the eyelid may be single (Fig. 2–23A), multiple, broad-based, multilobulated, or pedunculated in character. A papillary conjunctivitis and a sectoral epithelial keratitis (Fig. 2–23B) may be produced by the papovaviral infection if the verruca involves the lid margin.

Herpes simplex infections of the lid and lid margin begin as erythematous macules, which vesiculate, crust (Figs. 2–24A, 2–24B), and then heal (Darougar et al., 1985; Jakobiec et al., 1979; Egerer and Stary, 1980). Scarring of the skin is unusual in herpes simplex infections, unless secondary infection supervenes. A scraping of the base of the lesion often demonstrates multinucleated giant cells (Fig. 2–24C).

The skin of the eyelid is frequently involved in the skin eruption of primary varicella (Jordan et al., 1984), and the individual lesions are similar to those found in other parts of the body (Fig. 2–25). In ophthalmic zoster, the skin eruptions usually involve the upper eyelid (Fig. 2–26A) because of involvement of the ophthalmic division of the trigeminal nerve; involvement of the maxillary branch usually causes skin eruptions on the lower eyelid (Fig. 2–26B). In younger patients, the skin and lid lesions of ophthalmic zoster may be localized to a small area and limited to a few vesicles. In immunosuppressed patients or in aging patients, herpes zoster may disseminate (Fig. 2–26C). Dissemination occurs during the secondary viremia and should not be confused with the few lesions that can occur in other areas of the body during the primary viremia.

Scarring frequently supervenes in both primary and secondary varicella (Fig. 2–27). Multinucleated giant cells, identical to those seen in herpes simplex infections, are found in scrapings of the base of the skin lesions of herpes zoster or chicken pox.

Molluscum contagiosum may infect the skin of the lid or lid margin (Fig. 2–28A) and may simulate trachoma by causing a follicular conjunctivitis, a superior epithelial keratitis, and pannus. The molluscum nodule is elevated, dome-shaped, pearly white in color, and has an umbilicated center. The nodule may be macerated, however, and therefore may go unrecognized. Biopsy of the lesion reveals eosinophilic (Feulgen-positive), hyaline-like masses within the prickle cells of the malpighian cell layer. The virus inclusions gradually crowd the nuclei of the cells to one side as the infection progresses (Fig. 2–28B).

Orf (ecthyma contagiosum) is a pox-virus infection of sheep which rarely involves the lid or ocular adnexa in humans. The skin lesion begins as a red papule which quickly vesiculates, becomes hemorrhagic, pustulates, and crusts (Freeman et al., 1984). Regional adenopathy and a follicular conjunctivitis are commonly associated. Healing by scarring occurs within about five weeks.

Parasitic Infections

Although protozoan infections of the eyelid are very uncommon, leishmaniasis of the face affects the eyelid in about 2–5% of cases (Chu et al., 1983). The lateral canthal region is most frequently involved, but in some instances the medial canthus and lacrimal system may be involved. The infection produces a granuloma simulating a chalazion, a simple or phagedenic ulcer, or a fungating mass.

The metazoan parasite *Demodex folliculorum* commonly infects the eyelids. In most instances the infection is asymptomatic, but if organisms are present in large numbers, itching and redness of the eyelid may occur (English and Nutting, 1981). Infections by *Demodex* can be recognized by the finding of sleeves (tube-like processes) that arise from the skin and extend over the base of the eyelash for 0.5–1 mm (Fig. 2–29A). *Demodex* is an arachnid with eight jointed legs and a striated abdomen (Fig. 2–29B). It is readily recognized with the aid of a microscope when affected lashes are removed and examined.

The *Phthirus pubis* organism may also infect the eyelid (Couch et al., 1982; Baker and Feingold, 1984). Because of its size it is particularly suited to clinging to the widely spaced cilia of the lid. The adult organism, though having a distinctive appearance (Figs. 2–30A, 2–30B) is transparent and often is mistaken for fibrin on the lid margin unless the lid margin is carefully searched. The nits (Fig. 2–30C), when present in large numbers, are readily seen attached to the eyelashes. Other ectoparasites such as ticks can also attach at the lid margin (Fig. 2–31).

Allergic Reactions

Allergic conditions involving the eyelid include hay fever, atopic dermatitis, acute urticaria, and angioneurotic edema.

In hay fever conjunctivitis (Chapter 3) the eyelid becomes edematous (Fig. 2–32) and frequently becomes macerated because of the patient rubbing the eyes.

In the early stages of atopic dermatitis, the skin of the eyelid is erythematous, and exudative lesions are evident (Fig. 2–33A). Later, scaling and crusting develop, and in the late stages (usually in late childhood) the skin of the eyelid becomes pigmented and often lichenified (Fig. 2–33B); in rare instances the lichenification persists for life (Fig. 2–33C). Loss of lashes and staphylococcal blepharitis are common complications of atopic dermatitis (Garrity and Liesegang, 1984).

Contact dermatitis frequently involves the skin of the eyelid(s). The acute phase is manifested by symptoms of itching and findings of erythema, exudation of fibrin, edema, and vesiculation (Fig. 2–34A); the chronic phase is accompanied by thickening, fissuring, and lichenification (Fig. 2–34B). The dermatitis may be localized to a tiny area (as in contact hypersensitivity to nail polish), to one eyelid, or to all four eyelids, or it may be a generalized eruption. Acute infectious eczematoid dermatitis is a special form of contact dermatitis (see the earlier section on staphylococcal blepharitis).

Acute urticaria may involve the eyelids and is associated with erythematous weals which mainly affect the dermis (Fig. 2–35). Angioneurotic edema on the other hand, even though it is of sudden onset, is chronic in type. The edema involves primarily the subcutaneous tissue, producing lesions that are tense and round (Fig. 2–36) (Daxecker, 1980).

Miscellaneous Inflammations

Various inflammations of the eyelid may occur without well defined allergic or infectious causes. These include meibomitis, chalazion formation, erythema multiforme major (Stevens-Johnson syndrome), toxic epidermal necrolysis, alopecia areata, and alopecia totalis.

Meibomitis (meibomianitis) is characterized by an excessive secretion of meibomian oil and is associated with symptoms of periodic intense burning and a heavy feeling of the eyelids. Dilated and inspissated orifices of the meibomian gland (Fig. 2–37A) and meibomian froth (Fig. 2–37B) are prominent features. Meibomitis may result from prolonged irritation, as by an ill fitting contact lens, a chronic infection of the lid margin, keratoconjunctivitis sicca, or a primary oversecretion of oil such as occurs in seborrhea (Gutgesel et al., 1982; Seal et al., 1985).

A chalazion may occur with or without the presence of a staphylococcal blepharitis. The patient notes a hard lump (like a hailstone) in the eyelid (Figs. 2–38A, 2–38B, 2–38C, 2–38D) with minimal associated inflammation. Histologically a chalazion represents a lipogranuloma (Fig. 2–39).

The eyelid may be involved in the generalized skin eruption of erythema multiforme major or Stevens-Johnson syndrome; in some instances infection, drugs, or trauma serve as a trigger for the syndrome, while in other instances the trigger is unknown. The typical skin lesions are symmetrical and begin as a generalized erythema (Fig. 2–40A), followed by the formation of tense iris or target-like bullae. Mucous membrane involvement is an early manifestation of erythema multiforme major (Fig. 2–40B).

Toxic epidermal necrolysis may resemble erythema multiforme at onset, and some clinicians consider the two to be variants of a single condition. In many instances, they have similar triggers. However, the two entities differ histologically in several ways: Nikolsky's sign is a prominent feature of toxic epidermal necrolysis (Fig. 2–41A), and the scalded skin appearance (Fig. 2–41B), which frequently involves the eyelids, is quite distinctive for toxic epidermal necrolysis (Ostler et al., 1970).

The loss of eyelashes in alopecia areata and alopecia totalis (Fig. 2–42), though uncommon, is often very distressful to the patient. Fortunately, in most instances the eyelashes tend to regenerate after a few months.

References

Baker, RS, Feingold, M: *Phthirus pubis* (pubic louse) blepharitis. *Am. J. Dis. Child.* 138: 1079–1080, 1984.

Chappler, RR, Maibach, HI, Conant, MA: Mucocutaneous candidiasis or mucocutaneous microbiosis? *JAMA* 239: 428–429, 1978.

Chu, FC, Rodrigues, MM, Cogan, DG, Neva, FA: Leishmaniasis affecting the eyelids. *Arch. Ophthalmol.* 101: 84–91, 1983.

Couch, JM, Green, WR, Hirst, LW, de la Cruz, ZC: Diagnosing and treating *Phthirus pubis* palpebrum. *Surv. Ophthalmol.* 26: 219–225, 1982.

Darougar, S, Wishart, MS, Viswalingam, ND:

Epidemiological and clinical features of primary herpes simplex virus ocular infection. *Br. J. Ophthalmol.* 69: 2–6, 1985.

Daxecker, F: Komplementdefekt beim hereditaren Angioödem als Ursache von Lidödemen. *Klin. Monatsbl. Augenheilkd.* 177: 390–393, 1980.

Dougherty, JM, McCulley, JP: Comparative bacteriology of chronic blepharitis. *Br. J. Ophthalmol.* 68: 524–528, 1984.

Egerer, I, Stary, A: Erosive-ulcerative herpes simplex blepharitis. *Arch. Ophthalmol.* 98: 1760–1763, 1980.

English, FP, Nutting, WB: Demodicosis of ophthalmic concern. *Am. J. Ophthalmol.* 91: 362–372, 1981.

Freeman, G, Bron, AJ, Juel-Jensen, B: Ocular infection with orf virus. *Am. J. Ophthalmol.* 97: 601–604, 1984.

Garrity, JA, Liesegang, TH: Ocular complications of atopic dermatitis. *Can. J. Ophthalmol.* 19: 21–24, 1984.

Gutgesel, VJ, Stern, GA, Hood, CI: Histopathology of meibomian gland dysfunction. *Am. J. Ophthalmol.* 94: 383–387, 1982.

Jakobiec, FA, Srinivasan, BD, Gamoa, ET: Recurrent herpetic angular blepharitis in an adult. *Am. J. Ophthalmol.* 88: 744–747, 1979.

Jordan, DR, Noel, LP, Clarke, WN: Ocular involvement in varicella. *Clin. Pediatr.* 23: 434–436, 1984.

Ostler, HB, Conant, MA, Groundwater, J: Lyell's disease, the Stevens-Johnson syndrome, and exfoliative dermatitis. *Trans. Am. Acad. Ophthalmol. Otolaryngol.* 74: 1254–1265, 1970.

Ostler, HB, Okumoto, M, Halde, C: Dermatophytosis affecting the periorbital region. *Am. J. Ophthalmol.* 72: 934–938, 1971.

Prevost, E, Kreutner, A Jr, Vallotton, WW, Walker, EM Jr: Conjunctival lesion caused by *Rhinosporidium seeberi. South. Med. J.* 3: 1077–1079, 1980.

Seal, DV, McGill, JI, Jacobs, P, Liakos, GM, Goulding, NJ: Microbial and immunological investigations of chronic non-ulcerative blepharitis and meibomianitis. *Br. J. Ophthalmol.* 69: 604–611, 1985.

Smolin, G, Okumoto, M: Staphylococcal blepharitis. *Arch. Ophthalmol.* 95: 812–816, 1977.

Valenton, MJ, Okumoto, M: The toxin-producing strains of *Staphylococcus epidermidis* (albus). Isolates from patients with staphylococcic blepharoconjunctivitis. *Arch. Ophthalmol.* 89: 186–189, 1973.

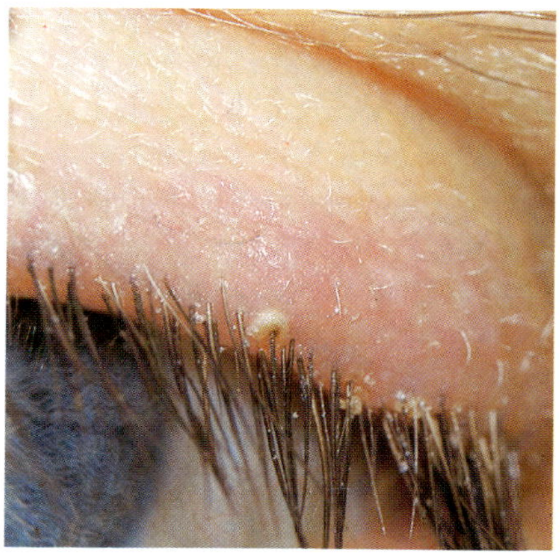

2–1 Folliculitis. A superficial folliculitis involving the lash follicle often occurs from staphylococcal infection. The folliculitis is characterized by symptoms of tenderness, and the findings of erythema, edema, and pustulation at or near the orifice of the follicle. An ulcer usually supervenes which is quickly covered by fibrin. A folliculitis, ulceration, loss of eyelashes, and erythema are all visible in this 27-year-old male.

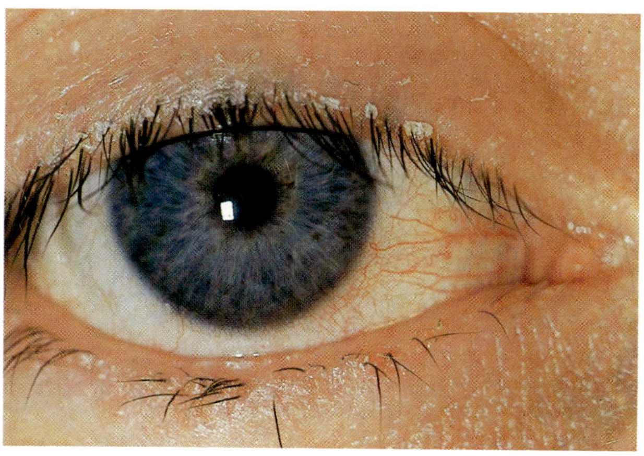

2–2A Collarettes of the lid margin. A collarette develops following pustulation (superficial folliculitis) and ulceration. It is formed by the fibrin exuding from the ulcer and is carried away from the lid margin as the eyelash grows. The fibrin crust often encircles the lash and appears like a piece of paper impaled upon a stick. In this patient, multiple collarettes are present on the upper eyelid. Erythema of the lid and small misdirected eyelashes are evident inferiorly. A tiny area of superficial folliculitis is also noted on the lower eyelid nasally.

2–2B Collarettes of the lid margin. In this photograph, many collarettes can be seen on the eyelashes. Erythema of the eyelid and fibrin on the lid margin are also evident.

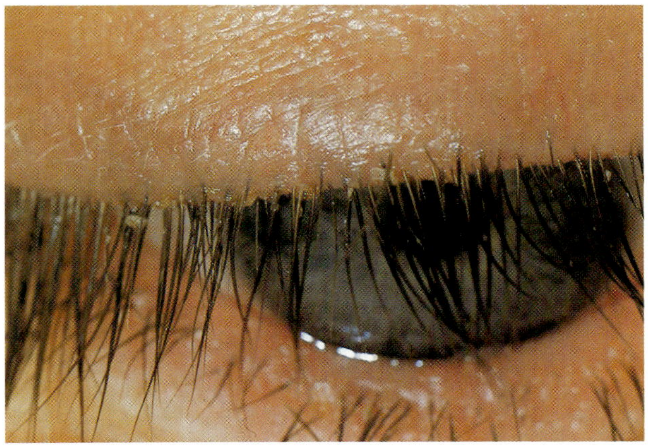

2–3 Ulcerative blepharitis. An ulcerative blepharitis frequently occurs in staphylococcal blepharitis. The ulcers may be quite large, suggesting an erosion of the skin, and they may be covered by fibrin. In this 28-year-old female with severe staphylococcal blepharitis, ulceration of the lid margin, erythema, loss of eyelashes, and exudation of fibrin, which covers several of the ulcerated areas, are readily evident.

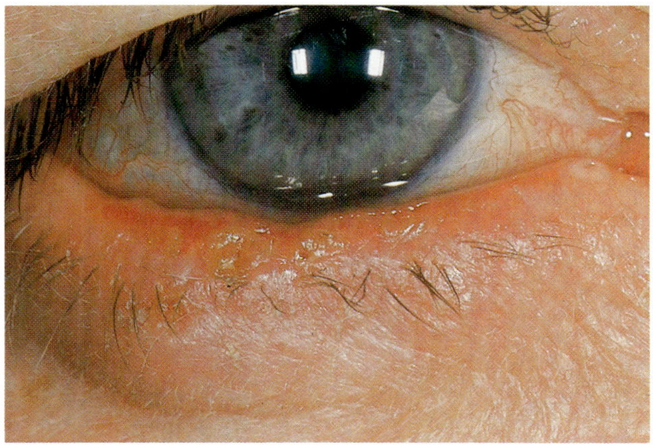

2–4 External hordeolum. A stye or external hordeolum is an acute, purulent inflammation of a gland of Zeis or gland of Moll caused by a staphylococcal infection. The stye is associated with pain, tenderness, edema, erythema, and pustule formation within the gland. This patient complained of pain and swelling of the eyelid. Erythema, edema of the surrounding area, and early pointing of purulent material are evident.

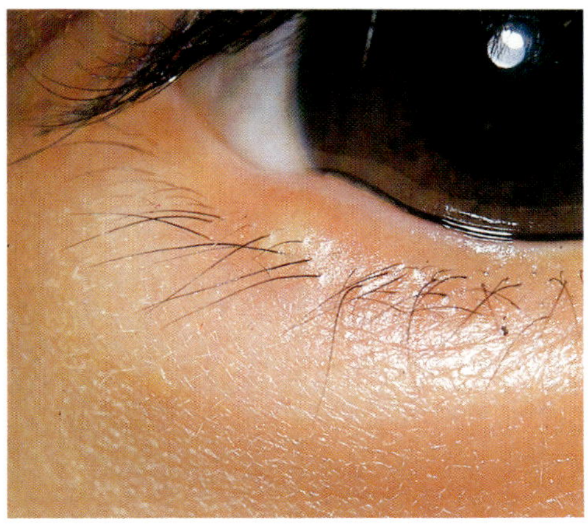

2–5A Marginal corneal infiltrate. A marginal (catarrhal) infiltrate represents an antigen-antibody reaction with fixation of complement and chemotaxis of neutrophils. It occurs as a complication of staphylococcal blepharitis and occasionally of *Haemophilis aegyptius* conjunctivitis of the adult. The infiltrate appears white, is well demarcated, and is adjacent to the limbus with a small lucid interval interposed between the infiltrate and the limbus. The infiltrate usually occurs at the 2:00, 4:00, 8:00, or 10:00 positions, areas where the lid and the staphylococcal or *H. aegyptius* antigen contained within the tear meniscus cross the limbus. If the infiltrate is untreated, the epithelium overlying a marginal infiltrate may break down to become a marginal ulcer.

In this patient, a small corneal infiltrate is evident at the 8:00 position and is associated with marked hyperemia of the adjacent conjunctiva and neovascularization of the cornea. Conjunctival hyperemia is also visible at the 4:00 position. Note the hyperemia of the eyelid and crusting at the lateral aspect of the lower eyelid, as well as a small superficial folliculitis of the upper eyelid.

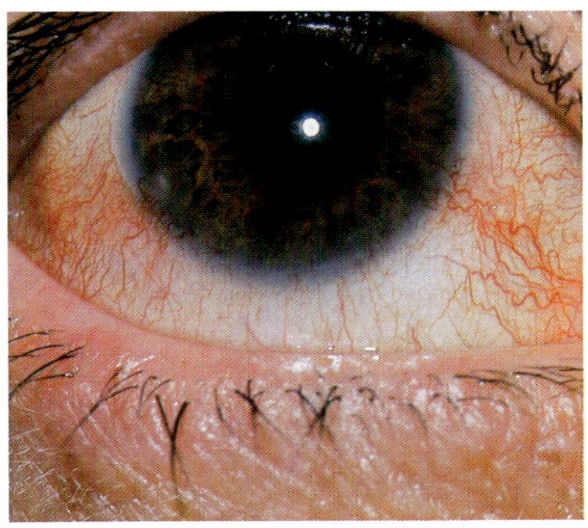

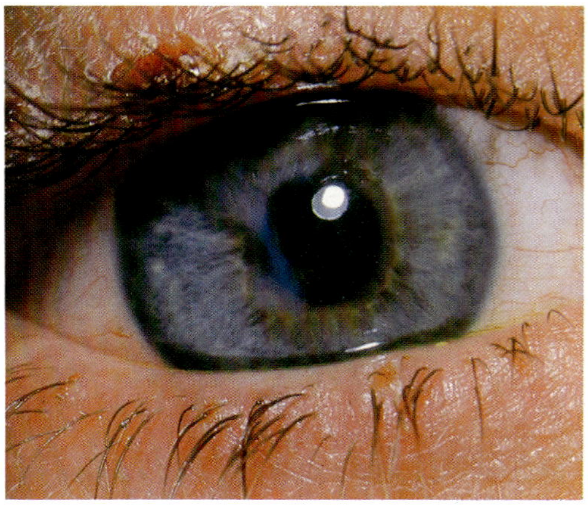

2–5B Erythema, ulceration with fibrin formation, and thickening of the lid margin along with a fascicular keratitis due to staphylococcal blepharokeratitis. In some instances a corneal infiltrate attracts new vessels into the cornea, these in turn are followed by the development of new infiltrates more centrally. Finally a leash of vessels, which may even cross the visual axis, is brought into the corneaas noted in this patient with severe staphylococcal blepharitis. Ulceration of the lid margin, infectious eczematoid dermatitis, and thickening of the lid margin are all present.

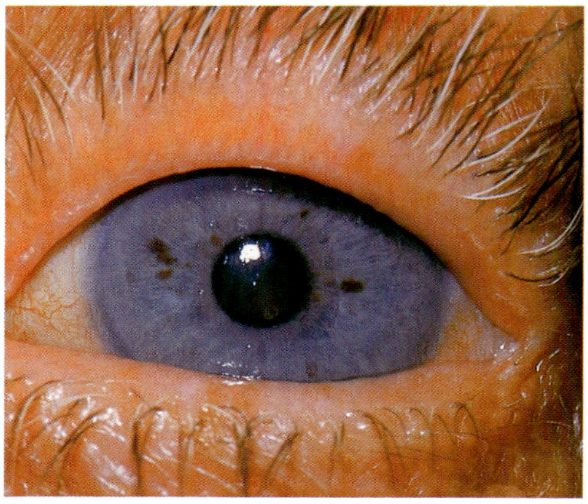

2–6 Poliosis of the eyelashes. Whitening of the eyelashes as well as missing, misdirected, and broken eyelashes are frequent sequelae of staphylococcal blepharitis and arise from damage to the lash follicle by the staphylococcal infection. Many white eyelashes, erythema, and thickening of the lid margin are present in this patient, along with irregularity of the corneal epithelium, filament formation, and decreased tear meniscus. These findings have developed because of a combination of staphylococcal blepharitis and keratoconjunctivitis sicca.

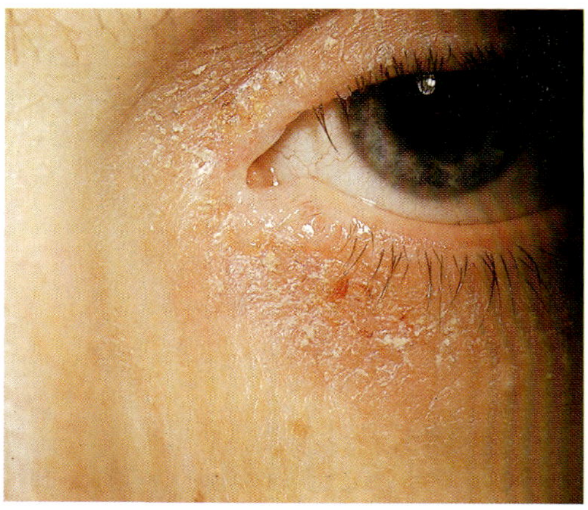

2–7 Infectious eczematoid dermatitis. This is an uncommon finding in staphylococcal blepharitis, but when found is significant. This 12-year-old female had been treated for more than two years with topical glucocorticoids for a contact hypersensitivity, without relief of symptoms. When seen, she had lichenification and erythema of the upper and lower eyelids of each eye, and lid cultures revealed many colonies of *Staphylococcus aureus*. Topical treatment of the lid margins resulted in marked improvement of symptoms, although the authors have been obliged to continue therapy at periodic intervals for the past five years to maintain the patient without symptoms.

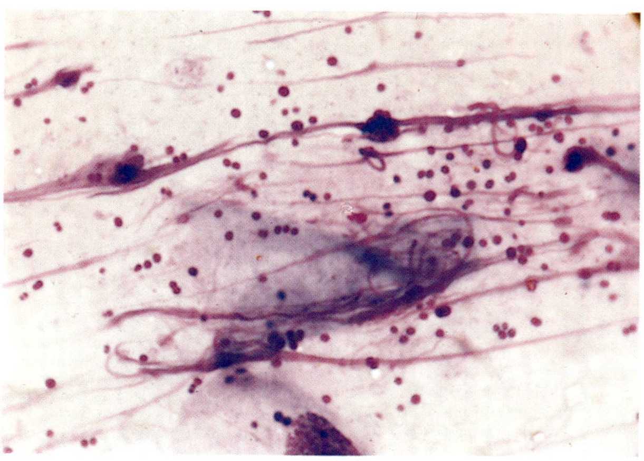

2–8 Scraping of the lid margin in staphylococcal blepharitis. Scrapings of the lid margin in staphylococcal blepharitis usually demonstrate many Gram-positive cocci; when large numbers are present they are probably causing disease. (A few Gram-positive cocci, however, may or may not be significant.) The keratinized and keratinizing cells are normal findings in smears of the lid margin. Giemsa stain, × 1000.

2–9 Seborrhea of the scalp showing dry branny flakes. The scalp, eyebrows, glabellar region, the area behind the ears, and the lid margin are commonly involved in seborrhea. The involved skin is erythematous and oily and may be covered with dry branny flakes (scurf or dandruff) if the condition is mild, or may be covered with greasy scales if the condition is severe. In this patient, dry branny flakes are evident in the region of the forehead. In the region of the eyelids, he was noted to have greasy crusts (Fig. 2–10).

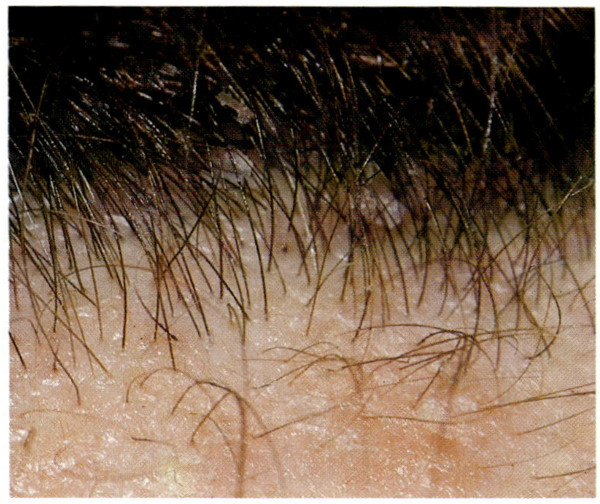

2–10 Greasy crusts in seborrhea. Because of the adhesiveness of the oil, the yellow greasy crusts of seborrhea cling to the eyelashes and appear thick, and in some instances cling to the side of or surround the eyelash, as occurs with the fibrin in staphylococcal infections (see Figs. 2–2A and 2–2B). The greasy crusts of seborrhea are evident in this photograph of a patient with seborrheic blepharitis who complained of a heavy feeling of the eyelids and periodic burning of the eyes.

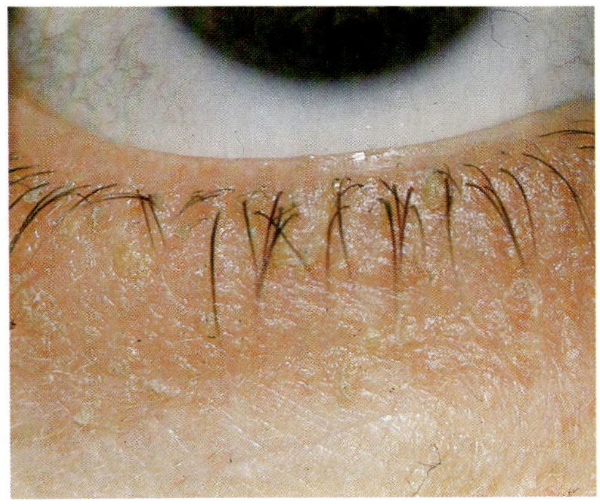

2–11 *Pityrosporum orbiculare* and *Pityrosporum ovale* in a scraping of the lid margin in seborrhea. *P. orbiculare* and *P. ovale* are commonly present in smears of the lid margin in seborrheic blepharitis. These saphrophytic, yeast-like organisms require fatty acids, and hence are common in seborrhea and possibly contribute to inflammation through production of breakdown products of the fatty acids. Giemsa stain, ×400.

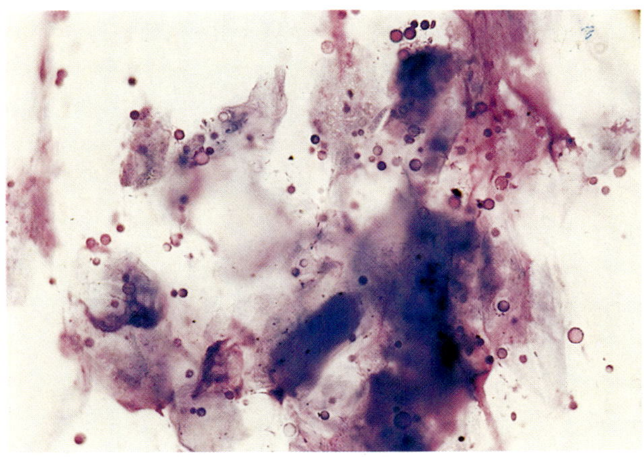

2–12 Mixed blepharitis. This common condition represents a combination of staphylococcal changes (e.g., collarettes, poliosis, and ulceration at the base of the eyelashes) with the greasy scales of seborrhea. In this patient, both the greasy scales of seborrhea and the collarettes of staphylococcal infection are evident.

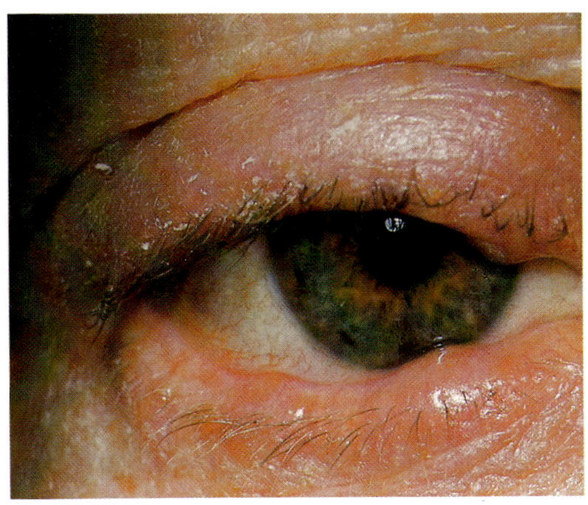

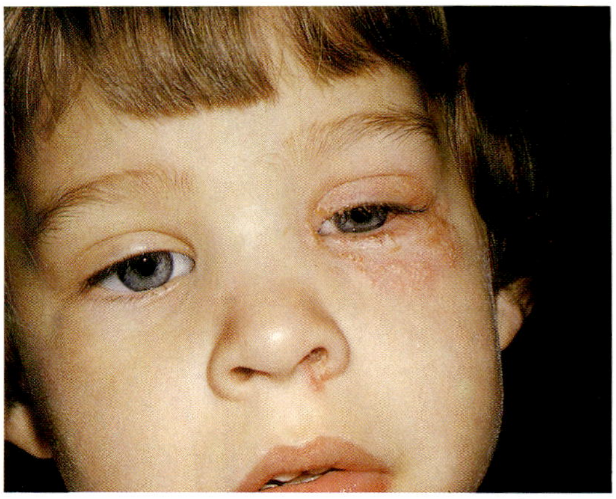

2–13 Impetigo contagiosum. Impetigo contagiosum of the face and eyelids may occur from group A beta hemolytic streptococci, coagulase-positive *Staphylococcus aureus*, or a combination of the two organisms. Bullous impetigo is caused by *S. aureus;* the impetigo caused by streptococci or a combination of streptococci and staphylococci is usually nonbullous in type. In this 3-year-old female, a mixed skin infection due to infection with *Staphylococcus aureus* and *Streptococcus pyogenes* is present. The upper and lower eyelid are erythematous with some crusting; the left nostril is also affected because of spread by drainage of the infectious material into the nose by way of the nasolacrimal duct.

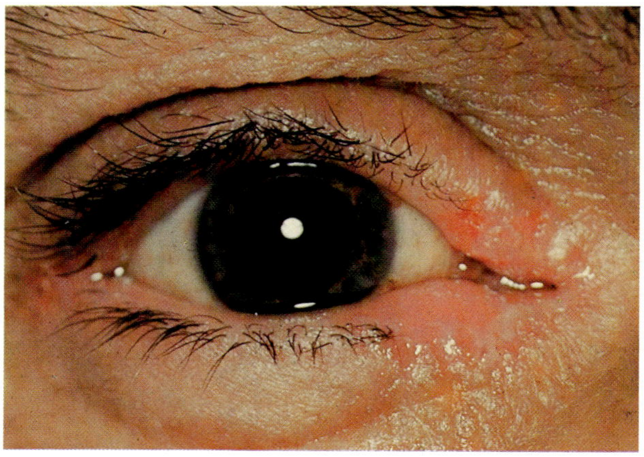

2–14 Angular blepharitis due to *Moraxella lacunata*. Angular blepharitis is typically caused by *M. lacunata*, but may also be caused by a staphylococcal infection of the lid margin. It is characterized by erythema, crusting, fissuring, and an angular conjunctivitis. This 28-year-old female developed pain and tearing that was especially marked when she opened her eyes. Maceration, erythema, and discharge of the medial and lateral canthus are evident in this photograph, taken after several days of topical antibiotic treatment. (Photograph courtesy of Dr. Phillips Thygeson.)

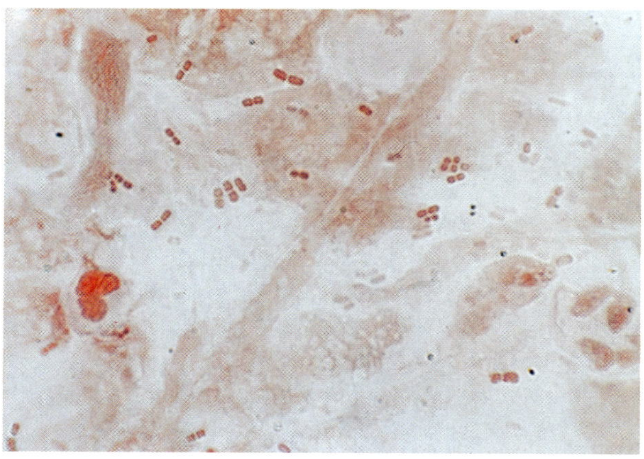

2–15 Scraping from moraxella angular blepharitis. *Moraxella* organisms are readily found in scrapings from moraxella angular blepharitis. The organisms are distinctive in appearance, being large, square-ended Gram-negative diplobacilli. This is a nonpyogenic bacterium and few polymorphonuclear leukocytes are seen. Gram stain, $\times 1000$.

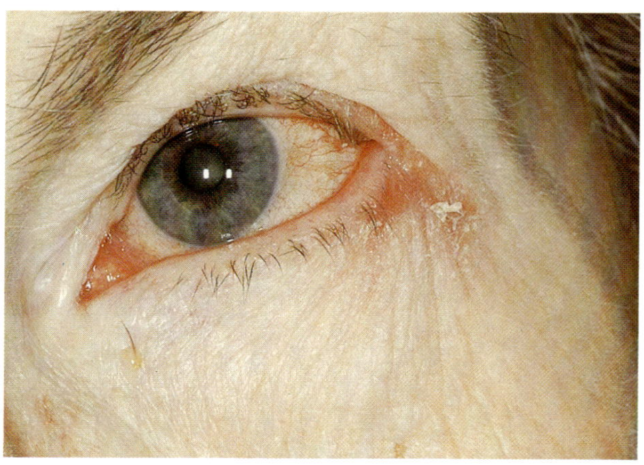

2–16 Angular blepharitis due to *Staphylococcus aureus*. An angular blepharitis may be caused by the staphylococcus or by *Moraxella* spp. The blepharitis may involve either the medial or the lateral aspect of the eyelids and is often associated with an angular conjunctivitis. In this 74-year-old female, an angular blepharitis is noted in the lateral canthal region. The crusting and fissuring are characteristic of an angular blepharitis.

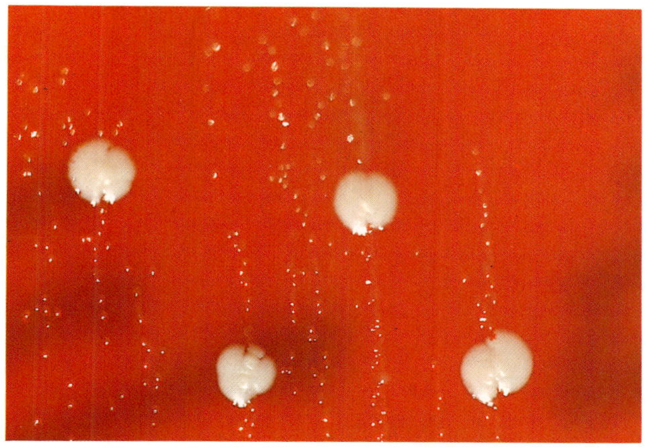

2–17 Culture on blood agar showing both *Moraxella lacunata* and *Staphylococcus epidermidis*. Many colonies of *M. lacunata* are shown. They are typically tiny, translucent, and nonhemolytic in contrast to the *S. epidermidis* colonies, which are many times larger and opaque.

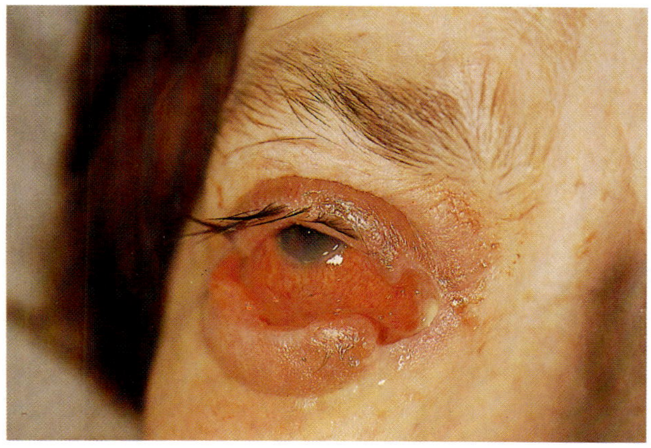

2–18 Necrotizing cellulitis of the eyelid due to *Pseudomonas aeruginosa*. Gram-negative infections of the eyelid usually cause minimal or no signs of infection unless the patient is immunosuppressed, such as this patient who developed necrotizing cellulitis of the eyelid due to *P. aeruginosa*. The infection did not respond to therapy until the agranulocytosis resulting from an idiosyncratic reaction to methimazole was reversed. *P. aeruginosa* was readily cultured from the areas of infection and from the bloodstream. Note the necrosis of the medial aspect of the eyelids and the center of the lower eyelid. At one time, the medial canthal ligament and the lacrimal sac region were exposed by destruction of tissue. Loss of corneal epithelium and moderate infiltration of the superficial corneal stroma are also present.

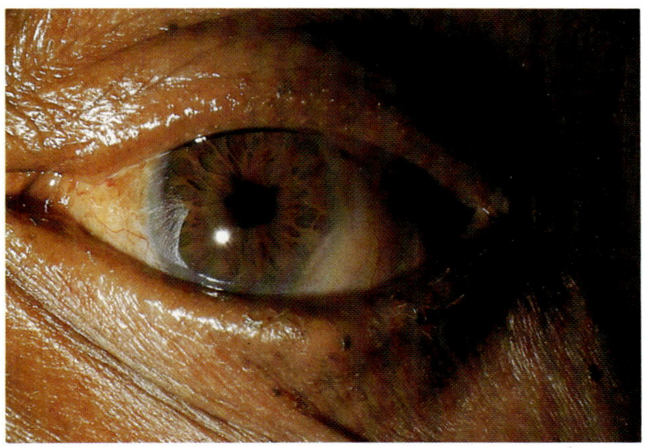

2–19 Loss of eyelashes in Hansen's disease. Thinning, or partial or complete loss of the eyelashes and/or eyebrows may occur in Hansen's disease. The loss is permanent, and arises from infiltration of the hair follicles by *Mycobacterium leprae*. In this patient, marked loss of eyelashes is present, together with posterior synechiae nasally and two large lepromas in the chamber angle, which have arisen from the ciliary body.

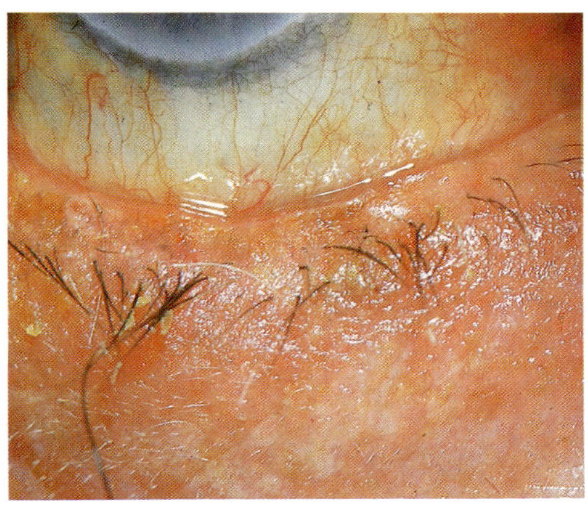

2–20A Candidal blepharitis. In many respects candidal blepharitis simulates staphylococcal blepharitis: it produces folliculitis of the lash follicles with ulceration and collarettes, and loss, misdirection, and poliosis of the eyelashes. Tiny granulomas of the lid margin are distinctive however, and should alert the clinician to the possibility of a candidal blepharitis. In this patient with a candidal blepharitis, erythema and thickening of the eyelid are evident along with loss of lashes, misdirection of lashes, poliosis, and crusting.

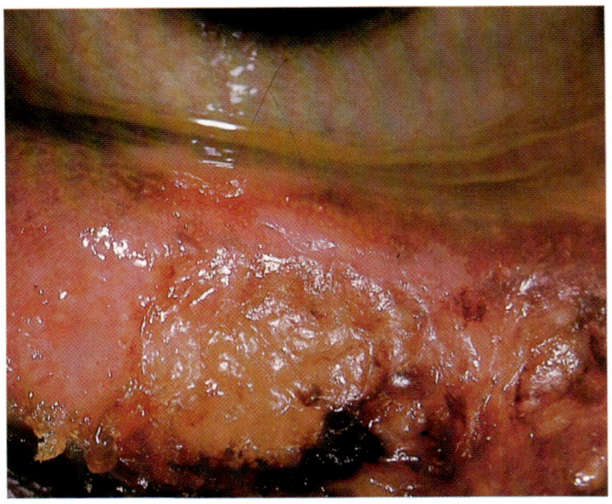

2–20B Candidal blepharitis in a patient with mucocutaneous candidosis. In contrast to most instances of mucocutaneous candidosis, in which staphylococcal blepharitis usually occurs (Chappler et al., 1978), this patient had severe candidal blepharitis. (Photograph courtesy of Dr. Phillips Thygeson.)

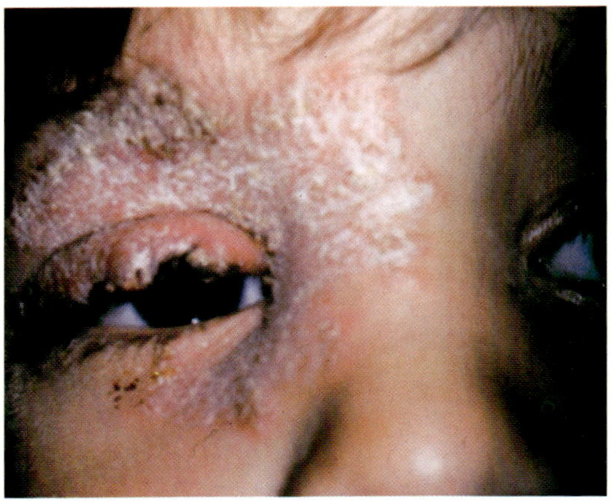

2–21A Dermatophytosis of the eyelids. Like dermatophytosis in other areas of the skin, superficial ringworm of the eyelid begins as flat reddish papules that spread peripherally while healing centrally. The infection may begin on the eyelid or spread to the eyelid from the glabrous regions of the face. The eyebrow and eyelashes, if involved, may be temporarily lost in such infections. In this child, the infection at first simulated a pyoderma (see Fig. 2–21B); later, as the disease progressed, the characteristic ringworm appearance developed. (Reprinted with permission from the *American Journal of Ophthalmology.*)

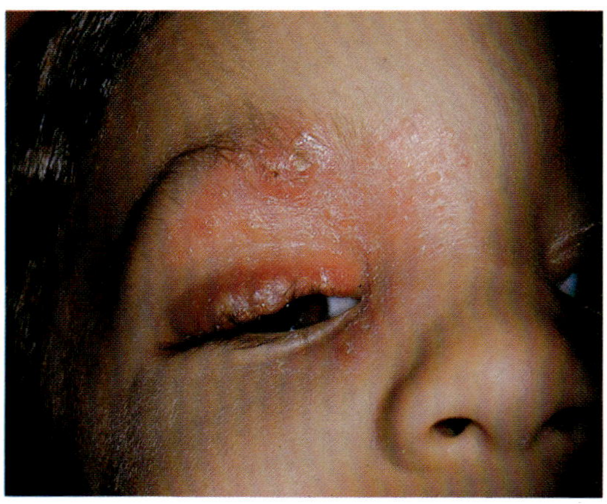

2–21B Dermatophytosis of the eyelids. At onset, dermatophytosis of the eyelid may simulate a pyoderma, as is seen in this child who developed a *Trichophyton mentagophytes* infection. The lesion later became more distinctive for ringworm infection (see Fig. 2–21A). (Reprinted with permission from the *American Journal of Ophthalmology.*)

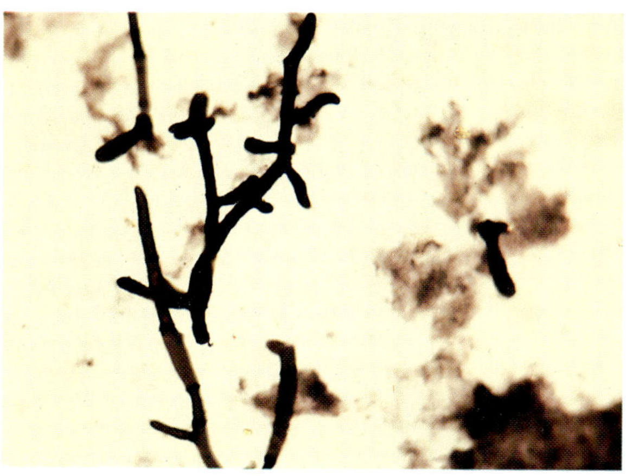

2–21C Scraping of the eyelid of the patient in Figs. 2–21A and 2–21B, showing *Trichophyton mentagrophytes.* The etiological organism is usually readily demonstrated in scrapings or cultures of the affected area in dermatophytosis. Methenamine silver stain, ×400.

2–22 Biopsy of rhinosporidiosis of the lid margin. Biopsy of a pedunculated tumor arising from rhinosporidiosis revealed the thick-walled cyst-like sporangia filled with endospores of *Rhinosporidium seeberi*. Hematoxylin and eosin, × 100.

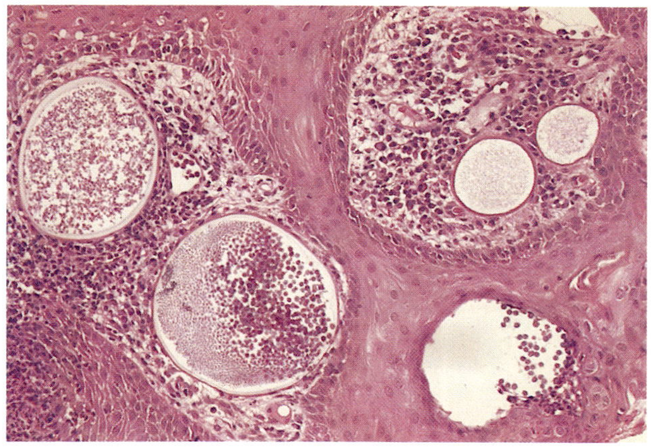

2–23A Verruca of the lid margin. Verrucae frequently occur on the lid and lid margin. They are similar to verrucae found in other areas of the body and may be single or multiple. The lesion in this patient is a large filiform verruca. Within one of the "fingers" of the lesion a central vessel is visible, which serves to supply the verruca with blood.

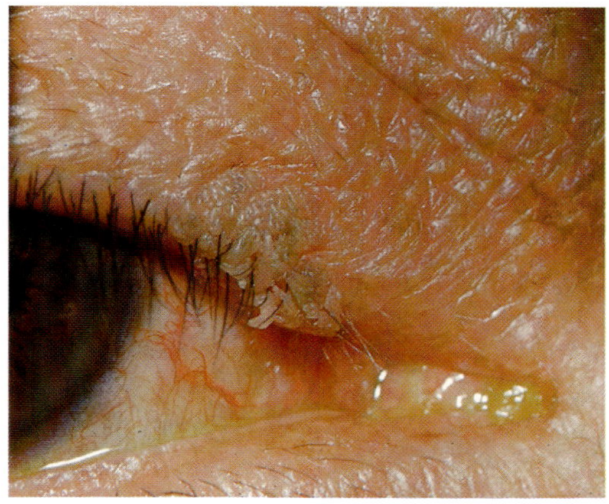

2–23B Epithelial keratitis due to verruca of the lid margin. Verrucae often produce a papillary conjunctivitis and a segmental keratitis, such as is evident in this patient's cornea. The keratitis can be seen in the pupillary area and has taken up some fluorescein. (The verruca itself is not evident in this photograph.)

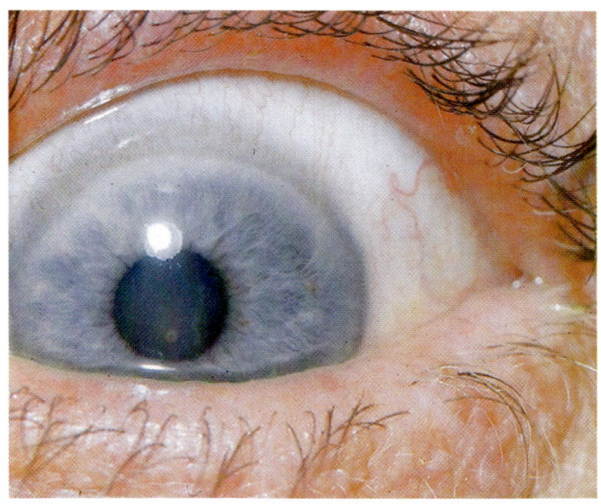

2–24A Herpes simplex infection of the eyelid. Lid infections occur in both primary and recurrent herpes simplex. The lesions begin as vesicles which later crust and heal. Erythema, edema, and vesicles that are beginning to crust are evident on both eyelids in this child with primary herpes simplex infection.

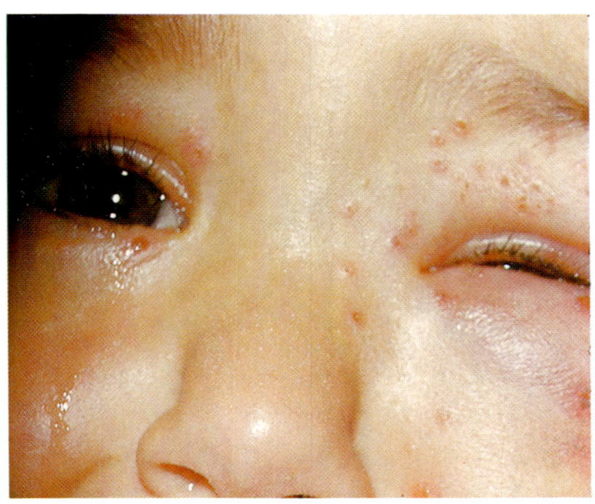

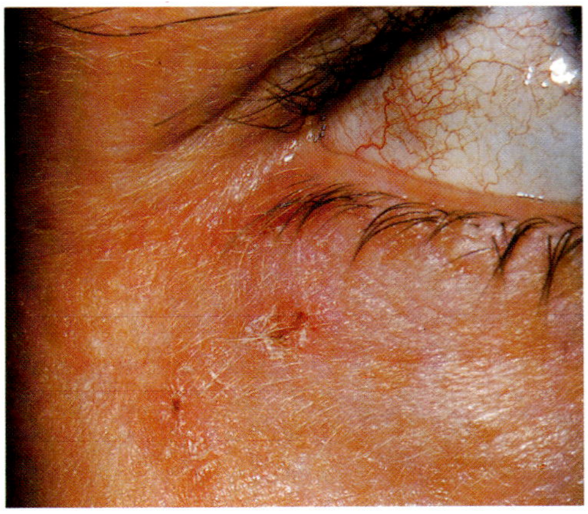

2–24B Crusting of herpetic lesions on the lateral canthal region. Erythema of the lateral canthal region along with crusting of herpetic vesicles are evident in this patient with recurrent herpes simplex infection of the eyelid. As noted here, a conjunctivitis in recurrent herpes simplex infections of the eyelid is uncommon, whereas a conjunctivitis is commonly associated with a primary herpes simplex lid infection.

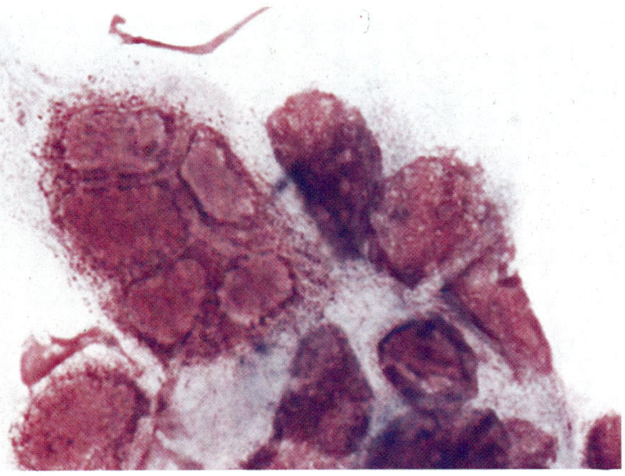

2–24C Multinucleated giant cells from herpes simplex. These cells are characteristically found in scrapings of active herpes simplex lesions. They cannot be differentiated, however, from the multinucleated giant cells found in scrapings of primary or secondary varicella. This Giemsa stained scraping from a dendrite shows a giant cell with five nuclei. Giemsa stain, ×1000.

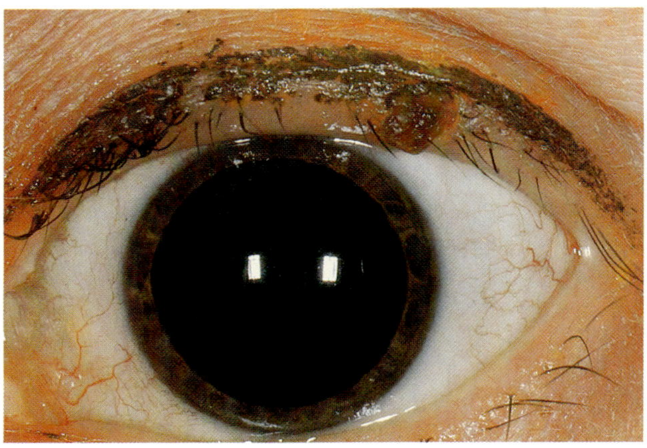

2–25 Skin eruption of primary varicella (chicken pox). The eyelid may be involved in the generalized skin eruption of primary varicella. The typical lesion begins as a papule which becomes vesicular then crusts. Since additional lesions develop during the course of chicken pox, lesions in varying stages may be found on the face. In this 17-year-old female with varicella, a lesion on the upper lid margin is in the crusting phase. The pupil has been pharmacologically dilated because of a nongranulomatous iritis that developed two weeks after onset of the skin rash.

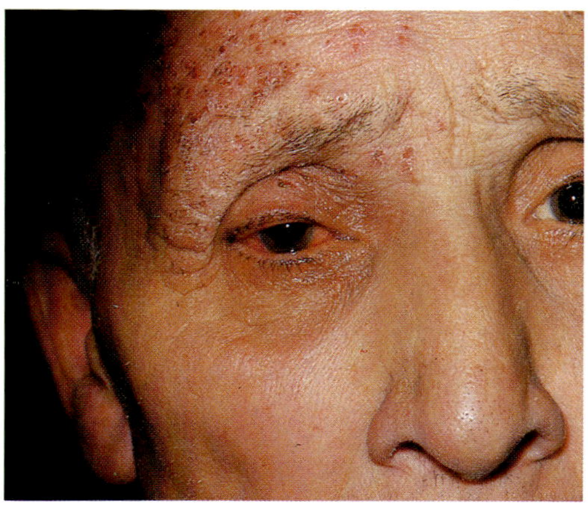

2–26A Herpes zoster ophthalmicus skin eruption. Secondary varicella (herpes zoster) frequently involves the dermatomal distribution of the ophthalmic branch of the trigeminal nerve. The individual lesions are similar to those of primary varicella, but the dermatomal eruption and the past history of chicken pox are sufficient to eliminate varicella as the cause of the eruption. This 63-year-old male developed a vesicular eruption of the ophthalmic branch of the right trigeminal nerve seven days previously. Crusting of the lesions on his forehead and on the lateral aspect of his nose are evident; loss of the eyebrow has also occurred.

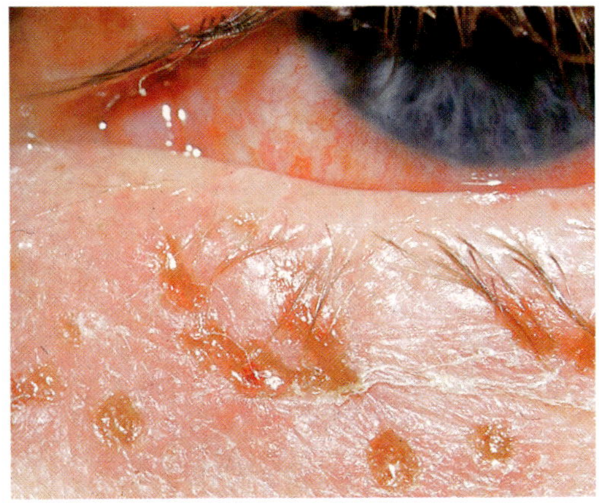

2–26B Crusting of lower eyelid due to herpes zoster involvement of the maxillary branch of the trigeminal nerve. When the maxillary branch of the trigeminal nerve is involved in secondary varicella, typical erythematous macules, which go on to vesiculation and crusting, are commonly found on the lower eyelid, as is seen in this 3-year-old female who developed herpes zoster of the ophthalmic and maxillary branches.

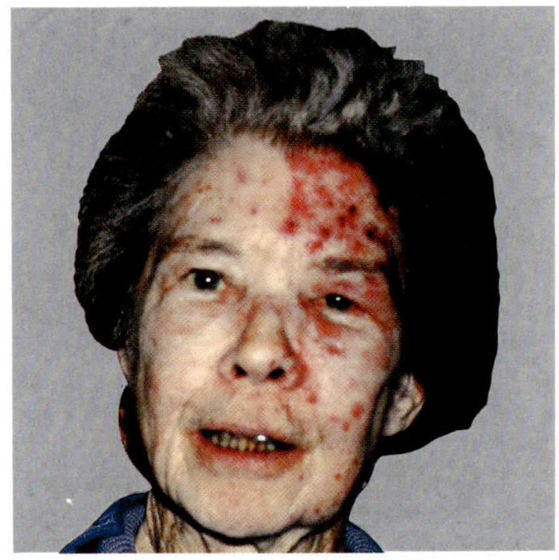

2–26C Disseminated herpes zoster. The varicella zoster virus may disseminate in aging or otherwise immunosuppressed patients, as in this 79-year-old woman who developed herpes zoster ophthalmicus five days prior to noting further eruptions on her body. The lesions are evident on the opposite side of her forehead and in the maxillary area; they were also present on her trunk and legs.

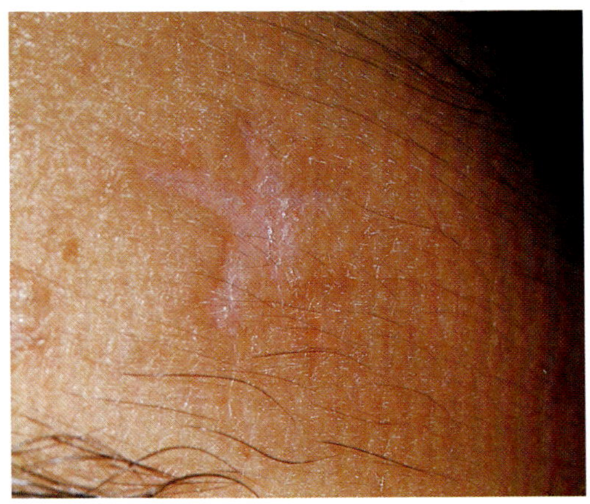

2–27 Scarring of the skin from herpes zoster. Unlike skin infections due to herpes simplex, both primary and secondary varicella commonly result in scarring.This 47-year-old male developed a skin eruption that involved the ophthalmic branch of the left trigeminal nerve. Several lesions healed with moderate scarring, as seen here. The stellate shape of the scar is not typical but is interesting because the epithelial lesions in the cornea usually have a branching character.

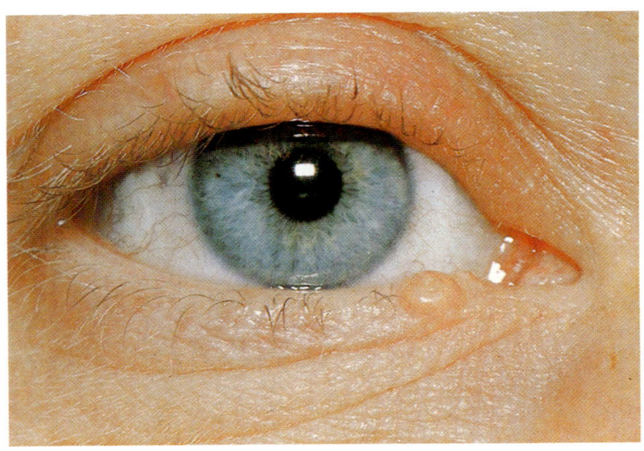

2–28A Molluscum contagiosum nodule of eyelid. The typical molluscum contagiosum nodule is pearly white, dome-shaped, and has a central dimple. In many instances, however, the nodule is macerated and can be missed. This 24-year-old female had a chronic unilateral conjunctivitis for more than four months. She was noted to have a mild follicular conjunctivitis associated with the large molluscum contagiosum nodule on the lower lid margin. Removal of the molluscum nodule gave her complete relief of symptoms.

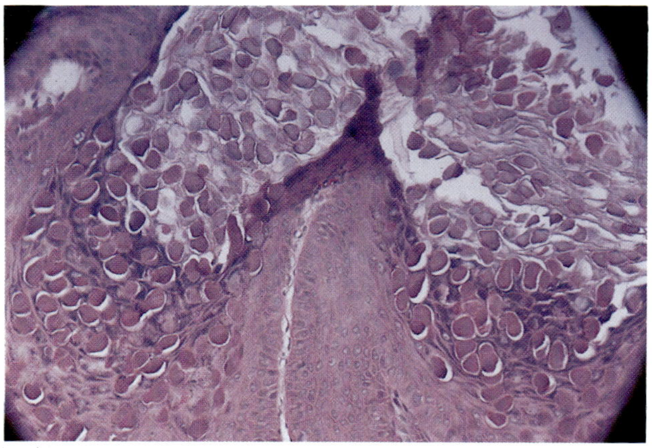

2–28B Histology of molluscum contagiosum nodule. Eosinophilic, hyaline-like masses, which represent the viral inclusions of molluscum contagiosum, are evident within the prickle cells of the malpighian cell layer. As the inclusion matures, the nucleus of the cell is pushed to one side. × 100.

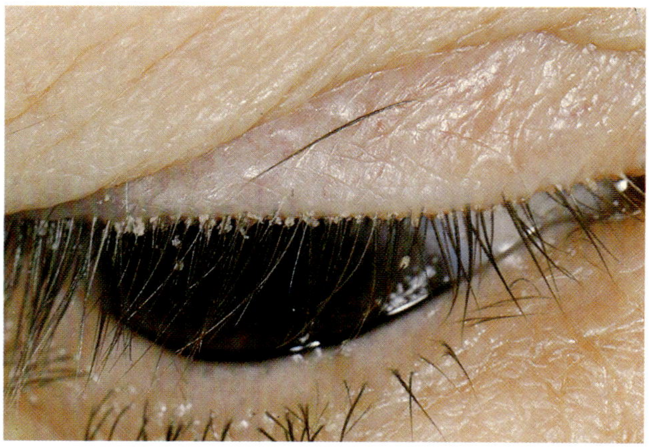

2–29A Sleeves on lid margin due to *Demodex*. The finding of sleeves on the lid margin are almost pathognomonic for *Demodex*. Sleeves consist of small clear extensions of the epithelium of the skin for 1–2 mm along the eyelashes. They resemble the sleeve of a short-sleeved shirt. In this 49-year-old female, many sleeves are noted on the upper eyelid.

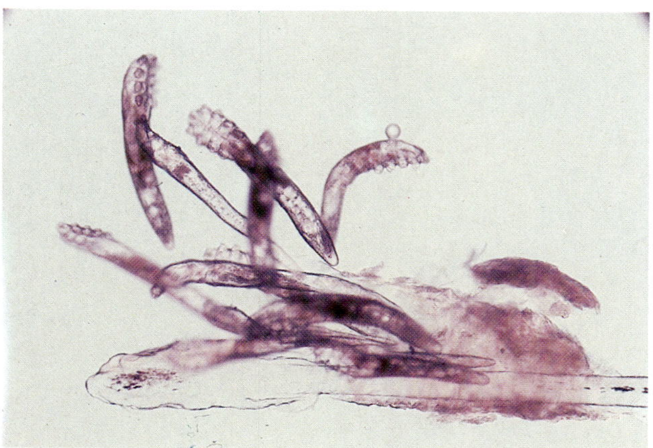

2–29B *Demodex folliculorum*. The eight-legged *D. folliculorum* commonly infects the lid margin. The parasite may act as a vector in staphylococcal infections by carrying the cocci on its abdomen into the lash and oil gland orifices of the lid. The organism is readily found if an infected lash is examined under the low power of the microscope. Its eight jointed legs and abdominal striations are distinctive. *Demodex* is usually found clinging to the base of the eyelash; this photo shows eleven mites on one lash. Giemsa stain, × 63.

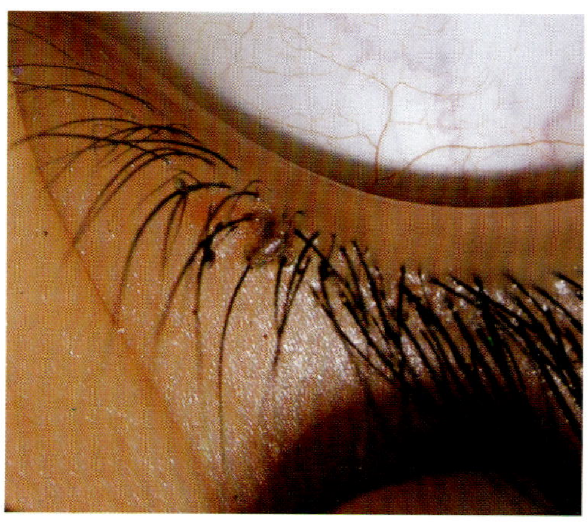

2–30A *Phthirus pubis* on the lid margin. *P. pubis* may be easily missed or mistaken for fibrin on the lid margin because it is semitransparent. Careful examination of the lid margin will usually reveal the organism clinging to the eyelashes. The organism may have a small amount of blood in its gastrointestinal tract which will help the clinician to recognize its presence. This 24-year-old female suffered from itching and irritation of the eye for two weeks. The body of a *Phthirus pubis* can be seen attached to an eyelash. On the outer aspect of the eyelid, several small nits can be seen.

2–30B *Phthirus pubis* organism. This organism is quite distinctive when viewed under the dissecting microscope, as seen in this photograph of an organism taken from a 22-year-old male. This parasite has claws and jointed legs resembling a crab and is commonly called the crab louse. ×25.

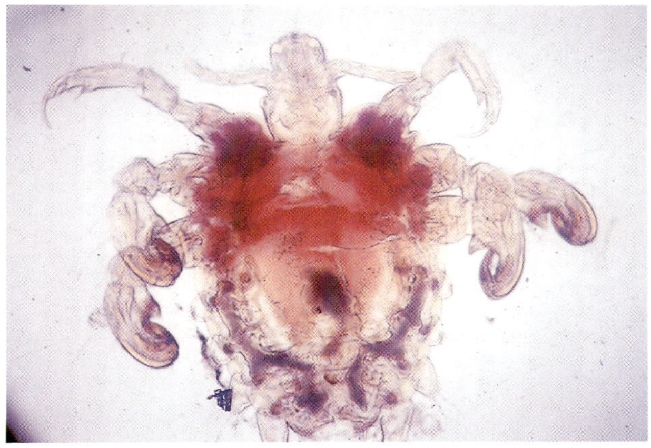

2–30C Nits of *Phthirus pubis* organism. These are easily distinguished when they occur in large numbers on the eyelashes. The nits represent the cases of eggs which are cemented to the eyelash. ×63.

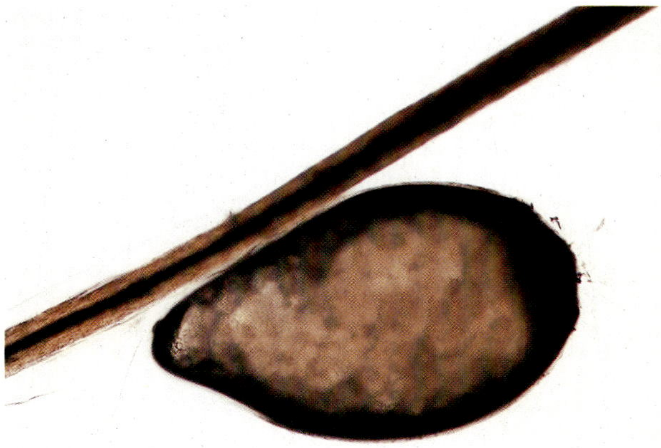

2–31 Soft shelled tick on eyelid. This 16-year-old male was noted to have a soft-shelled tick attached to the eyelid after hiking in the hills. It was easily removed and surprisingly caused no symptoms.

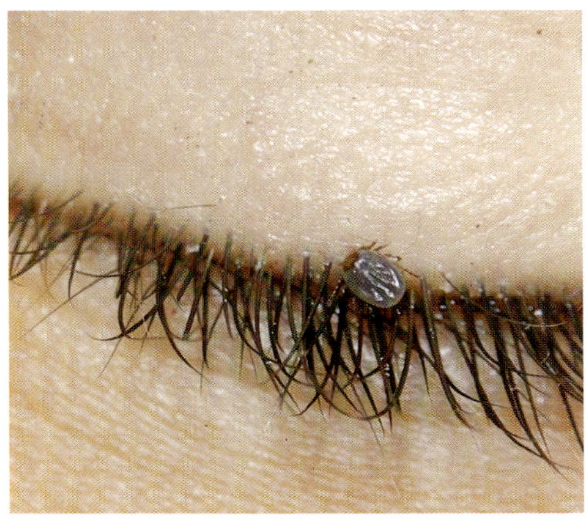

2–32 Edema and erythema of eyelid due to hay fever conjunctivitis. Edema and erythema of the eyelid may occur in hay fever conjunctivitis, as is seen in this 44-year-old laboratory technician who was sensitive to guinea pig dander. Because of the itching, a patient often rubs the eyes excessively, which produces an eczematoid reaction.

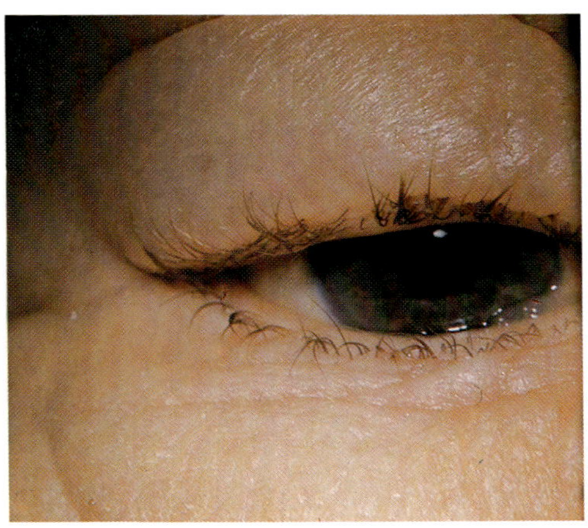

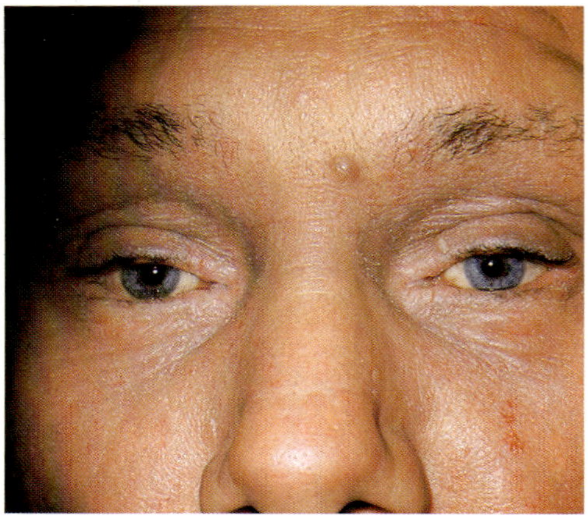

2–33A Eyelid in atopic keratoconjunctivitis. During the early stages of atopic keratoconjunctivitis, erythema and an eczematoid reaction characterized by vesicles, edema, erythema, and exudation may occur on the eyelids. This 22-year-old male was noted to have eczema at eight months of age; the eyelids were affected by about 2 years of age. Erythema, scaling of the skin, and some loss of eyelashes are evident.

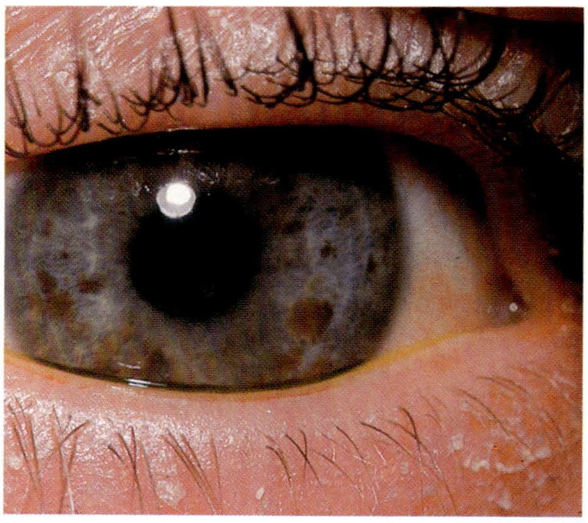

2–33B Atopic dermatitis (late stage). In the late stages of atopic dermatitis, lichenification and pigmentation of the eyelids frequently occur. In this 49-year-old male, edema, lichenification of the eyelids, hyperpigmentation, and excoriation of the lower eyelids and cheek are evident.

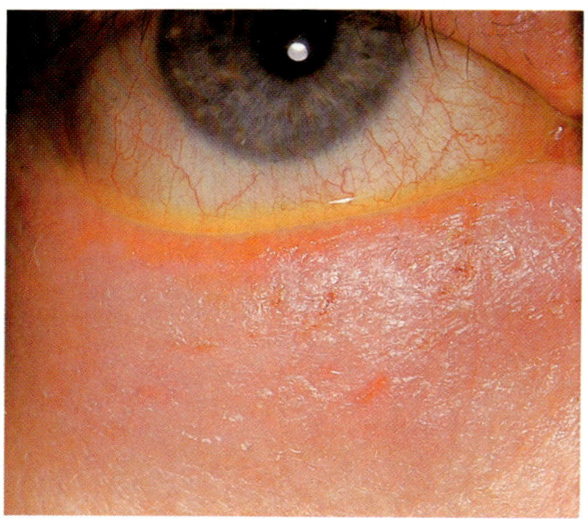

2–33C Atopic dermatitis of the eyelids (late stage), with secondary staphylococcal blepharitis. Loss of lashes, thickening of the eyelid, and lichenification are common findings of atopic blepharitis in the late stages of the disease, as is evident in this 37-year-old male.

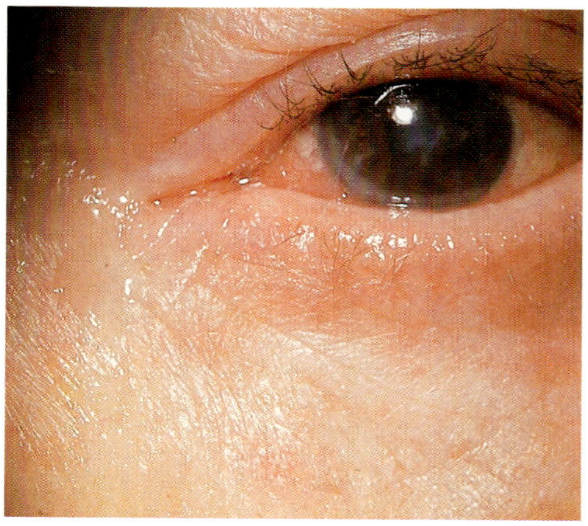

2–34A Contact dermatitis due to idoxuridine (IDU) hypersensitivity. Contact dermatitis may be localized to a small area or may involve the entire eyelid. The early lesions are characterized by erythema, edema, vesiculation, and exudation. This 65-year-old male was using IDU for the corneal dendrite evident in the photograph; he developed an acute allergic reaction to the IDU. Edema and hyperemia are evident, but vesiculation and exudation have not yet occurred.

2–34B Contact dermatitis of the eyelids. If a contact dermatitis is persistent, the skin of the eyelid becomes hypertrophied and there is evidence of fissuring and lichenification. In this 46-year-old male, a contact dermatitis of the eyelids and forehead is noted, with erythema, scaling, and edema being the primary findings. The contact dermatitis occurred from a hypersensitivity to Neosporin®. (The lesion on the forehead represents the original disease for which the patient was treated.)

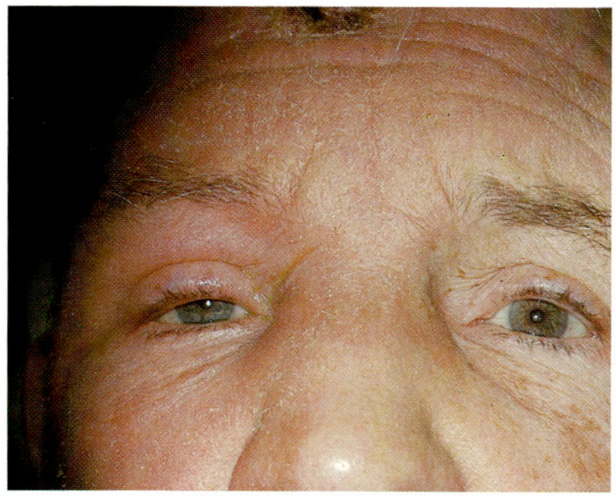

2–35 Acute urticaria of the eyelids and skin of face. An acute urticaria is usually of acute onset and is associated with erythematous weals. It frequently involves the skin of the face and the eyelids. This patient developed an acute urticaria after consuming nuts.

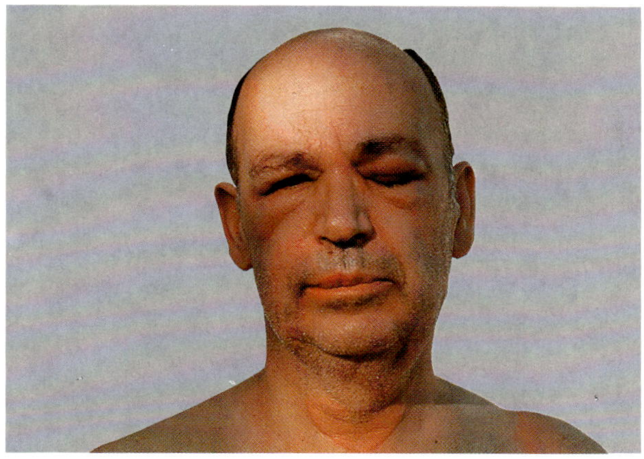

2–36 Angioedema (angioneurotic edema). Because of involvement of the subcutaneous tissues, the lesions of angioneurotic edema are tense, round, and poorly demarcated. Angioedema is often recurrent. In this man from central Africa, the angioedema was thought to be related to a systemic parasitic infection.

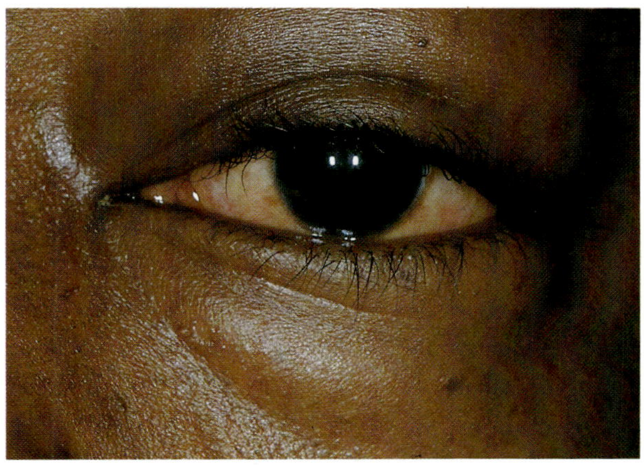

2–37A Meibomitis. A meibomitis or meibomianitis is characterized by dilated and inspissated orifices of the meibomian glands and excessive secretion of the meibomian glands. It may occur for several reasons including irritation, infection of the meibomian glands, a chronic or severe conjunctivitis, keratoconjunctivitis sicca, and seborrhea. This patient, a 36-year-old female, had developed a follicular conjunctivitis eight weeks previously due to inclusion conjunctivitis. She was noted to have inspissation of the meibomian glands and excessive meibomian secretion in association with the follicular conjunctivitis.

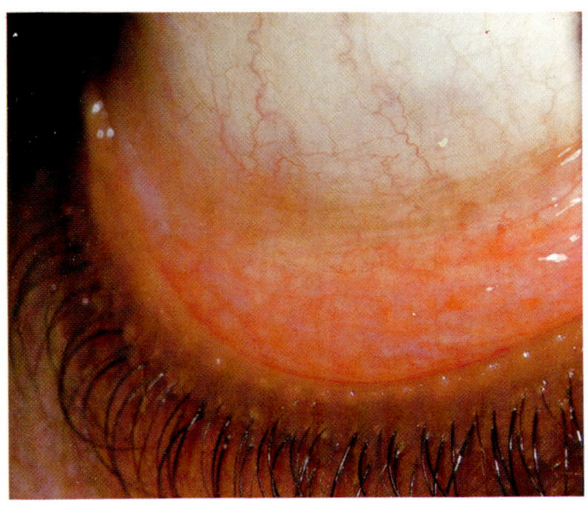

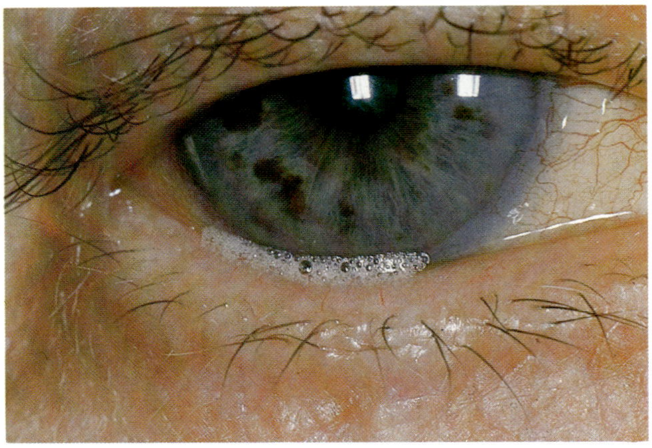

2–37B Meibomian froth. This arises when excess oil secreted by the meibomian glands is whipped into a froth by the movement of the eyelids. Its presence suggests excessive secretion from the meibomian glands and can be seen in any chronic conjunctivitis and with those factors that cause a meibomitis (see Fig. 2–37A). This patient, a 67-year-old male, had a chronic blepharoconjunctivitis due to staphylococcal infection. An epithelial keratitis and telangiectasis of the lid margin are also evident.

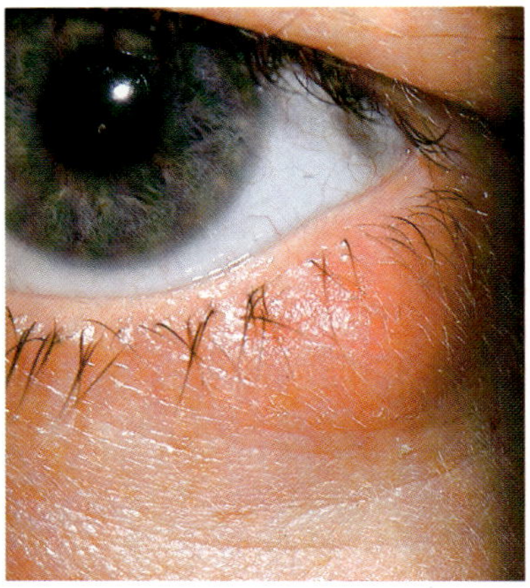

2–38A Chalazion. A chalazion is a small tumefaction of the eyelid that occurs from distension of a meibomian gland. The lesion is usually painless, evolves slowly, and eventually forms a lipogranuloma. It is hard like a hailstone, from which its name is derived. In this patient, who was seen with the complaint of a hard lump and swelling of the eyelid, edema, mild erythema, and a swollen appearance to the external eyelid in the region of the chalazion are evident.

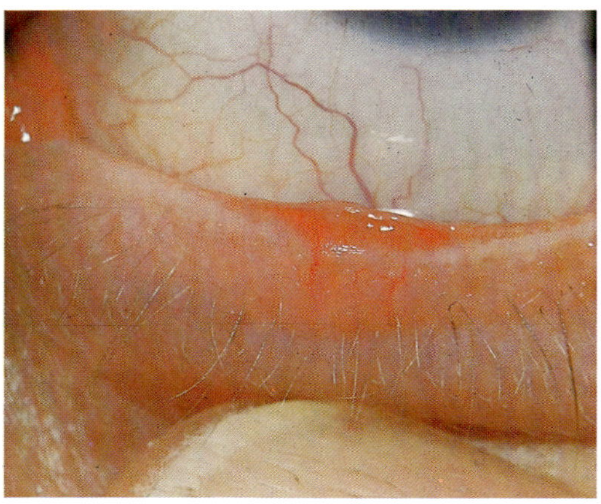

2–38B Marginal chalazion. The inflammation and tumefaction of the eyelid may involve the neck of the meibomian gland, producing a marginal chalazion. This 48-year-old female noted redness and swelling of the lid margin three weeks previously. The lid is red and swollen and has been everted slightly to demonstrate the more pronounced redness and swelling on the conjunctival side of the lesion.

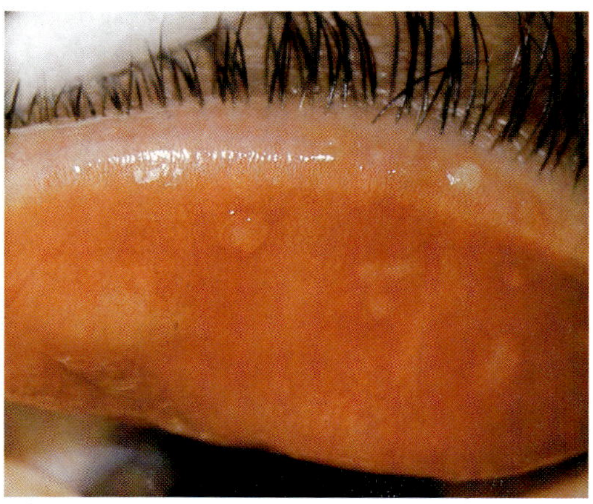

2–38C Chalazion. Multiple and/or recurrent chalazia are frequently caused by staphylococcal infections of the eyelid. In this 58-year-old male, multiple and recurrent chalazia are evident within the tarsus and at the lid margin of the eyelid. An inspissated orifice of one of the meibomian glands is prominent.

2–38D Chalazion. In many instances a chalazion ruptures through the tarsus to form a granuloma on the conjunctiva, as noted in this 34-year-old female who developed a pedunculated granuloma from an inflammatory reaction to the lipid material contained in the meibomian gland.

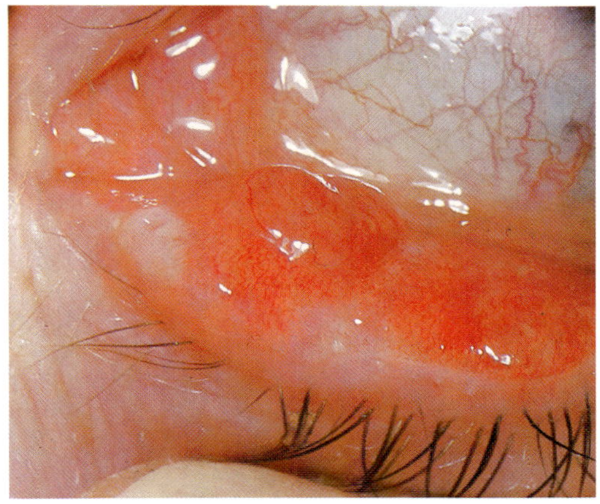

2–39 Histologic section of chalazion. A chalazion represents a lipogranuloma resulting from a granulomatous reaction to meibomian oil. It is a focal granuloma with abscess formation around fat. The granuloma is composed of foreign-body type giant cells, epithelioid cells, lymphocytes, and plasma cells. Hematoxylin and eosin, ×63.

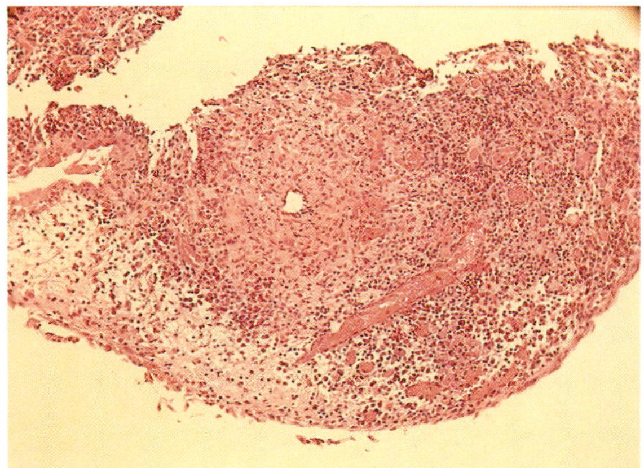

2–40A Erythema multiforme skin eruption. The skin eruption of erythema multiforme major frequently begins with an erythema, such as is evident in this 18-year-old female who developed a generalized skin eruption with involvement of the eyes and mouth following exposure to sulfonamides. Marked erythema of the skin of the nose and a ruptured bulla near the nose are evident.

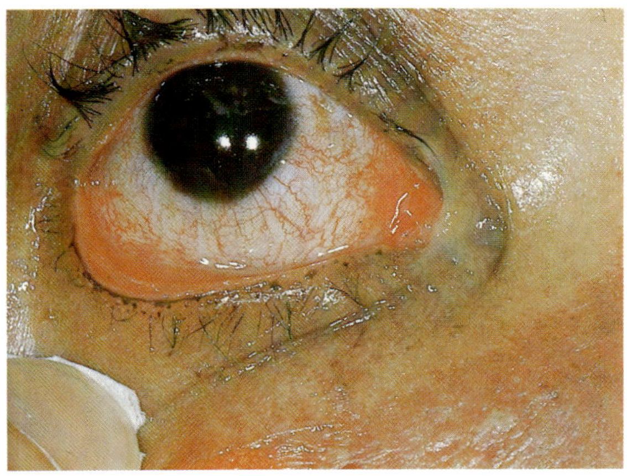

2–40B Erythema multiforme skin lesions. The erythematous lesions of erythema multiforme major progress rapidly to form typical target-like lesions. The skin eruption may involve the face and eyelids and is symmetrical in form. The mouth and often the nose are involved (Stevens-Johnson syndrome). In this 24-year-old male, ulceration of the lips with crusting, ulceration of the tongue, and dried blood that has exuded from a lesion in the nostril can be seen.

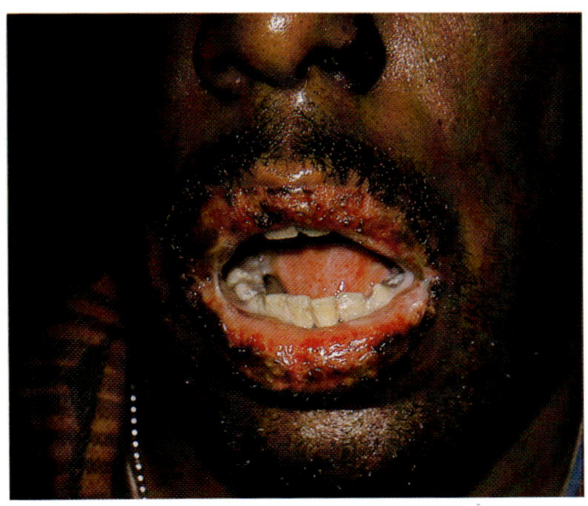

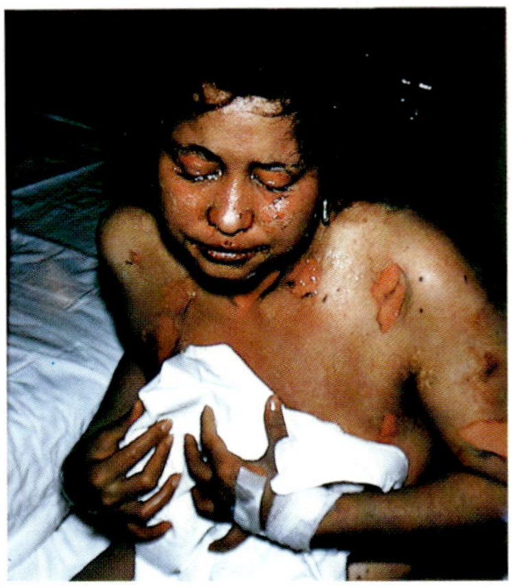

2–41 A Nikolsky's sign in toxic epidermal necrolysis. A typical Nikolsky's sign occurs in toxic epidermal necrolysis. It is characterized by the tendency of normal epidermis to be stripped away from underlying dermis when tangential pressure is applied to the skin. The skin on the shoulder of this patient appeared normal before pressure was exerted to test for a Nikolsky sign. (Reprinted with permission from *Transactions of the American Academy of Ophthalmology and Otolaryngology.)*

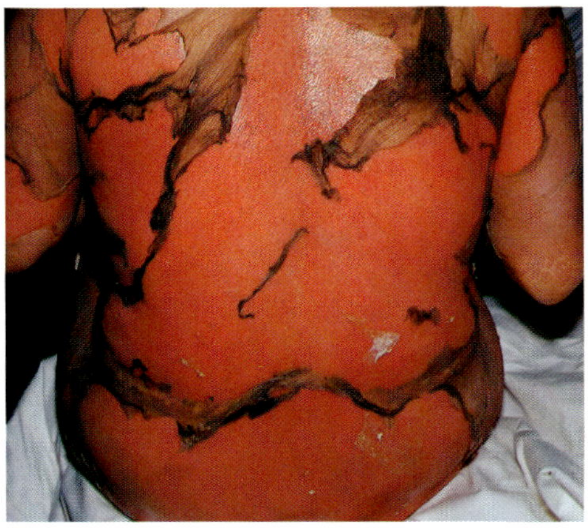

2–41 B Skin in toxic epidermal necrolysis. Toxic epidermal necrolysis is also called the scalded skin syndrome because of the appearance of scalded skin in involved areas. As in patients with third degree burns, exudation of fluids frequently occurs into the flaccid bullae of toxic epidermal necrolysis, which complicates therapy. This photograph is of the same woman pictured in Fig. 2–41 A. The eruption was triggered by the use of phenylbutazoladine. (Reprinted with permission from *Transactions of the American Academy of Ophthalmology and Otolaryngology.)*

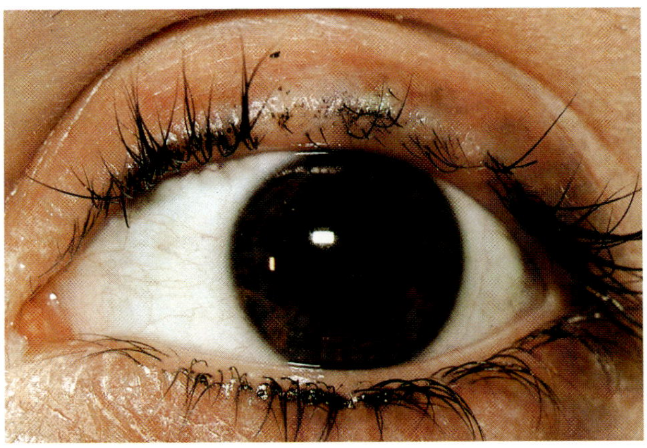

2–42 Alopecia areata involving eyelashes. Alopecia areata or alopecia totalis rarely involve the eyelashes or eyebrows. However, when the eyelashes and eyebrows are involved, the hair usually regenerates. Loss of the central area of eyelashes of the upper eyelid are evident in this photograph of a 27-year-old female.

Chapter 3

Infections and Inflammations of the Conjunctiva

The clinician can often narrow the possible cause of a conjunctivitis by carefully evaluating the patient's symptoms (such as itching), the duration of the disease (acute or chronic), and the type of conjunctival exudate (purulent or watery). These findings can be used to help in selection of appropriate specific laboratory studies, and the results of these studies can then be used to direct or modify therapy.

Papillae

Papillae and diffuse infiltration are the hallmarks of allergic and bacterial conjunctivitis (Ostler and Braley, 1954; Thygeson, 1947). Papillae are nipple-shaped projections of the conjunctival surface, which develop from the infiltration of cells (lymphocytes, granulocytes, and plasma cells) into the conjunctiva around dilated capillaries. They occur in areas where the conjunctiva is firmly attached by fine fibrils to the underlying tissue (tarsus, limbus, and semilunar fold). Fine, almost microscopic, papillae develop in acute and subacute conjunctival infections and give a velvety appearance to the conjunctiva (Figs. 3–1, 3–2). On slit-lamp examination, each papilla appears to be centered around a small tuft of vessels located within its core, which runs perpendicularly toward the surface of the conjunctiva, then branches subepithelially like the framework of an umbrella over the surface of the papilla. In areas where the conjunctiva is not firmly attached to the underlying tissues (e.g., inferior cul-de-sac), a similar diffuse infiltration of inflammatory cells produces rugae.

In prolonged or severe inflammations such as vernal keratoconjunctivitis or gonorrheal conjunctivitis, many of the conjunctival fibrils are broken by the intense cellular infiltration and giant papillae are formed (Figs. 3–3, 3–4). The giant papillae are polygonal and flat-topped. Because a giant papilla arises from the fusion of several fine papillae, several tufts of vessels course through the papilla to reach its surface before branching. In conjunctival inflammation, thickening also occurs because of diffuse infiltration. This obscures the normal deep vessels of the upper tarsus so that the vessels appear fuzzy or are completely hidden.

Lymphoid Follicles

Lymphoid follicles develop in the conjunctival cul-de-sac and at the edge of the tarsus in many inflammatory conditions of the eye, especially in young children. However, follicles occurring in the tarsal or limbal conjunctiva or on the semilunar fold are characteristic of a chlamydial or viral infection or occasionally a "toxic" reaction (Fig. 3–5). Follicles represent lymphoid tissue and consist of pale-staining, immature lymphocytes and macrophages surrounded by a peripheral zone of lymphocytes (Figs. 3–6A, 3–6B). Necrosis of the central zone of the follicle produces conjunctival scarring. Follicles are round, avascular structures, 0.2–2 mm in diameter, and white or gray in color (Fig. 3–6C). By slit-lamp observation, small blood vessels can be seen encircling a follicle and forming superficial vascular tufts that project toward the center of the follicle.

Granulomas

Granulomatous infiltration of the conjunctiva is uncommon but may occur in various infectious processes, as a reaction to retained foreign bodies (including suspensions of steroids or a ruptured chalazion), or in several diseases of unknown etiology. Granulomas are formed by collections of lymphocytes, plasma cells, epithelioid cells, and giant cells which surround budding capillaries within the substance of the granuloma. They vary in size, are yellow or red in color, and appear semiopaque or opaque (Fig. 3–7). The adjacent conjunctiva is markedly inflamed and infiltrated, resulting in a papillary or follicular hypertrophy. A granuloma also may become necrotic and ulcerate, which in turn accentuates the inflammation and inflammatory exudate.

Edema

Edema fluid produces a clear, translucent swelling of the bulbar conjunctiva (chemosis) and/or a milky appearance of the palpebral conjunctiva. Edema is often accompanied by hyperemia, and is most apparent in the bulbar conjunctiva and in the fornices where large amounts of fluid can cause the conjunctiva to protrude through the lids and even over the cornea. Conjunctival edema and chemosis may result from acute inflammation of the lids, conjunctiva, and orbit, from allergic and hypersensitive reactions due to intrinsic conditions such as angioedema, from blocked venous or lymphatic drainage of the orbit (e.g., carotid and cavernous fistulae), and from endocrine exophthalmus.

Bacterial Infections

Purulent Conjunctivitis

A purulent or hyperacute conjunctivitis is characterized by copious secretion of pus (Fig. 3–8 A), edema of the eyelids, marked papillary hypertrophy (Fig. 3–8 B), and in many cases ulceration of the peripheral cornea. The major causative organism of a purulent conjunctivitis is *Neisseria gonorrhoeae,* but other causes include *Neiserria meningitidis* infection or improper treatment of any bacterial conjunctivitis, such as the use of a pressure dressing. Scraping of the conjunctiva in *N. gonorrhoeae* infection reveals many Gram-negative intracellular diplococci (Figs. 3–9 A, 3–9 B). However, culture and sugar utilization studies are necessary to differentiate *N. gonorrhoeae* from *N. meningitidis* (Figs. 3–10 A, 3–10 B).

Membranous and Pseudomembranous Conjunctivitis

Membranous and pseudomembranous bacterial conjunctivitis are characterized by the appearance of a fibrinous exudate, which may be extensive, and involve most of the tarsal and in some instances the bulbar conjunctiva; alternatively, the fibrinous exudate may be localized and occur in patches on the tarsal or bulbar conjunctiva. The major bacterial causes of a membranous or pseudomembranous conjunctivitis are *Streptococcus pyogenes* and *Corynebacterium diphtheriae.* A membranous conjunctivitis is differentiated from a pseudomembranous conjunctivitis by the tendency for the base of a membrane to bleed if it is removed from the conjunctiva. In most instances, a true membranous conjunctivitis results from ulceration or necrosis of the conjunctiva with transudation of fibrin and inflammatory cells into the conjunctiva. A pseudomembrane, on the other hand, can be removed relatively easily from the underlying surface leaving only a few or no bleeding points. It represents transudation of fibrin and inflammatory cells onto the surface of the conjunctiva.

Acute Catarrhal Conjunctivitis

An acute catarrhal or mucopurulent conjunctivitis is characterized by hyperemia and a mucopurulent discharge. It often occurs in epidemic form and is commonly called "pinkeye" because both the bulbar and the tarsal conjunctiva are injected. The discharge is serous or watery at first but becomes mucopurulent. Among the common causes of acute catarrhal conjunctivitis are *Streptococcus pneumoniae* (Figs. 3–11 A, 3–11 B, 3–11 C) and *Haemophilus influenzae* biotype 2 *(H. aegyptius)* (Figs. 3–12 A, 3–12 B, 3–12 C) (Dawson, 1960). Scraping from the conjunctiva usually reveals the offending organism (Figs. 3–11 B, 3–12 B), and the findings can be verified by culture (Figs. 3–11 C, 3–12 C).

Subacute Catarrhal Conjunctivitis

A subacute catarrhal conjunctivitis is characterized by a watery or flocculant discharge and is usually caused by *Haemophilus influenzae.* The hyperemia is most marked in the conjunctival fornices and on the tarsal conjunctiva (Fig. 3–13 A). The conjunctivitis, like the acute catarrhal conjunctivitides, occurs in epidemic form. Scrapings of the conjunctiva reveal tiny, Gram-negative coccobacilli (Fig. 3–13 B), which are frequently missed because of their size. Cultures are helpful to verify the presence of the organism (Fig. 3–13 C).

Chronic Catarrhal Conjunctivitis

In chronic catarrhal conjunctivitis, the conjunctival inflammation is prolonged and discharge is minimal. The major symptoms are foreign body sensation, burning, and in some instances itching. The clinical findings are usually minimal, and the discrepancy between symptoms and findings are the major characteristics of this form of conjunctivitis. The common causes of a chronic catarrhal conjunctivitis are chronic staphylococcal blepharitis (Chapter 2) (Fig. 3–14), seborrhea, keratoconjunctivitis sicca (Chapter 6) (Fig. 3–15), and excessive use of medications.

Granulomatous Conjunctivitis

Conjunctivitis caused by other bacterial infections is uncommon, and is often characterized by the presence of granulomas in the conjunctiva and greatly enlarged preauricular and/or submandibular lymph nodes. (See the section on oculoglandular syndromes).

Chlamydial Infections

There are two species of chlamydia, *Chlamydia trachomatis* and *Chlamydia psittaci,* and both infect the human conjunctiva; *C. trachomatis* causes trachoma, lymphogranuloma venereum, and inclusion conjunctivitis; *C. psittaci* causes psittacosis and feline pneumonitis. The *C. trachomatis* strains (or biovars) are almost all human pathogens, whereas the *C. psittaci* strains primarily infect other vertebrate species and only occasionally infect humans; in those humans who are infected, the conjunctiva is only very rarely involved.

The *C. trachomatis* strains are classified by immunological methods into 15 serotypes. Classic endemic trachoma is almost always associated with serotypes A, B, Ba and C. Serotypes D through K, on the other hand, are usually associated with sexual transmission. Strains A through K infect the mucous epithelia in humans, but do not invade the deeper tissues; they are often referred to as TRIC strains (Trachoma-Inclusion Conjunctivitis). Lymphogranuloma venereum strains are designated as L1, L2, or L3. They differ biologically from the TRIC strains in a number of ways including failure to infect epithelium, a tendency to invade the cells of the lymphatic system, and a tendency to rapidly kill embryonated hens' eggs and mice on first inoculation. *C. trachomatis* strains are susceptible to the tetracyclines, erythromycin, and sulfonamides.

Most cases of chlamydial conjunctivitis, with the exception of inclusion conjunctivitis of the newborn and lymphogranuloma venereum, are characterized by follicle formation in the tarsal conjunctiva. However, in inclusion conjunctivitis of the newborn, a papillary conjunctivitis develops, followed by a follicular conjunctivitis if the infection persists longer than six to eight weeks.

Scoring of Follicles and Papillae

The World Health Organization has identified four signs to be used for identifying trachoma: tarsal follicles, typical conjunctival scarring, vascular pannus, and Herbert's pits. If two or more of these signs are present, a diagnosis of trachoma can be made.

In order to standardize the diagnosis of trachoma and its severity, it is recommended that the inflammation (papillary and follicular reaction) be classified according to the recommendations of the World Health Committee for Trachoma (Figs. 3–16A, 3–16B, 3–16C) (Dawson et al., 1981). In many industrially developing countries, flies serve as a major vector for the trachoma organism (Fig. 3–17).

Trachoma

Trachoma is the most common cause of preventable blindness in the world. This chronic follicular conjunctivitis is characterized by follicles on the tarsal conjunctiva (Figs. 3–16A, 3–16B, 3–16C), superficial neovascular infiltration of the cornea (pannus), epithelial keratitis, and corneal and conjunctival scarring. Follicles may also occur at the limbus (Fig. 3–18A); on resolving, these follicles leave clear areas or depressions (Herbert's pits) (Fig. 3–18B), a pathognomonic sign of trachoma.

Varying degrees of scarring of the conjunctiva occur in trachoma, but in many patients, the scarring and pannus formation are minor and do not lead to further problems (Fig. 3–19A). In some patients, however, the scarring is severe (Fig. 3–19B), and the scars may gradually contract (Fig. 3–19C) causing the lashes and lid margin to turn in (trichiasis) (Fig. 3–20A); this may cause individual cilia to constantly abrade the cornea. The trichiasis and the resultant corneal abrasion may in turn lead to corneal ulceration and loss of vision (Fig. 3–20B).

Trachoma is an endemic disease of the poorer rural populations of developing countries. The infection is acquired in childhood, and the infectious phase resolves as the child reaches adolescence. The conjunctival scarring that develops during the childhood infection may many years later (in adult life) produce trichiasis/entropion and corneal opacities.

Although the diagnosis of trachoma may be made on clinical grounds, the Microtrac test has been developed recently as an aid in the diagnosis of chlamydial infections such as trachoma and is widely available for use. Typical chlamydial inclusion bodies may also be seen (Figs. 3–21A, 3–21B). Care should be taken, however, not to confuse pigment granules with intracytoplasmic inclusions (Fig. 3–22). Bacteria may also be seen in conjunctival scrapings of patients with trachoma (Fig. 3–23) and these should not be confused with inclusion bodies.

Inclusion Conjunctivitis

In adults, inclusion conjunctivitis usually presents as an acute follicular conjunctivitis with mucopurulent discharge and preauricular lymphadenopathy (Fig. 3–24). If untreated, the conjunctivitis may persist for many months. In patients with chronic inclusion conjunctivitis, epithelial and subepithelial keratitis and minor degrees of pannus formation are very common. In addition, conjunctival scarring has been reported to occur in adults with inclusion conjunctivitis in the

United Kingdom; however, the disease does not lead to permanent visual loss.

Neonatal inclusion conjunctivitis (inclusion blennorrhea) is caused by infection of the newborn's conjunctiva with *C. trachomatis* arising from the genital tract of the mother. If not appropriately treated, the infection may persist for months. Conjunctival scarring and minor degrees of pannus formation are common in untreated patients.

Neonatal inclusion conjunctivitis is characterized by hyperemia, diffuse infiltration and papillary hypertrophy, swelling of the conjunctiva, and moderate mucopurulent discharge (Fig. 3–25). Conjunctival follicles become a prominent sign of the inclusion conjunctivitis if the disease persists longer than six to eight weeks. Scraping of the conjunctiva reveals many polymorphonuclear leukocytes and a few intraepithelial inclusion bodies (Fig. 3–26), which are identical to those seen in trachoma (Figs. 3–21A, 3–21B).

About 15% of infants exposed during birth to their mother's *C. trachomatis* genital-tract infection develop chlamydial interstitial pneumonia; moreover, exposed infants may shed the agent from the gastrointestinal tract. Thus, treatment of inclusion blennorrhea must include systemic antibiotics and not be limited to the topical application of antibiotics to the eye. The current recommended treatment regimen is erythromycin in a pediatric suspension for oral use (40 mg/kg day in four divided doses) for two to three weeks.

Lymphogranuloma Venereum

A conjunctivitis caused by lymphogranuloma venereum is very rare and presents as a Parinaud's oculoglandular syndrome with grossly enlarged preauricular or submandibular lymph nodes (see the section on Parinaud's syndrome). There is diffuse hyperemia, swelling, infiltration of the conjunctiva, and granulomata (Fig. 3–27). The conjunctival scraping from lymphogranuloma venereum reveals many polymorphonuclear leukocytes but no epithelial inclusions.

Chlamydia psittaci Conjunctivitis

C. psittaci occasionally causes a follicular conjunctivitis. Humans have developed conjunctivitis after both natural and laboratory exposure to psittacosis, and after natural exposure to feline pneumonitis. The conjunctivitis caused by these infections resembles inclusion conjunctivitis (Ostler et al., 1969). (Fig. 3–28), but the infection is more resistant to therapy and may require oral tetracycline for six to eight weeks. Epidemiologically, these patients have been exposed to infected psittacine birds or to infected cats. Systemic manifestations, particularly pulmonary involvement, may also occur in psittacosis.

Rickettsial Infections

Rickettsial infections of the conjunctiva are rare, although the conjunctiva may serve as the portal of entry for rickettsia. With few exceptions (Q-fever and epidemic typhus) the conjunctivitis is mild.

Viral Infections

Lymphoid follicles are the hallmark of viral conjunctivitis, except in particularly severe cases that present as a membranous or pseudomembranous conjunctivitis. Corneal involvement is also common.

Viral infections of the conjunctiva include the following:

1. Adenoviruses 3 and 7, the common causes of pharyngoconjunctival fever (Fig. 3–29);
2. Adenoviruses 8 and 19, the common causes of epidemic keratoconjunctivitis (Jawetz et al., 1957) (Figs. 3–30A, 3–30B, 3–30C);
3. Enterovirus 70 and coxsackievirus A24, the causes of acute hemorrhagic conjunctivitis (Fig. 3–31);
4. Conjunctivitis resulting from a molluscum contagiosum infection of the lid margin (Fig. 3–32);
5. Keratoconjunctivitis due to Newcastle's disease virus;
6. Oculoglandular syndrome due to Epstein-Barr virus;
7. Conjunctivitis associated with primary and occasionally recurrent herpes simplex (Figs. 3–33A, 3–33B, 3–33C, 3–33D);
8. Keratoconjunctivitis occurring with ophthalmic zoster (Fig. 3–34);
9. Kaposi's sarcoma apparently resulting from infection with HTLV 3 virus (Fig. 3–35);
10. Keratoconjunctivitis associated with exanthema such as measles, mumps, rubella, and primary varicella.

A pseudomembranous conjunctivitis may occur instead of or in addition to follicle formation in some viral conjunctivitides, such as epidemic keratoconjunctivitis (Fig. 3–30D), primary and (rarely) secondary herpes simplex conjunctivitis, and the conjunctivitis associated with herpes zoster ophthalmicus.

A verruca of the conjunctiva differs from most viral infections of the conjunctiva; a papilloma (Fig. 3–36) or multiple papillomas are formed in place of the follicular or pseudomembranous conjunctivitis noted above.

Kaposi's sarcoma of the conjunctiva is often confused with a subconjunctival hemorrhage of the bulbar conjunctiva or the cul-de-sac (Fig. 3–35). The lesion, however, fails to resolve and usually increases in size over many weeks. In rare instances, Kaposi's sarcoma may be the presenting sign of the acquired immune deficiency syndrome (AIDS).

With the exception of the conjunctivitis resulting from a molluscum contagiosum infection of the lid margin and Kaposi's sarcoma, all viral conjunctivitis heals spontaneously within two to three weeks; this makes it possible for the clinician to differentiate a viral from a chlamydial conjunctivitis by history alone. Moreover, patients with viral conjunctivitis often have systemic manifestations of infection (e.g., pharyngitis and fever in adenoviral 3 and 7 infections, or regional adenopathy, malaise, and fever associated with ophthalmic zoster).

The inflammatory cells in conjunctival scrapings from a viral conjunctivitis characteristically are predominantly lymphocytes. This can be used to distinguish a viral follicular conjunctivitis from a chlamydial conjunctivitis: the polymorphonuclear granulocytes and lymphocytes occur in equal numbers in chlamydial infections. The one exception to this rule is a pseudomembranous or membranous conjunctivitis of any origin, in which the predominant inflammatory reaction consists of polymorphonuclear granulocytes.

Fungal Infections

The most common fungal infection of the conjunctiva is due to *Candida* spp. It is characterized by the appearance of a soft, white, slightly elevated plaque, which when scraped from the surface of the conjunctiva leaves a raw bleeding surface. Smears of the plaque show that it consists of a mass of pseudohyphal organisms. Candidal infections of the conjunctiva are found most commonly in newborn children and in immunocompromised patients.

Other fungal infections such as *Sporothrix schenckii, Rhinosporidium seeberi* (Prevost et al., 1980), and *Coccidioides immitis* (Wood, 1967) produce granulomata of the conjunctiva together with grossly visible regional lymphadenitis (oculoglandular syndrome), as discussed below.

Metazoal Infections

Many metazoa may infect the conjunctiva, such as *Thelazia californiensis,* which causes a mild conjunctivitis with symptoms of irritation and redness; *Trichinella spiralis,* which during the systemic stage of the illness produces a yellow discoloration and chemosis of the conjunctiva, most prominent overlying the rectus muscles; *Onchocerca volvulus,* which produces mild injection, chemosis, and swelling of the limbus; *Loa loa,* which during its aimless wandering throughout the body and orbit produces conjunctival chemosis, burning and irritation; and American leishmaniasis, which produces an ulcerating granuloma of the conjunctiva and eyelid.

A severe irritative form of conjunctivitis may develop from the tissue juices of *Taenia solium* entering the eye, as may occur during the cutting of heavily infected meat when the juices squirt into the eye. A mild irritative form of conjunctivitis may occur from maggots of flies (e.g., larvae of *Oestrus ovis* and *Hypoderma bovis*), which develop after the eggs are deposited in the conjunctival sac. This form of conjunctivitis is accompanied by symptoms of itching, burning, and tearing, and should be distinguished from the effects of fly maggots on the orbit (Chapter 7).

In young children and adolescents, a follicular conjunctivitis may be associated with a *Phthirus pubis* lid infection and is probably the result of the propensity of the child to produce follicles when even mildly stimulated antigenicly.

Parinaud's Oculoglandular Syndrome

Parinaud's oculoglandular syndrome is characterized by the presence of conjunctival granulomata (Fig. 3–37A) and a grossly visible regional (usually preauricular) lymphadenitis (Fig. 3–37B). Although follicles usually occur, they are not a mandatory part of the syndrome. The oculoglandular syndrome may be caused by bacterial, chlamydial, rickettsial, viral (Meisler et al., 1981), or fungal infections. (Table

Table 3–1 Etiology of Parinaud's Oculoglandular Syndrome

Bacteria	*Leptotrichia* spp. *Mycobacterium tuberculosis* (Fig. 3–38) *Treponema pallidum* *Francisella tularensis* (Figs. 3–39 A, 3–39 B)
Chlamydia	*Chlamydia trachomatis* (Lymphogranuloma venereum) (Fig. 3–27)
Rickettsia	*Rickettsia conorii* (boutonneuse fever)
Virus	Epstein-Barr virus (infectious mononucleosis) (Fig. 3–40)
Fungus	*Coccidioides immitis* (coccidioidomycosis) (Fig. 3–41)
Unknown etiology	Cat scratch disease (Figs. 3–37 A, 3–37 B), Sarcoid (Fig. 3–42)

3–1). As can be seen from the list of causes, many of the infections are systemic in nature with the eye playing a predominant role in symptomatology.

Noninfectious Inflammations

Not all forms of conjunctival inflammation are caused by microbial or parasitic organisms. While the exact causes of these noninfectious forms of conjunctivitis are unknown, the natural history and appearance of the conditions have been well characterized.

Pterygium

A pterygium is a hyperplastic overgrowth of a small patch of conjunctiva onto the cornea. Pterygia usually arise in the exposed bulbar conjunctiva and extend from the nasal limbus, and less commonly from the temporal limbus, over the peripheral cornea. The growth has a fan shape, in which the smaller portion (head) is located on the cornea, and the wider, fleshy vascular portion (base) extends into the medial or lateral bulbar conjunctiva (Fig. 3–43).

A pterygium is often associated with a pinguecula (see below), and both pterygia and pinguecula probably represent conjunctival degenerative changes occurring in response to chronic solar radiation. An active pterygium continues to grow toward the center of the cornea and occasionally impinges on the visual axis. It is frequently inflamed and may be confused with a conjunctivitis. Pterygia are not true neoplasms, but are proliferative degenerations composed of thickened and degenerative connective tissue and elastic fibers. In the cornea, anterior to the head of the pterygium, a faint clouding in Bowman's membrane and islands of superficial opacity may occur during periods of clinical activity.

A pseudopterygium is composed of a tongue of conjunctiva adherent to the cornea. It occurs most often in response to a marginal ulcer or other corneal inflammation and can occur at any point on the corneal limbus. Unlike true pterygia, pseudopterygia form a bridge over the limbus under which a probe may be passed

Pinguecula and Pingueculitis

A pinguecula is a yellow triangular patch of hypertrophic and degenerated connective tissue fibers, occurring close to the limbus in the interpalpebral fissure area on either side of the cornea. The name is derived from its yellow color and means fat (Fig. 3–44).

A pingueculitis is an inflammation of a pinguecula and is considered by some to be a form of episcleritis. Although the etiology of a pinguecula is unknown, chronic exposure to sunlight appears to be a common factor; these conditions are more frequent in the aging population. Pingueculae are localized to the subepithelial and episcleral connective tissue.

Superior Limbic Keratoconjunctivitis

Superior limbic keratoconjunctivitis (SLK) is a condition of unknown etiology (Thygeson, 1963; Theodore, 1963). It is manifested by inflammation of the upper tarsal conjunctiva (diffuse fine papillary hypertrophy) (Fig. 3–45 A); thickening, flaccidity, and inflammation of the upper bulbar conjunctiva (Fig. 3–45 B); and fine superficial epithelial keratitis, filament formation, and micropannus in the upper one-third of the cornea. The condition is commonly associated with some form of thyroid abnormality (hyper- or hypothyroidism). It occurs in all age groups and is usually bilateral.

Toxic Follicular Conjunctivitis

A chronic follicular conjunctivitis (Fig. 3–46) may occur from the prolonged use of many topical ocular medications, including atropine, idoxuridine, and other antivirals, and carbachol and other antiglaucoma medications. This syndrome may lead to the formation of conjunctival scars, epithelial keratitis, and vascular pannus. Because of the mode of presentation it has been called "pseudotrachoma" (Thygeson and Dawson, 1971).

Erythema Multiforme Major (Stevens-Johnson Syndrome)

Erythema multiforme major is a systemic illness that usually begins with acute malaise and fever followed within days by a skin eruption consisting of macules, papules, vesicles, and then bullae. There is an ulcerative stomatitis and a conjunctivitis which may be catarrhal, purulent, or pseudomembranous (Fig. 3–47A). The conjunctivitis usually heals with scarring (Fig. 3–47B). Although the etiology is frequently not determined, many cases of erythema multiforme major are associated with the ingestion or topical administration of drugs such as antibiotics, exposure to radiation, or onset of infections such as herpes simplex.

Ligneous Conjunctivitis

Ligneous conjunctivitis is a rare, chronic form of conjunctivitis of unknown etiology, most commonly seen in young girls (Fig. 3–48). It is manifested by the presence of a persistent, thick, white membrane on the upper and, less commonly, the lower tarsal conjunctiva, which imparts a woody hardness to the eyelid. The membrane may also involve the bulbar conjunctiva. Although beta-hemolytic streptococci are often found beneath the membrane, their role in etiology is not clear.

Vitamin A Deficiency (Hypovitaminosis A)

Vitamin A deficiency in its early stages is characterized by wrinkling, redness, loss of luster and pigmentation of the conjunctiva, and a Bitot's spot (Fig. 3–49), which appears as a thickened, foamy area of the temporal or medial exposed conjunctiva. Other early clinical signs include night blindness, blepharitis, meibomitis, lengthening of eyelashes, hyperkeratosis of the forehead, and a hyperkeratotic skin rash. Lack of wetting of the cornea and conjunctiva also occurs because of loss of the goblet cells. Clinical signs in the conjunctiva and cornea are manifestations of the keratinizing metaplasia produced by the deficiency of vitamin A.

Keratoconjunctivitis Sicca (Dry Eye)

Keratoconjunctivitis sicca includes a number of disease entities in which there is deficient tear flow. Patients with this syndrome characteristically have symptoms of burning that becomes more marked later in the day. The tear meniscus is decreased or absent, and shreds of mucus are present in the tear film. Epithelial filaments covered with shreds of mucus are often seen clinging to the cornea (Chapter 6).

Allergic Conjunctivitis

The major symptom of an allergic conjunctivitis is itching. The conjunctiva itself appears pale red, and the tarsal conjunctival inflammation is associated with small punctate papillae in hay fever conjunctivitis or with giant papillae in vernal and atopic keratoconjunctivitis. In conjunctival smears, eosinophils and free eosinophilic granules are often present in large numbers (Fig. 3–50).

Hay Fever Conjunctivitis

Hay fever conjunctivitis is a short-lived conjunctivitis characterized by symptoms of intense itching, photophobia, redness, tearing, and scant ropy discharge. During an acute attack, severe chemosis of the bulbar conjunctiva is a common sign (Fig. 3–51).

Atopic Keratoconjunctivitis

Atopic keratoconjunctivitis is usually associated with an atopic dermatitis, in which there is an eczematoid reaction involving the forehead, cheeks, and flexor surfaces of the arms and legs, or occasionally the entire body. The skin eruption is associated with marked itching, and there is usually a history of exacerbations and remissions over many years.

The skin of the eyelids is involved by erythematous and exudative lesions followed by scaling and crusting as the disease progresses. In the late stages, the skin of the eyelid may become pigmented and is often lichenified (Chapter 2).

Conjunctival involvement is characterized by symptoms of itching, stringy discharge, and redness. The conjunctiva is hyperemic and edematous, and there is a papillary hypertrophy associated with a stringy mucoid discharge. The hyperemia is of a pale nature and is best described as milky in color. In some instances giant papillae occur on both the inferior (Fig. 3–52) and superior tarsal conjunctiva, whereas in vernal keratoconjunctivitis (see below) the giant papillae are preferentially located on the upper tarsal conjunctiva. Limbal giant papillae may also occur, most frequently at the upper limbus (Fig. 3–53), but sometimes also in the area of the interpalpebral fissure. Trantas' dots may also be seen in atopic keratoconjunctivitis. These are chalky concretions composed of eosinophils, usually found at the limbus in areas where giant papillae are present (Fig. 3–54), but also occurring on the tarsal and bulbar conjunctiva. Superficial and linear scarring of the tarsal conjunctiva and mild shrinkage of the inferior cul-de-sac may also occur.

Corneal involvement in atopic keratoconjunctivitis takes several forms:

1. A commonly occurring fine epithelial keratitis in the inferior part of the cornea. This form of keratitis frequently arises from staphylococcal lid infection which often complicates atopic keratoconjunctivitis, but it may also occur without the infection.
2. Superficial vascularization, usually in the form of a micropannus. In some instances the vessels extend large distances into the cornea.
3. Subepithelial opacities, which form during the inflammatory phase of the disease and persist when it resolves. These opacities are superficial, diffuse, and grayish in appearance.
4. Keratoconus. About 11% of patients with keratoconus have been found to have atopic dermatitis.
5. A pseudogeronotoxin. This may occur in atopic keratoconjunctivitis (Fig. 3–55) and many years after the disease has subsided may be the only clue to eye involvement. It is similar to a small segment of an arcus senilis.

Other findings in atopic keratoconjunctivitis include cataract, occurring as a posterior subcapsular or an anterior shield-like opacity (Fig. 3–56), and retinal detachment.

Vernal Keratoconjunctivitis

Vernal keratoconjunctivitis is a chronic condition characterized by symptoms of extreme itching, redness, photophobia, and a ropy discharge. The findings include a milky appearance of the conjunctiva, and the presence of giant papillae on the upper tarsus (palpebral vernal keratoconjunctivitis) (Fig. 3–57) or on the limbus (limbal vernal keratoconjunctivitis) (Fig. 3–58). In some cases, both the tarsal and limbal conjunctiva are involved (mixed vernal). The tarsal giant papillae are polygonal and flat topped with tufts of capillaries within their substance. The limbal giant papillae have a gelatinous appearance, but also contain tufts of capillaries. In vernal keratoconjunctivitis, if the lid is everted to expose the tarsal conjunctiva to air, a fine pseudomembrane may develop over its surface (Maxwell-Lyon's sign). Unlike atopic keratoconjunctivitis, vernal keratoconjunctivitis does not lead to scarring of the conjunctiva unless the patient is treated by methods that cause scarring, such as surgical removal of the papillae, cryotherapy, or irradiation.

Micropannus commonly develops in both palpebral and limbal vernal keratoconjunctivitis, but total pannus is very rare. A pseudogeronotoxin commonly develops adjacent to limbal giant papillae as a result of the increased vascularity at the limbus; in many instances this is the only evidence of previous disease (see above). Trantas' dots are characteristic of vernal keratoconjunctivitis, usually occurring at the limbus in conjunction with giant papillae (see section on atopic keratoconjunctivitis).

A superior fine, epithelial keratitis may occur in vernal keratoconjunctivitis. Gray amorphous opacities with areas of epithelial cell loss are also seen; these lesions may coalesce to form a syncytium. In some instances, a superficial horizontally oval corneal ulcer occurs, which may appear elevated because of the deposition of mucus or a plaque of epithelium within the defect. The mucus or epithelial plaque appears gray and retards healing. The underlying superficial stroma is scarred, resulting in a moderate decrease of vision after the ulcer heals.

Giant Papillary Conjunctivitis

Giant papillary conjunctivitis may occur as a response to the chronic use of hard or soft contact lenses and prostheses. It has been suggested that papillae arise from a reaction to antigens or protein absorbed on or material that leaches from the lens or prosthesis, or to an ill-fitting lens or prosthesis.

The conjunctivitis is characterized by the presence of redness, discharge, and discomfort whenever the contact lens or prosthesis is worn. Giant and fine papillae are present over the upper tarsal conjunctiva and are associated with a milky color (Fig. 3–59). Scrapings reveal polymorphonuclear leukocytes and in some instances a few eosinophils.

Cicatrizing Conjunctivitis

Scarring of the conjunctiva may be caused by:

1. A complication of a membranous or pseudomembranous conjunctivitis (Fig. 3–60);
2. A complication of the late stages of trachoma;
3. A complication of hypovitaminosis A;
4. Atopic keratoconjunctivitis;
5. Direct chemical injury to the conjunctiva;
6. A complication of cicatricial pemphigoid, Stevens-Johnson syndrome, toxic epidermal necrolysis, dermatitis herpetiformis, epidermolysis bullosa, or lymphogranuloma venereum;
7. An idiosyncratic reaction to oral medications such as practolol;
8. The prolonged use of various topical medications;
9. Molluscum contagiosum infection of the lid margin (Thygeson and Dawson, 1971).

Cicatricial Pemphigoid

Cicatricial or ocular pemphigoid (benign mucous membrane pemphigoid) is an autoimmune disease usually affecting patients over the age of 45 years. It causes scarring of the conjunctiva and other mucous membranes of the body including the oral, genital, and anal mucosa; the skin, nose, and larynx may also be involved. Deposition of immunoglobulins (IgG, IgM, and IgA) and complement in the basement membrane of the mucosal epithelium can be demonstrated by direct immunofluorescence. Conjunctival involvement in cicatricial pemphigoid usually begins insidiously, often resembling a nonspecific or subacute catarrhal conjunctivitis. Later in the course of the disease conjunctival vesicles and ulcerations develop, followed by shrinkage of the inferior conjunctival fornices. In rare instances the onset may be of an acute nature, with edema of the eyelids, marked conjunctival hyperemia, and rapid development of conjunctival scarring. Late in the course of cicatricial pemphigoid, extensive conjunctival scarring, symblepharon formation, and trichiasis/entropion may occur (Fig. 3–61). The cornea is involved secondarily as a result of loss of goblet cells, exposure, and lack of lid surfacing.

Erythema Multiforme Major

Extensive scarring of the conjunctiva may occur in erythema multiforme major, as noted previously (Figs. 3–47A, 3–47B).

Toxic Epidermal Necrolysis

With several major exceptions, toxic epidermal necrolysis is similar to erythema multiforme major (Fig. 3–62). The similarities include the prodrome and onset of skin eruption with erythema and bullae formation, and the oral and ocular findings. The major differences include the development of flaccid bullae; a positive Nikolsky's sign in which the normal-appearing epidermis can be easily stripped from the underlying dermis by applying tangential pressure to the skin; and the histological findings of loss of the epidermis and absence of inflammatory cells within the dermis (as opposed to erythema multiforme major in which inflammatory cells are located predominantly within the dermis and the epidermis appears intact). Moreover, the eruption of toxic epidermal necrolysis reaches its peak within 24 to 48 hours, after which healing occurs, whereas in erythema multiforme major, several cycles of eruptions occur over a four to six week period.

Ritter's disease is a form of toxic epidermal necrolysis resulting from a septicemic infection with group II *Staphylococcus aureus,* especially phage type 71. The skin reaction results from the action of the staphylococcus dermatonecrotoxin on immature skin. It occurs almost exclusively in young children and clinically resembles toxic epidermal necrolysis in the adult. It can be differentiated pathologically from toxic epidermal necrolysis because cleavage and the resultant bullae formation occur in the granular layer instead of the basal layer of the epidermis.

The ocular complications of toxic epidermal necrolysis and Ritter's disease are similar to those of erythema multiforme major: entropion/trichiasis, conjunctival shrinkage and scarring, decrease in tear formation, and secondary corneal changes including ulceration, vascularization, and perforation.

Drug-Induced Cicatrization of the Conjunctiva

Cicatrization of the conjunctiva may occur following the prolonged topical use of many medications, either because of the medications themselves or the preservatives in the medications. The authors have found it to occur following the use of most antiglaucoma medications, the antivirals (especially idoxuridine), and eye medications with preservatives (even paraben preservatives).

In drug-induced cicatrization, conjunctival shrinkage and even symblepharon formation occur, but total shrinkage of the cul-de-sac does not occur and scarring may be limited to the area of the tarsal sulcus. Scarring of the lower punctum is usually seen and should make the clinician suspect a drug-induced cicatrization.

References

Anderson, R: Oculoglandular tularemia. *J. Iowa Med. Soc.* 60: 21–24, 1970.

Dawson, CR, Jones, BR, and Tarizzo, ML: *Guide to Trachoma Control.* World Health Organization, Geneva, 1981.

Dawson, CR: Epidemic Koch-Weeks conjunctivitis and trachoma. *Am. J. Ophthalmol.* 49: 801–808, 1960.

Jawetz, E, Thygeson, P, Hanna, L, Nicholas, A, and Kimura, SJ: The etiology of epidemic keratoconjunctivitis. *Am. J. Ophthalmol.* 43: 79–82 (suppl.), 1957.

Meisler, DM, Bosworth, DE, and Krachmer, JH: Ocular infectious mononucleosis manifested as Parinaud's oculoglandular syndrome. *Am. J. Ophthalmol.* 92: 722–726, 1981.

Ostler, HB, and Braley, AE: Conjunctivitis: Its etiologic diagnosis and treatment. *J. Iowa Med. Soc.* 44: 427–436, 1954.

Ostler, HB, Schachter, J, and Dawson, CR: Acute follicular conjunctivitis of epizootic origin: Feline pneumonitis. *Arch. Ophthalmol.* 82: 587–591, 1969.

Prevost, E, Kreutner, A Jr, Valotton, WW, and Walker, EM Jr: Conjunctival lesion caused by *Rhinosporidium seeberi. South. Med. J.* 73: 1077–1079, 1980.

Theodore, FH: Superior limbic keratoconjunctivitis. *Eye Ear Nose Throat Monthly* 42: 25–28, 1963.

Thygeson, P: Clinical signs of diagnostic importance in conjunctivitis. *JAMA* 33: 437–441, 1947.

Thygeson, P: Observations on filamentary keratitis. In: *Trans. Am. Med. Assoc. Section on Ophthalmology, 112th Annual Meeting.* American Medical Association, Chicago, 1963, pp. 49–55.

Thygeson, P, and Dawson, CR: Pseudotrachoma caused by molluscum contagiosum virus and various chemical irritants. XXI Concilium Ophthalmologicum, Mexico, Acta, Pars II: 1894–1897, 1971. *Excerpta Medica,* Amsterdam, 1971.

Wood, TR: Ocular coccidioidomycosis. Report of a case presenting as Parinaud's oculoglandular syndrome. *Am. J. Ophthalmol.* 64: 587–590, 1967.

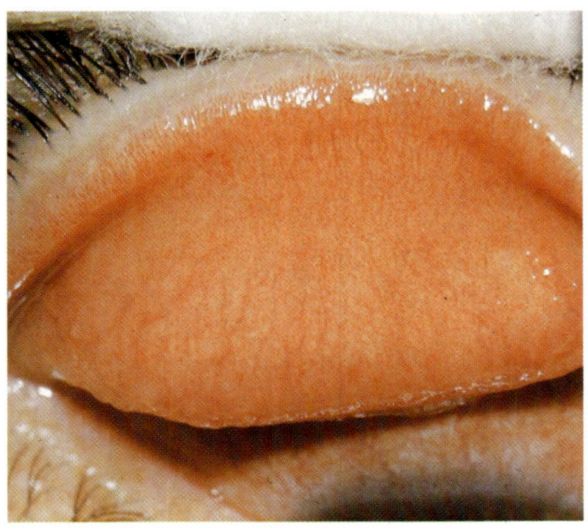

3–1 Papillary conjunctival reaction. Most bacterial conjunctivitides cause a fine papillary reaction in the upper and lower tarsal conjunctiva, which gives a red, velvety appearance to the conjunctiva. Papillae occur only in areas where the conjunctiva is firmly attached to an underlying structure by firm fibrous bands, i.e., the tarsus, the semilunar fold, and the limbus. When severe conjunctival inflammation occurs, other conjunctival areas are also involved, such as the cul-de-sac, which is thrown into rugae. Histologically, a papilla consist of polymorphonuclear leukocytes, a few lymphocytes, and a vascular tuft contained within the papilla. The boundary of the papillae is distinctly outlined by fibrous bands which attach the conjunctiva to the tarsus.
In this patient with superior limbic keratoconjunctivitis (SLK), a marked papillary conjunctivitis is noted in the superior tarsal conjunctiva. The fine papillae appear like small red dots, which represent the edges of the tufts of vessels growing perpendicular to the surface of the conjunctiva. The papillae are so numerous that they partially obscure the underlying vessels. The reaction in this patient would be graded as a grade two (P2) papillary conjunctivitis because of the partial obscuration of the underlying conjunctival vessels. The hyperemia and thickening of the superior limbal conjunctiva seen in this photograph are also characteristic of superior limbic keratoconjunctivitis.

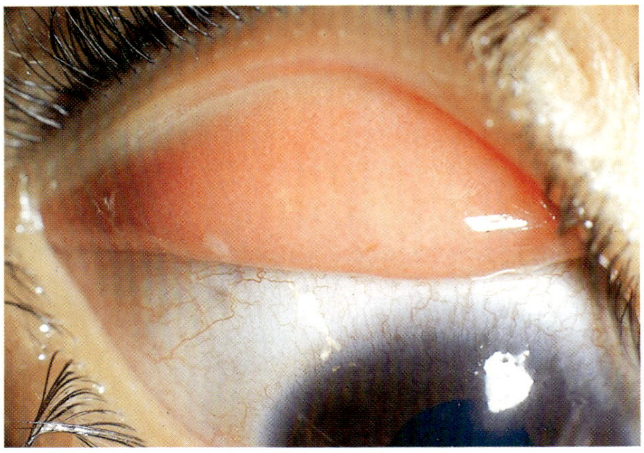

3–2 Velvety papillae in trachoma. In this 8-year-old Tunisian child, a marked velvety appearance to the upper tarsal conjunctiva is prominent. The child was classified as having stage IIb trachoma.

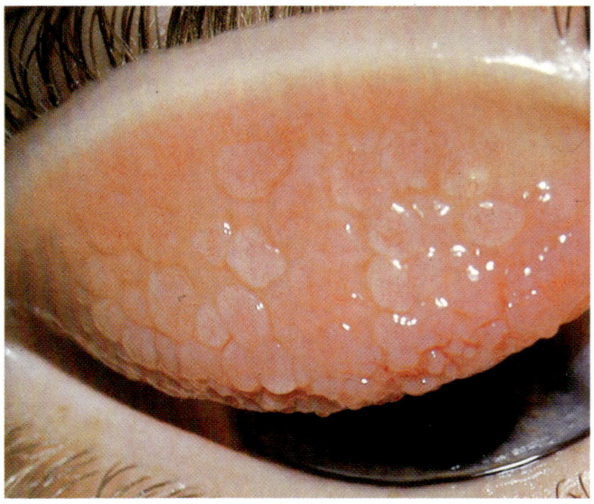

3–3 Giant papillae in vernal keratoconjunctivitis. Giant papillae occur in vernal keratoconjunctivitis, atopic keratoconjunctivitis, and giant papillary conjunctivitis. They are usually found on the upper tarsal conjunctiva (vernal keratoconjunctivitis), but may also be seen on the lower tarsal conjunctiva (atopic keratoconjunctivitis) and at the limbus. Giant papillae are flat-topped and polygonal in shape. Vessels course through the papillary substance to reach the surface, then branch to form an arborwork of vessels over the structure. Because of the associated edema fluid, giant papillae have a milky color. In some instances the papillae may become so large that the fibrous bands binding the conjunctiva to the underlying tarsus are broken, and the papillae assume irregular shapes on the tarsal conjunctiva, as is seen in this photograph. The milky color of the conjunctiva and the smaller papillae are also visible.

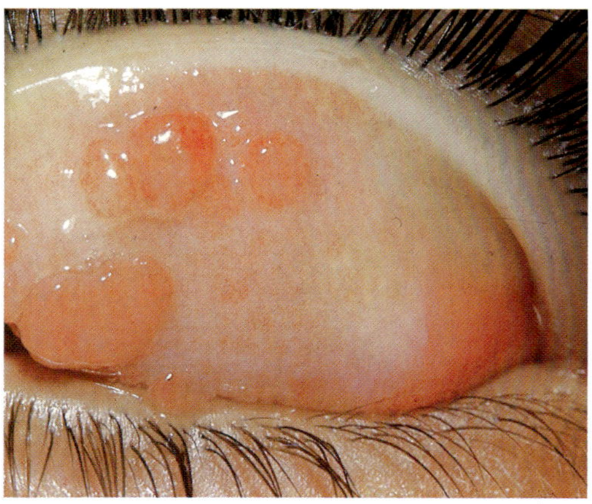

3–4 Giant papillae in vernal keratoconjunctivitis. In this patient with vernal keratoconjunctivitis, several giant papillae con be seen surrounded by many fine papillae. Note the milky color of the conjunctiva.

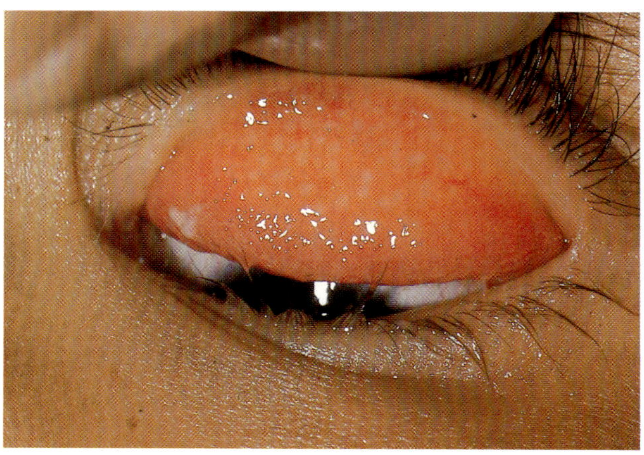

3–5 Conjunctival follicles. Follicles may occur on the tarsus, at the limbus, or on the bulbar conjunctiva. They are small, distinct, gray or white avascular structures. Blood vessels usually course upward around the edge of the follicles and branch to form a network over the surface of the follicles. In this patient with trachoma, the follicles appear as white, avascular areas separated by areas of papillary reaction. Some of the follicles are distinctly elevated, as is evident by the distorted light reflex. Note that the follicles are present in all areas of the upper tarsal conjunctiva.

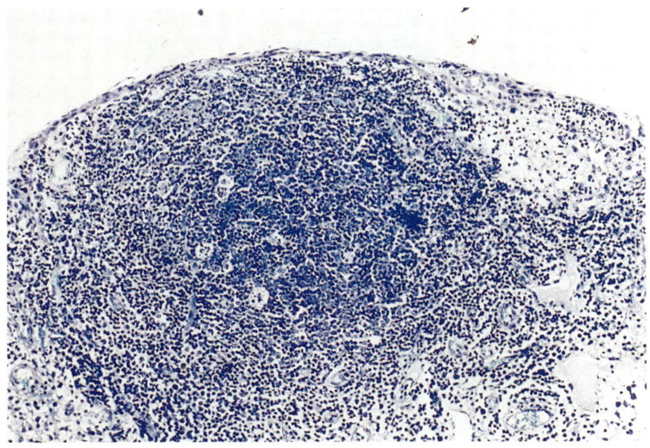

3–6A A lymphoid follicle in a section of a conjunctival biopsy from a patient with an acute *Chlamydia trachomatis* infection. Histologically, follicles are composed of a central zone of reticuloendothelial cells surrounded by a peripheral zone of lymphocytes. (Section supplied by Dr. Y. Mitsui, Tokoshima, Japan.)

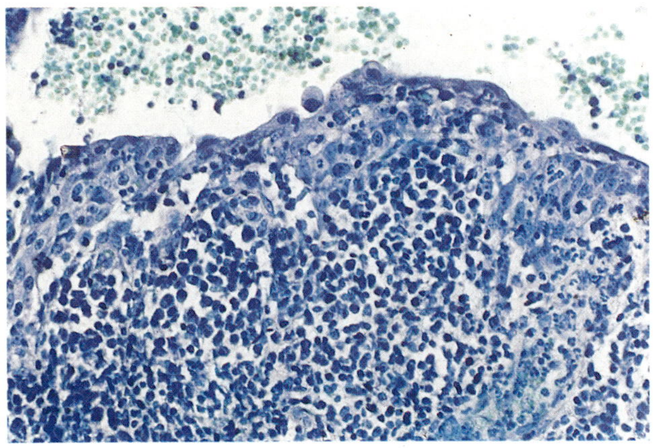

3–6B A high magnification of the same section shown in Fig. 3–6A, showing lymphocytic follicle beneath the epithelium. The epithelium itself is heavily infiltrated with polymorphonuclear leukocytes and lymphocytes. The epithelium is markedly thinned over the follicle.

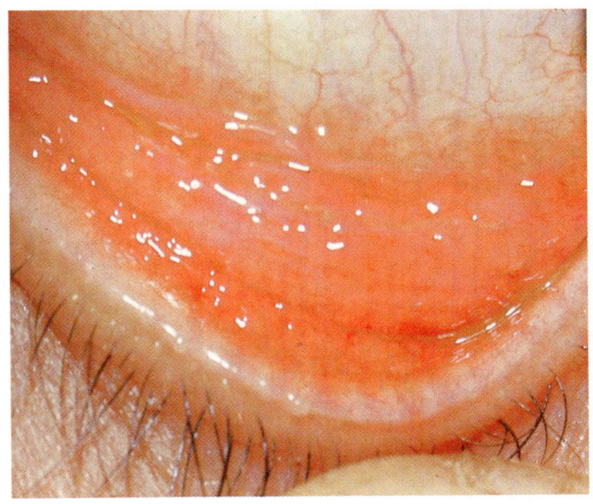

3–6C Follicles in the lower tarsal conjunctiva and cul-de-sac. In this patient with inclusion conjunctivitis, large follicles are evident in the cul-de-sac and in the inferior tarsal conjunctiva. The follicles are round and elevated and appear avascular.

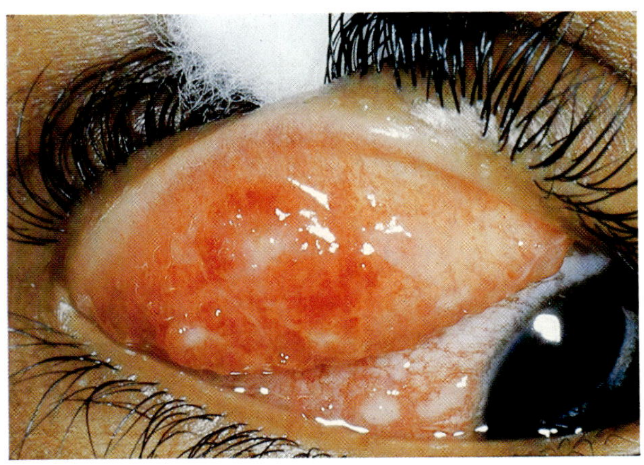

3–7 Granulomas of the conjunctiva. Granulomas may occur on the tarsal or bulbar conjunctiva and appear as protruberant, reddish, fleshy masses. They are composed of multinucleated giant cells and epithelioid cells which in turn are enclosed by a zone of lymphocytes and plasma cells. Granulomas are one of the hallmarks of Parinaud's oculoglandular syndrome. In this patient with Parinaud's oculoglandular syndrome due to cat scratch disease, multiple granulomas are located on the upper tarsal and bulbar conjunctiva. They are elevated and fleshy in appearance.

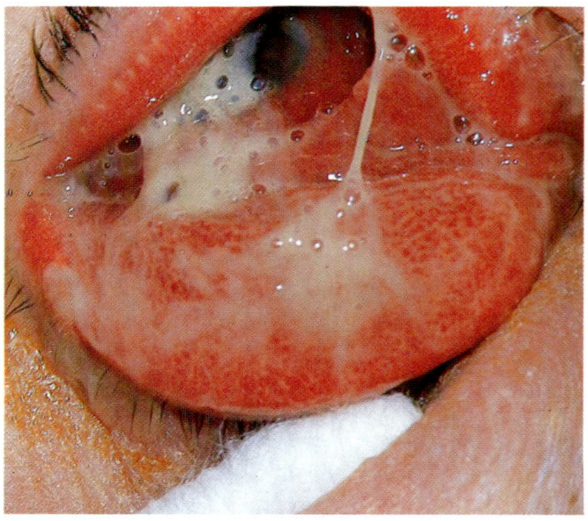

3–8A Hyperacute conjunctivitis of gonorrhea. The majority of cases of gonorrheal conjunctivitis are characterized by the copious secretion of pus associated with edema of the eyelid and conjunctiva. In many instances, peripheral corneal ulceration also occurs. (Photograph courtesy of Dr. Mario Valenton.)

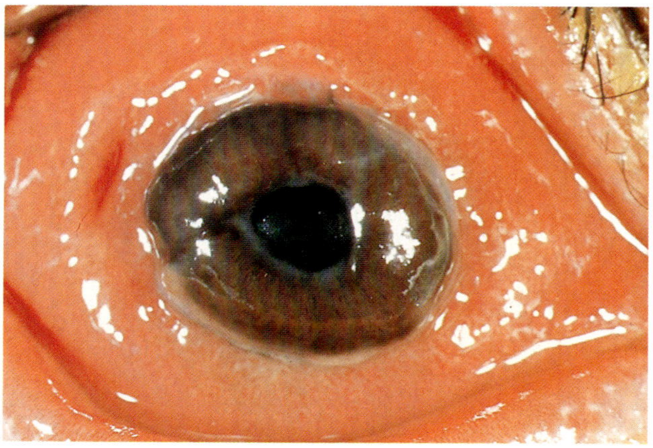

3–8B Severe papillary hypertrophy in gonorrheal conjunctivitis. In any acute form of conjunctivitis such as in gonorrhea, marked edema and infiltration of the conjunctiva occur, suggesting conjunctival hypertrophy. Even after control of the infection and subsidence of the purulent discharge, the edema and infiltration persist for weeks. This patient developed gonorrheal conjunctivitis from the injudicious use of contaminated urine as an eyewash. A marked papillary hypertrophy is evident, along with conjunctival edema and engorgement of the iris. (Photograph courtesy of Dr. Mario Valenton.)

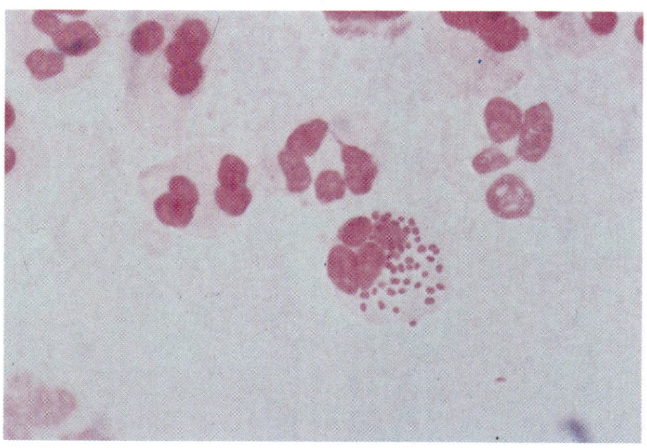

3–9A Conjunctival scraping from gonorrheal conjunctivitis. This scraping revealed many polymorphonuclear granulocytes loaded with bean-shaped Gram-negative diplococci. Gram's stain, × 1000.

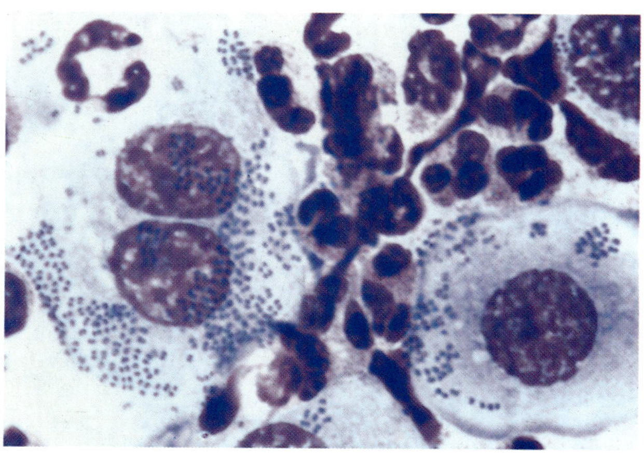

3–9B Neisseria gonorrhoeae. This conjunctival scraping shows many diplococci clustered on epithelial cells (epithelial tropism) and represents a useful diagnostic feature for pathogenic *Neisseria*. Note that this is a Giemsa stain which causes the diplococci to appear blue. Giemsa stain, × 1000.

3–10A Culture of *Neisseria gonorrhoeae. N. gonorrhoeae* grows readily on chocolate blood agar or Muller-Hinton agar under an atmosphere of 5–10% CO_2. The colonies are medium-sized and slightly translucent, but have no readily distinguishing features. An oxidase test is helpful for identifying the Neisseria species, which are all oxidase-positive. To differentiate *N. gonorrhoeae* from *N. meningitidis,* sugar utilization studies are useful (Fig. 3–10B).

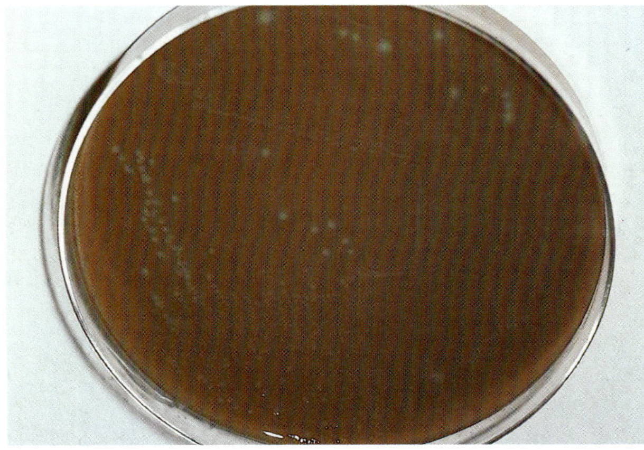

3–10B Sugar utilization by *N. gonorrhoeae. N. gonorrhoeae* is usually differentiated from *N. meningitidis* by sugar utilization studies. *N. gonorrhoeae* uses only glucose, whereas *N. meningitidis* uses both glucose and maltose. The organisms produce acid when the sugar is used, which causes the indicator in the media to turn yellow. This photograph demonstrates acid production from glucose by *N. gonorrhoeae* (left tube). There is no utilization of maltose or sucrose and therefore no color change in the maltose or sucrose tubes (center and right).

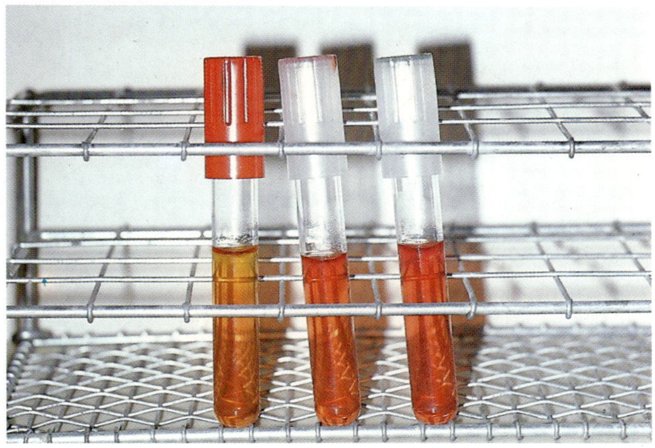

3–11A Acute catarrhal conjunctivitis due to *Streptococcus pneumoniae. S. pneumoniae* causes an acute catarrhal conjunctivitis. The conjunctivitis is commonly known as "pinkeye" because of its epidemic nature and because of the redness of the bulbar conjunctiva. A serous discharge is produced which rapidly becomes mucopurulent.

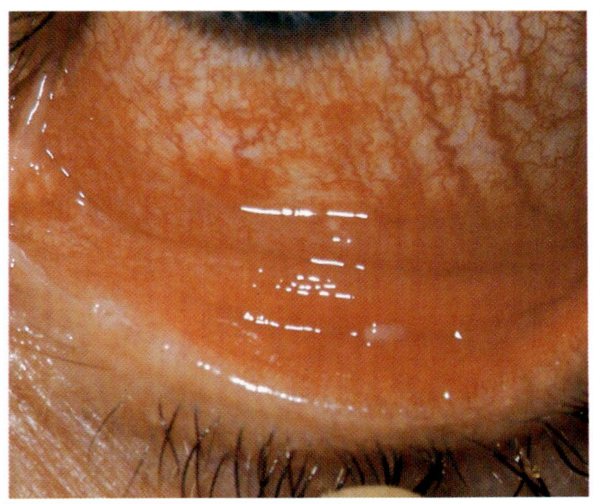

3–11B Scraping from *Streptococcus pneumoniae* conjunctivitis. This scraping shows a number of Gram-positive diplococci. In several of the organisms the distal ends are slightly tapered, which is a characteristic of the "lancet-shaped" *S. pneumoniae.* Gram's stain, ×1000.

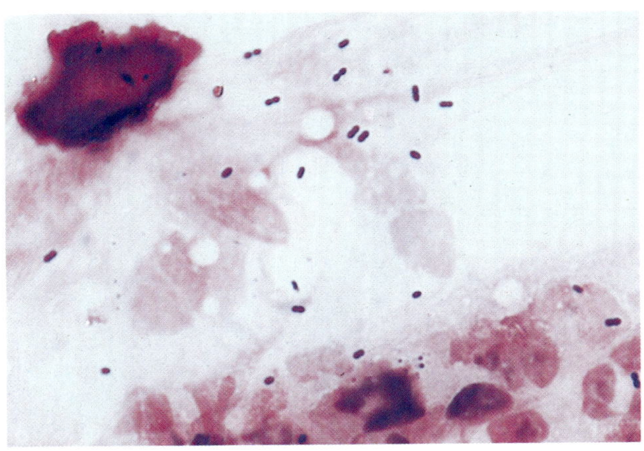

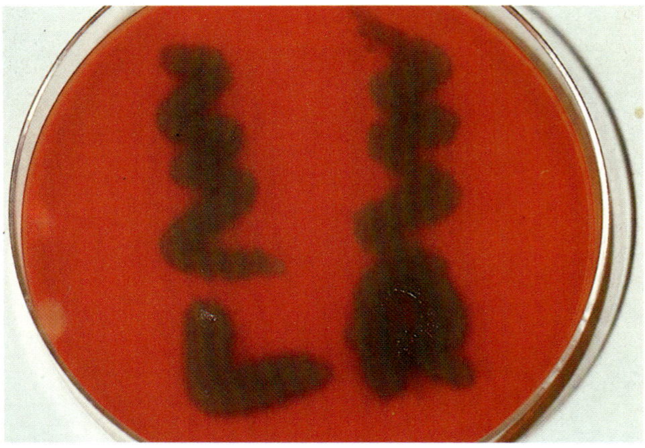

3–11C Culture of *Streptococcus pneumoniae. S. pneumoniae* grows readily on blood agar, causing alpha hemolysis. The colonies are differentiated from alpha-hemolytic streptococci by the fact that they are optochin positive. This photograph shows confluent growth of pneumococci from both the lids and the conjunctivae.

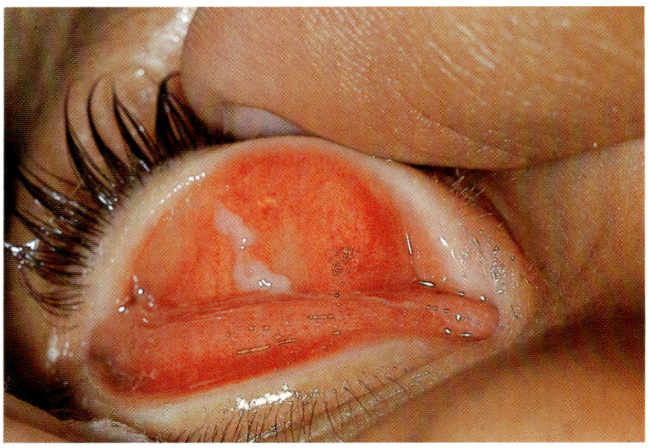

3–12A Acute catarrhal conjunctivitis due to *Haemophilus aegyptius*. An acute catarrhal conjunctivitis may occur from *H. aegyptius*. It is epidemic in form and similar in appearance to conjunctivitis caused by *S. pneumoniae* (Fig. 3–11A).

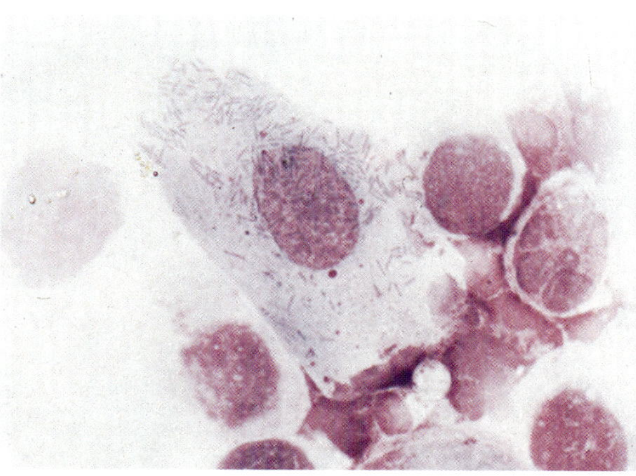

3–12B Scraping of acute catarrhal conjunctivitis due to *H. aegyptius*. In a Gram-stained smear, *H. aegyptius* are thin, long, Gram-negative rods that grow on epithelial cells (epithelial parasitism). *H. influenzae,* on the other hand, are short, Gram-negative coccobacilli that do not display epithelial parasitism (Fig. 3–13B). Giemsa stain, ×1000.

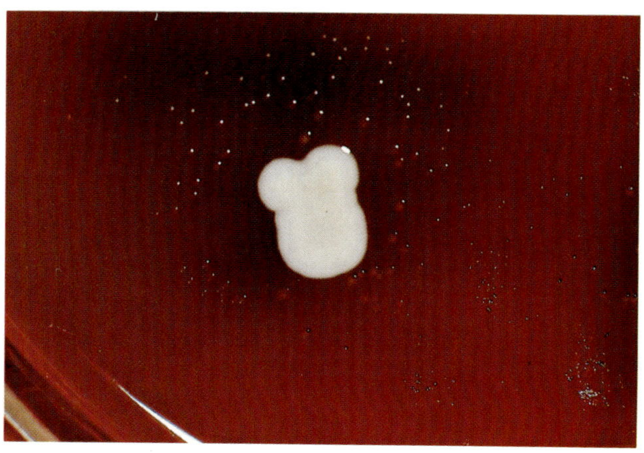

3–12C Culture of *H. aegyptius*. Cultures of *H. aegyptius* and *H. influenzae* appear similar (Fig. 3–13C). Furthermore, if a smear is made of either colony after the organism has been subcultured on artificial media, both organisms may appear as thin, long, Gram-negative bacilli or short, Gram-negative coccobacilli. Both organisms require special factors (X and V factors) for growth and do not grow on blood agar unless these factors have been added or staphylococci are also growing on the medium (staphylococci furnish the factors necessary for growth). The organisms also grow readily on chocolate blood agar. This photograph shows many *H. aegyptius* colonies "satelliting" around a *S. epidermidis* colony. The *Haemophilus* colonies demonstrate a gradation in size, with those closest to the staphylococcus being largest.

3–13A Subacute catarrhal conjunctivitis due to *Haemophilus influenzae. H. influenzae* cause a subacute catarrhal conjunctivitis that is often epidemic in nature. The conjunctivitis is characterized by a watery or flocculent discharge and a conjunctival hyperemia most marked on the tarsal conjunctiva and in the fornices and fading toward the limbus. The infection occurs most frequently in young children. This 6-year-old female developed a subacute catarrhal conjunctivitis with a mucoid discharge four days previously. The papillary conjunctivitis and a few early subconjunctival hemorrhages are visible on the upper tarsus.

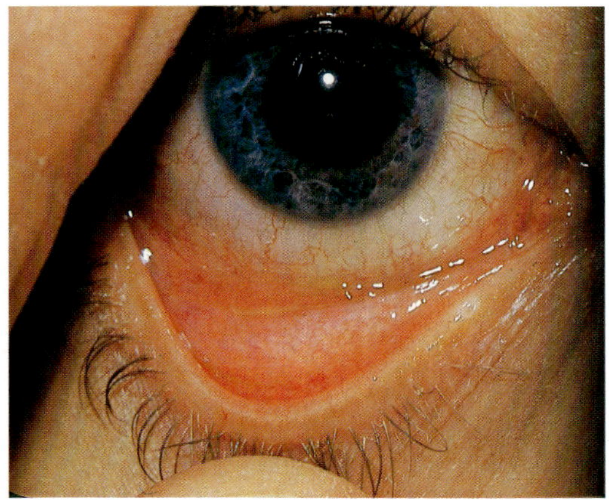

3–13B Scraping from subacute catarrhal conjunctivitis due to *H. influenzae.* Because of its size, the *H. influenzae* organism is often overlooked in a scraping of the conjunctiva. It appears as tiny, Gram-negative coccobacilli. Polymorphonuclear leukocytes are usually abundant. Gram's stain, ×1000.

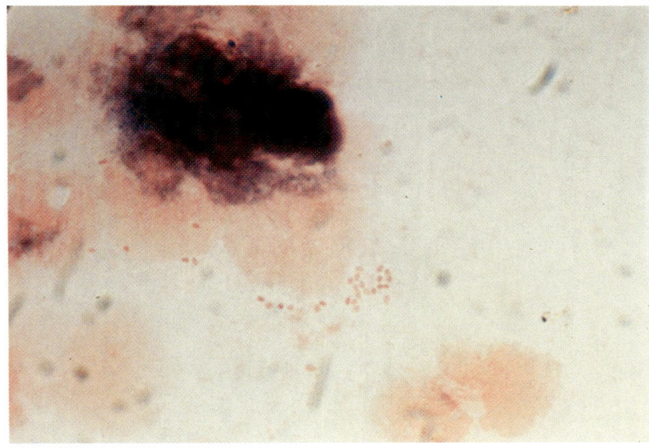

3–13C Culture from *H. influenzae* conjunctivitis. The culture shows numerous *H. influenzae* colonies "satelliting" around colonies of *S. epidermidis.* The appearance of *H. influenzae* colonies is essentially identical to that of *H. aegyptius* colonies (Fig. 3–12C).

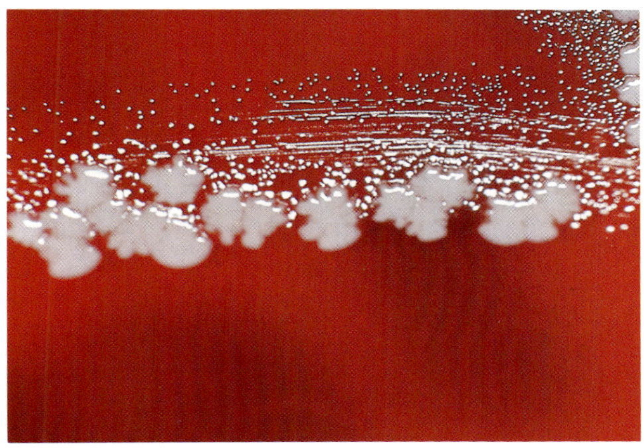

3–14 Staphylococcal conjunctivitis. The symptoms of chronic catarrhal conjunctivitis are foreign body sensation, burning, and occasionally itching, which are far out of proportion to the clinical findings. Mild hyperemia and infiltration of the tarsal conjunctiva are evident in this patient with a chronic staphylococcal blepharoconjunctivitis. Some poliosis of the eyelashes is evident, together with tearing.

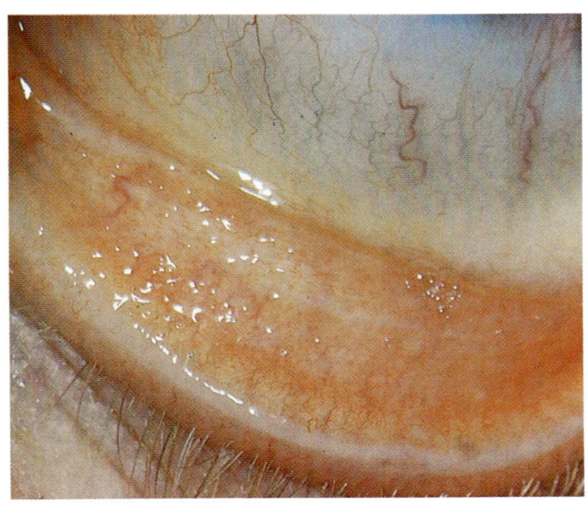

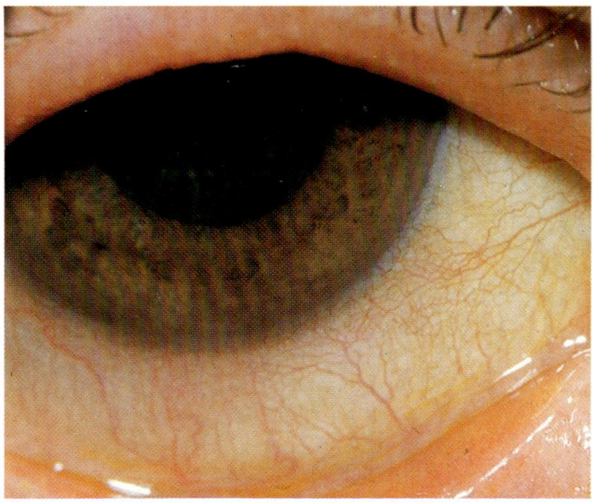

3–15 Keratoconjunctivitis sicca. This is a major cause of chronic conjunctivitis. A reduced tear meniscus, strands of mucus in the tear film, and mucous corneal filaments are common findings. A blotchy epithelial keratitis together with many strands of mucous corneal filaments are evident in the lower part of the cornea in this patient, together with mild bulbar injection and minimal papillary hypertrophy. The patient complained of marked symptoms of irritation and foreign body sensation. She also had dryness of the mouth and evidence of rheumatoid arthritis.

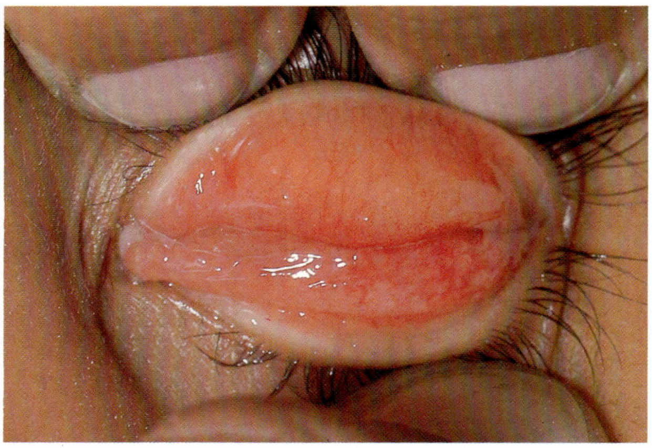

3–16A Mild intensity trachoma: acute trachoma with diffuse infiltration (P2) and less than ten follicles on the tarsal surface (F2). This mild intensity disease rarely leads to blinding complications. There is no conjunctival scarring.

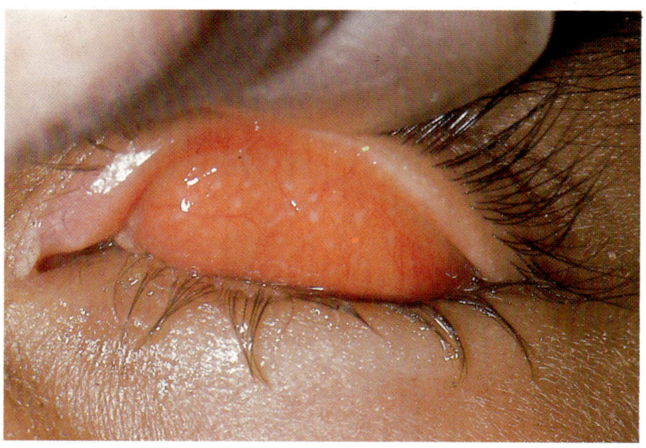

3–16B Moderate intensity trachoma with more than ten follicles on the tarsal plate (F3) and moderate papillary hypertrophy (P2). Avascular follicles stand out clearly against the diffuse infiltration and papillary hypertrophy. Large, opaque follicles such as these often rupture easily on light pressure, as indicated by the small subconjunctival hemmorrhages. Necrosis of these "mature" follicles is said to lead to conjunctival scarring. This case corresponds to McCallan stage IIa trachoma (mature follicles predominate).

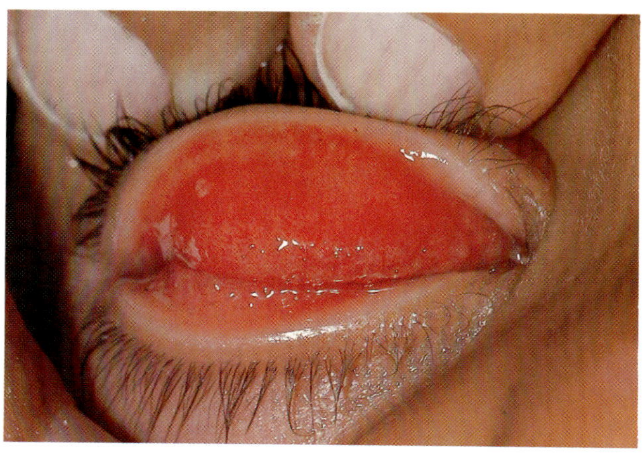

3–16C Severe intensity trachoma in a 2-year-old Egyptian child. The intense infiltration and papillary hypertrophy hide any follicles present on the tarsal surface, although follicles are seen at the edge of the tarsal plate (P3, F1). Chlamydial agent was detected in the conjunctival scrapings, tear swabs, and rectal swabs of this child.

3–17 A fly feeding on the conjunctival secretions of an Egyptian child with moderate intensity trachoma (F3, P2). In North Africa, flies frequently cluster on the nares and lids of children with ocular and nasal discharges and serve to effectively transfer infection from person to person.

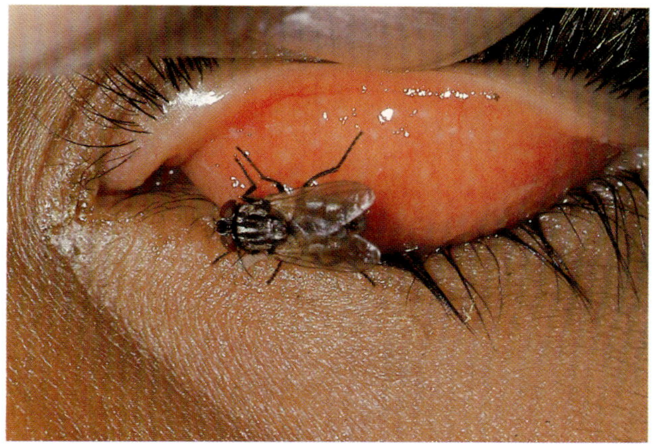

3–18 A Limbal follicles in a case of active trachoma. In this Tunisian child there are large succulent follicles at the limbal conjunctiva. Vessels can be seen coursing between them. As the follicles resolve, they leave depressions in the corneal scleral junction which are known as Herbert's peripheral pits. (The numbered label was used to identify this patient in a treatment study.)

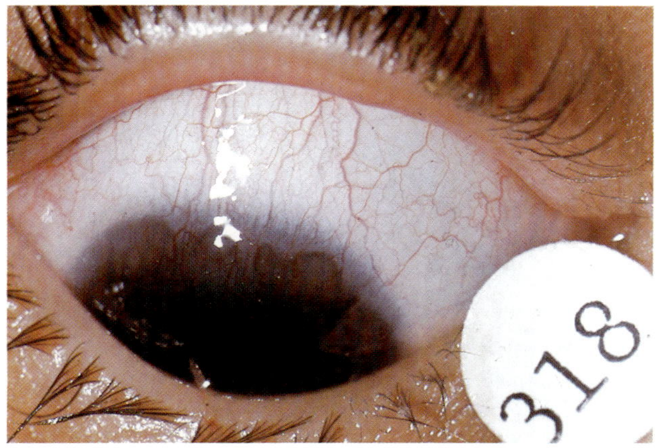

3–18 B The same patient shown in Fig. 3–18 A, six months later, following treatment. The limbal follicles seen in Fig. 3–18 A have disappeared and have left depressions (Herbert's pits). Superficial scarring of the cornea is evident between the Herbert's pits.

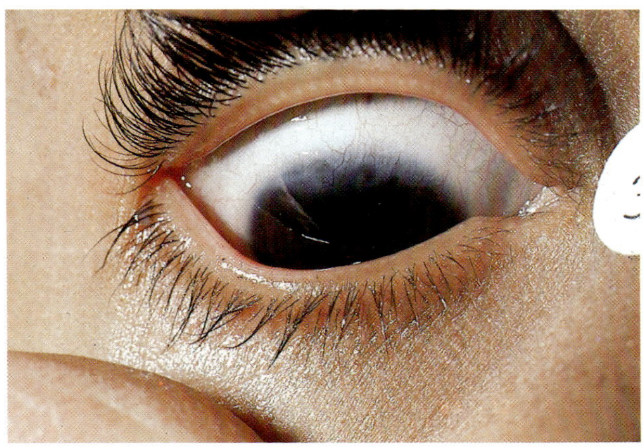

3–19 A Mild conjunctival scarring and follicles in a Tunisian child. The presence of round, avascular follicles and scarring is quite characteristic and is commonly seen in older children with trachoma. In this relatively mild case, it is unlikely that conjunctival scarring will later produce inturned eyelids.

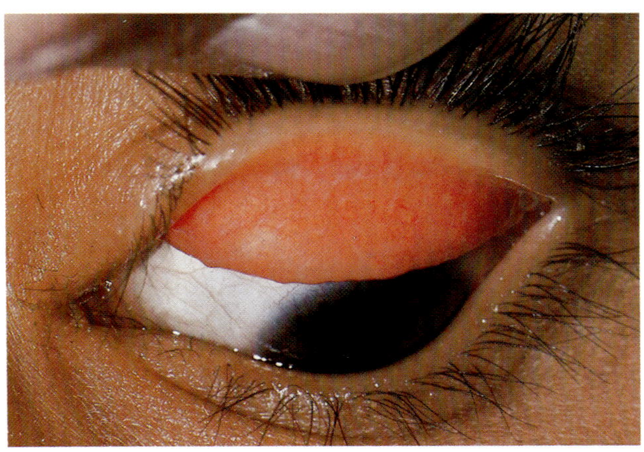

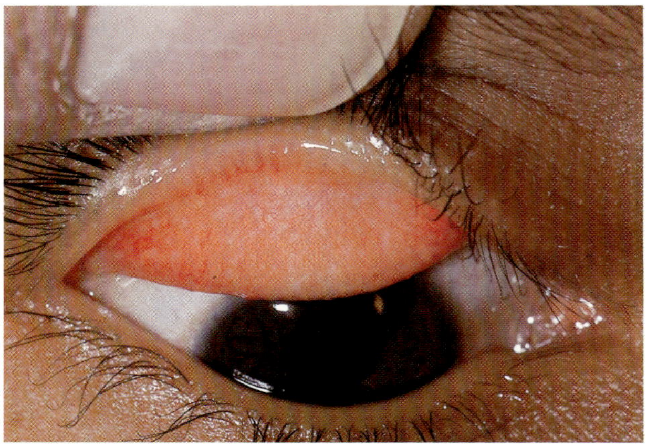

3–19B Marked conjunctival scarring and papillary hypertrophy in a patient with trachoma. The round scars in this patient can be distinguished from follicles by their angular outline. Despite the infiltration and papillary hypertrophy, the absence of follicles suggests that this case is not infectious.

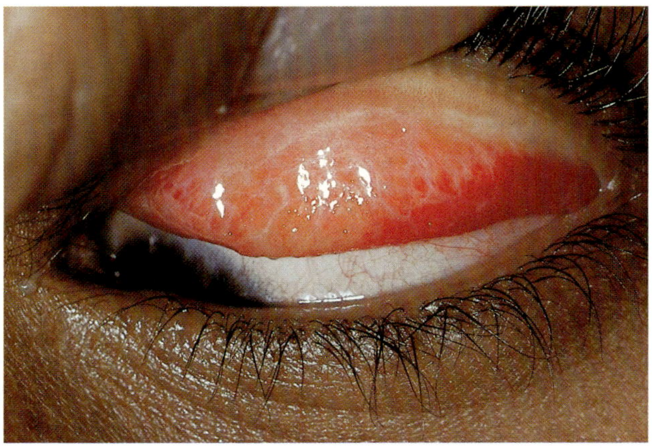

3–19C Severe distortion of the tarsal plate in a Tunisian adult. With prolonged and severe trachoma in childhood, intensive scarring of the conjunctiva develops, as seen in this case. The scarring near the lid margin probably produced distortion of the tarsal plate causing trichiasis. The conjunctiva is criss-crossed with scars. Histologically, the elevated islands of conjunctiva are diffusely infiltrated with lymphocytes but do not contain lymphoid follicles.

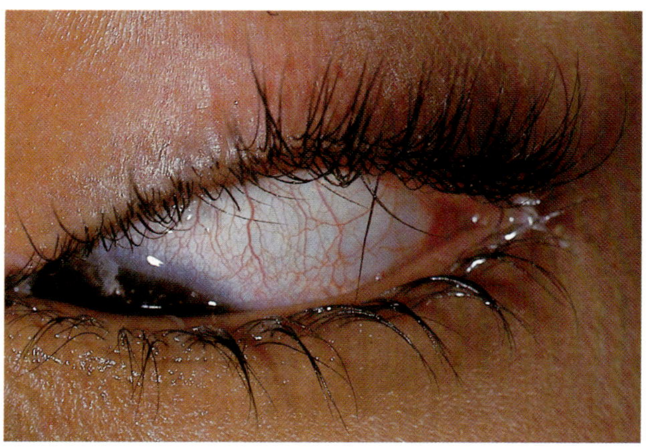

3–20A Trichiasis in a Tunisian patient with trachoma. Conjunctival scarring may produce trichiasis. In this patient, individual cilia are turned inward and rub against the eyeball causing irritation and loss of corneal epithelium.

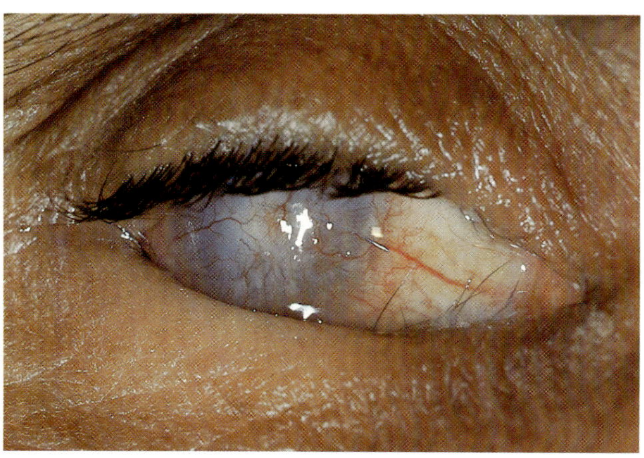

3–20B Trachomatous entropion and corneal scarring. Severe scarring of the upper tarsal plate may cause the entire lid margin to turn inward so that the lashes constantly abrade the cornea. In patients with trachoma, the loss of the mucous layer due to destruction of the goblet cells and the constant physical trauma from inturned lashes can lead to corneal scarring, as is evident in this patient.

3–21A A chlamydial inclusion and conjunctival epithelial cells in a case of trachoma. The cytoplasm of the epithelial cell has a typical chlamydial inclusion which contains both elementary bodies (small particles) and initial or reticulate bodies (larger blue particles). Giemsa stain, × 1000.

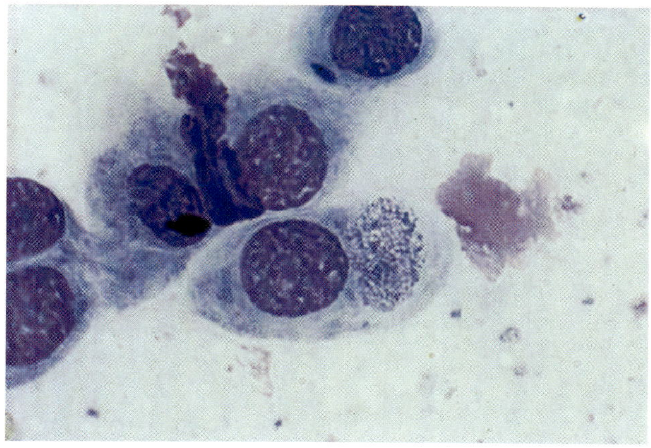

3–21B A late initial body chlamydial inclusion in a patient with trachoma. In the epithelial cell in the center of this photomicrograph, the large cluster of blue-stained particles represents a late initial body chlamydial inclusion. The size of the individual particles and their blue stain (with Giemsa stain) indicate that this inclusion consists primarily of the replicative form (the initial body) of chlamydia. A similar but much smaller inclusion can be seen in the adjacent cell. Giemsa stain, × 1000.

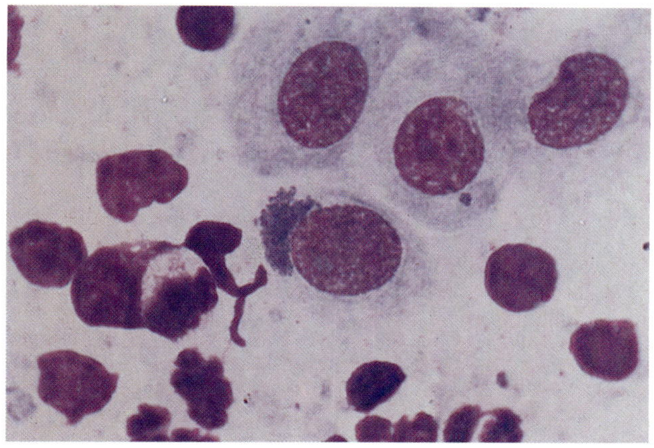

3–22 Melanin granules in conjunctival epithelial cells. This "pseudoinclusion" consists of black to green-black granules. In this case, the granules are distributed over the end of the nucleus forming a cap, much like a chlamydial inclusion. Melanin granules are often a source of confusion to the inexperienced cytologist. Giemsa stain, × 1000.

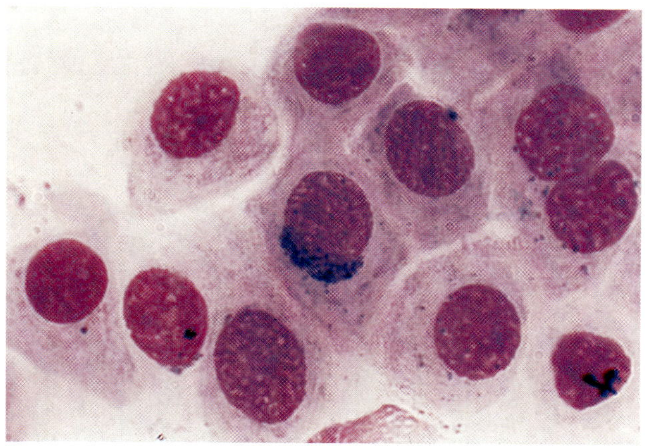

3–23 Koch-Weeks and *Neisseria*-like forms in a conjunctival scraping from an Egyptian child. The slender, faintly staining bacilli in the photomicrograph are characteristic of the Koch-Weeks bacillus or *Haemophilus aegyptius,* a common cause of epidemic conjunctivitis in trachomatous areas. The dark-staining pairs of cocci, on the other hand, are of a *Neisseria* species that causes more limited outbreaks of conjunctivitis and corneal ulceration in the Northern Mediterranean, Northern Africa, and the Middle Eastern countries. The *Neisseria* species has now been identified as a variant of *N. gonorrhoeae.* Both Koch-Weeks bacilli and *Neisseria* were described by Koch in 1886 in *Conjunctival Smears.* Giemsa stain, × 1000.

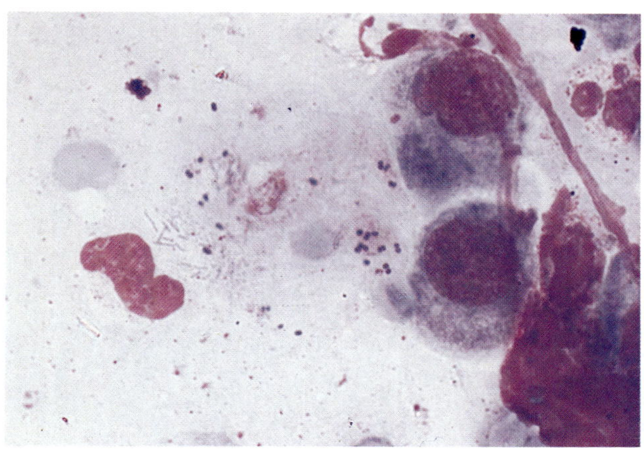

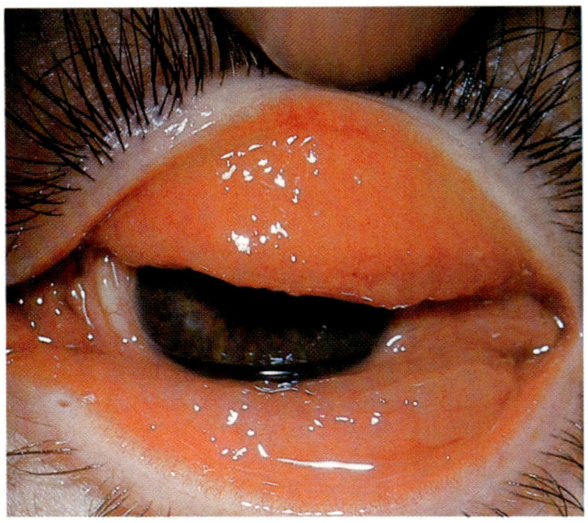

3–24 Inclusion conjunctivitis of the adult. Inclusion conjunctivitis in the child or adult causes a follicular reaction that is associated with mild to moderate mucopurulent discharge. The follicular reaction, together with a moderate papillary reaction, occurs on both upper and lower tarsi. An epithelial keratitis and micropannus may also develop. In this 16-year-old female, a marked follicular reaction is present in both the upper and lower tarsal conjunctiva. Although follicles are prominent in the inferior cul-de-sac, the upper and lower tarsi themselves are about equally involved.

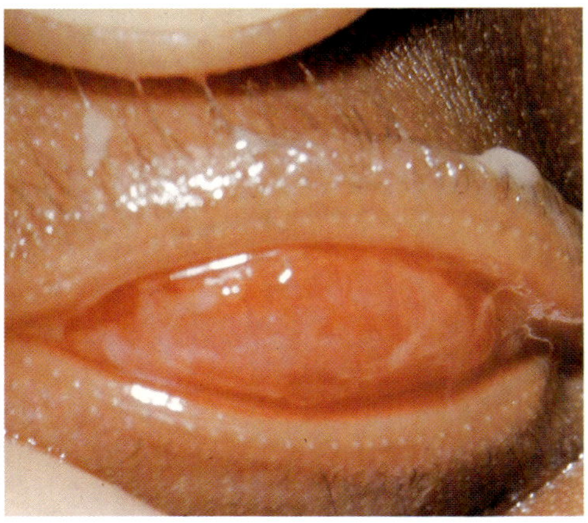

3–25 Inclusion conjunctivitis of newborn. Unlike the adult, the newborn has no adenoid layer to the conjunctiva and therefore does not produce follicles in response to inclusion conjunctivitis (unless the infection persists until the child is at least six weeks to two months old). The conjunctivitis is therefore papillary, or occasionally pseudomembranous, in nature. The pseudomembranous form of conjunctivitis may eventually cause nonspecific scarring unless treatment is initiated within twelve days. In this 7-day-old child, a pseudomembranous conjunctivitis developed two days previously. Scraping revealed many polymorphonuclear leukocytes together with several epithelial inclusion bodies. Note the mucopurulent discharge.

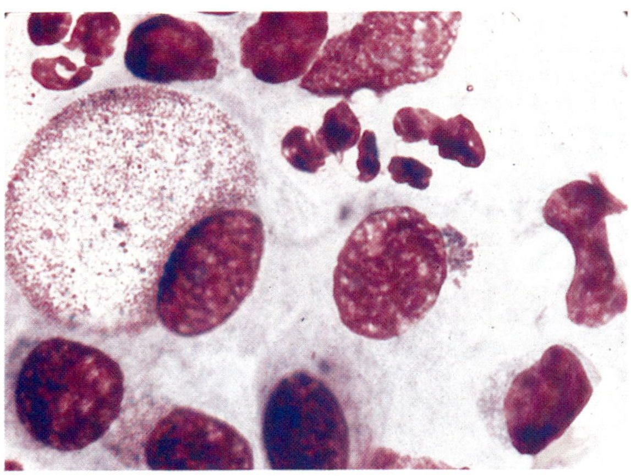

3–26 Scraping from an infant with inclusion conjunctivitis. This scraping shows a large inclusion body completely displacing the cytoplasm of the epithelial cell with its elementary bodies; a much smaller initial body inclusion is seen to its right. A cluster of initial bodies, which make up the inclusion, is seen capping the nucleus. Giemsa stain, $\times 1000$.

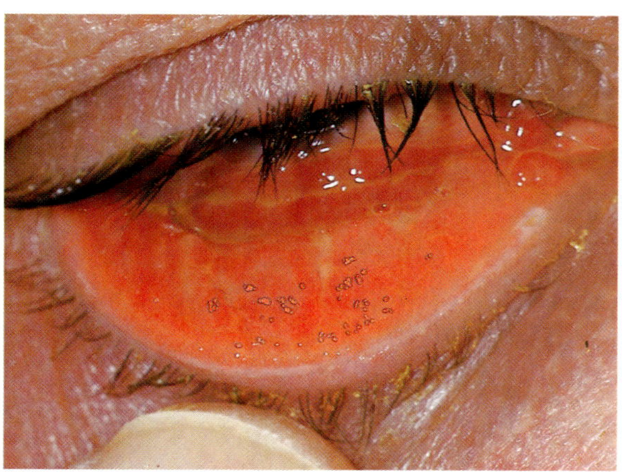

3–27 Lymphogranuloma venereum. Lymphogranuloma venereum occasionally infects the conjunctiva and is one of the causes of Parinaud's oculoglandular syndrome. It causes a grossly visible regional (usually preauricular) lymphadenopathy and multiple conjunctival granulomas. The conjunctival reaction in this patient suggested a follicular reaction, but biopsy of the lesions revealed a granulomatous reaction.

3–28 Feline pneumonitis in the adult. Feline pneumonitis, a chlamydial infection that usually infects the respiratory tract of newborn kittens, may occasionally cause a follicular conjunctivitis in humans. The clinical manifestations are similar to those of inclusion conjunctivitis of the child or adult, but the disease is more resistant to therapy. This man developed a follicular conjunctivitis after intimate exposure to his cat. His conjunctivitis responded only to prolonged systemic treatment with tetracycline. (Reprinted with permission from *Archives of Ophthalmology.*)

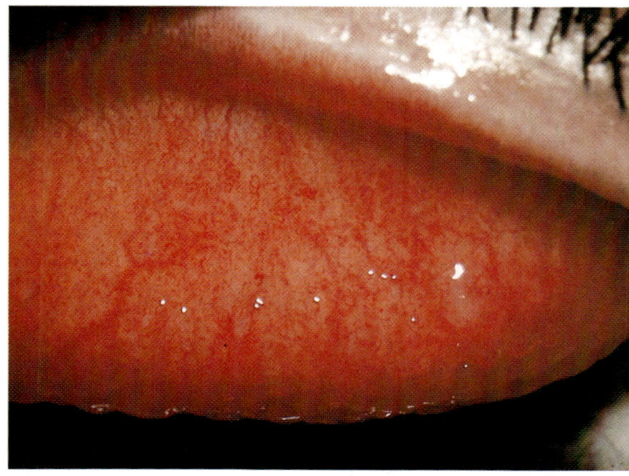

3–29 Adenovirus type 3 conjunctivitis (pharyngoconjunctival fever). Conjunctival infections with adenovirus (type 3 or type 7) commonly cause a follicular conjunctivitis. Because they are frequently associated with a sore throat and fever, they have also been termed pharyngoconjunctival fever. The conjunctivitis is follicular in type with tearing, but minimal or no true discharge is noted.

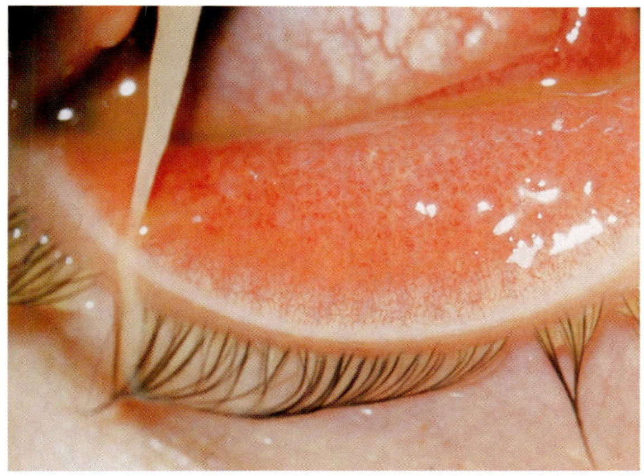

3–30A Epidemic keratoconjunctivitis (EKC); adenovirus type 8, follicular reaction. In adults, adenovirus types 8, 19, and 29 usually cause only a conjunctivitis, but in children, epidemic keratoconjunctivitis is frequently associated with diarrhea. In epidemics, most cases of the conjunctivitis are severe but a few cases are mild with minimal symptoms and signs of a conjunctivitis. EKC occurred in pandemic form in 1940 and was initially known as "shipyard conjunctivitis." When adenovirus type 8 was isolated the name epidemic keratoconjunctivitis was suggested and readily accepted by the scientific community; the name suggests the epidemic nature of the disease and the parts of the eye usually affected. The conjunctivitis is usually follicular in nature. There is some fibrinous discharge and tearing, but no purulent discharge. It resolves in 10–15 days.

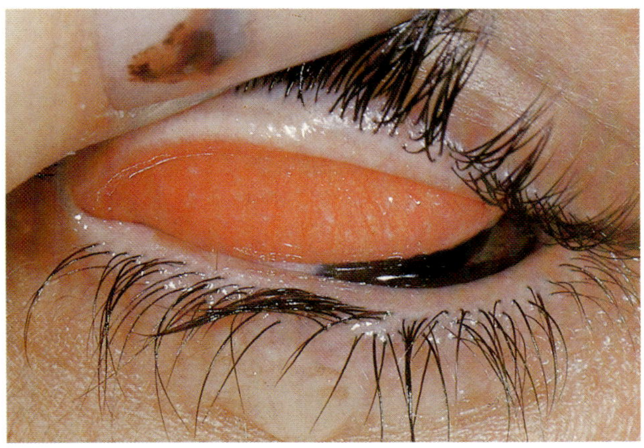

3–30B Epidemic keratoconjunctivitis; adenovirus type 8, pseudomembranous reaction. Adenovirus types 8 and 19 may cause a pseudomembranous conjunctivitis as well as a follicular conjunctivitis, as is evident in this patient with EKC. Moreover, the pseudomembranous reaction may lead to flat scars and even to symblepharon formation.

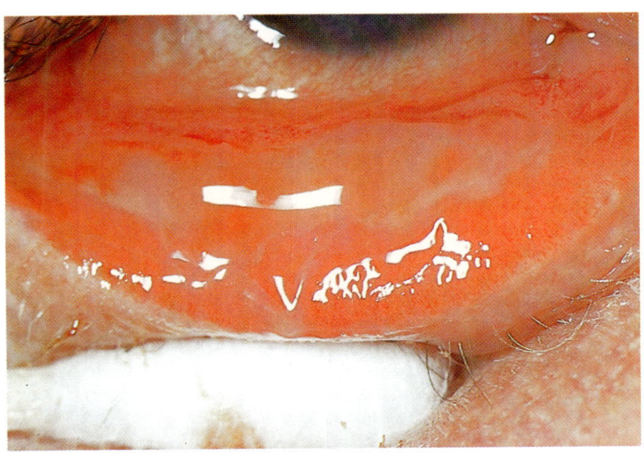

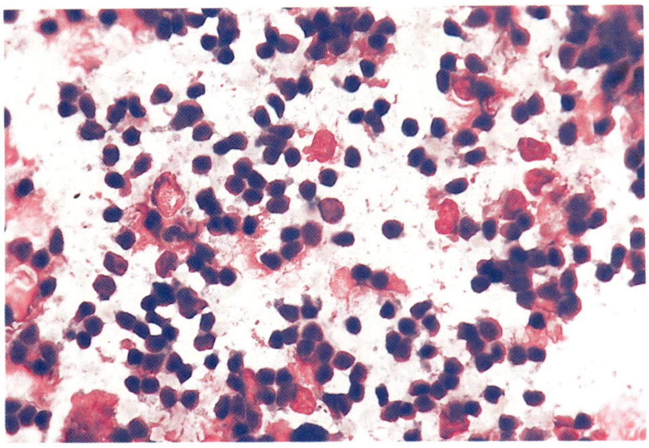

3–30C Conjunctival scraping from adenoviral conjunctivitis (EKC) showing numerous lymphocytes. A scraping from an adenoviral conjunctivitis reveals predominantly lymphocytes but if a pseudomembrane is present many polymorphonuclear leukocytes will also be found. Giemsa stain, ×400.

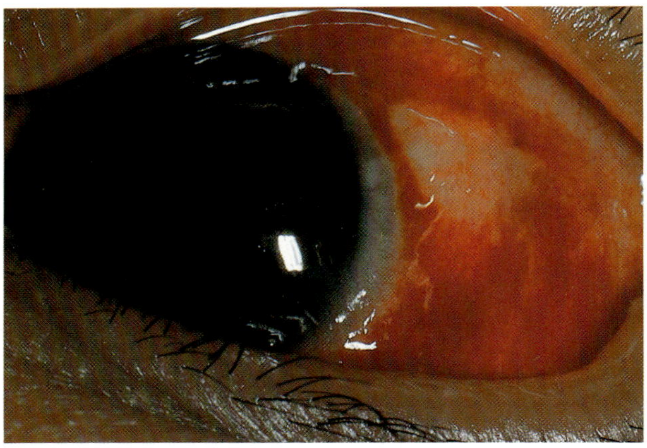

3–31 Acute hemorrhagic conjunctivitis. This type of conjunctivitis often occurs in pandemics and has been seen on all continents of the world. The infection is caused by enterovirus 70 and coxsackie virus A24. The conjunctivitis has a very short incubation period (18–30 hours) and runs a course of three to five days. It is associated with subconjunctival hemorrhages, as noted in this patient, and a fine epithelial keratitis.

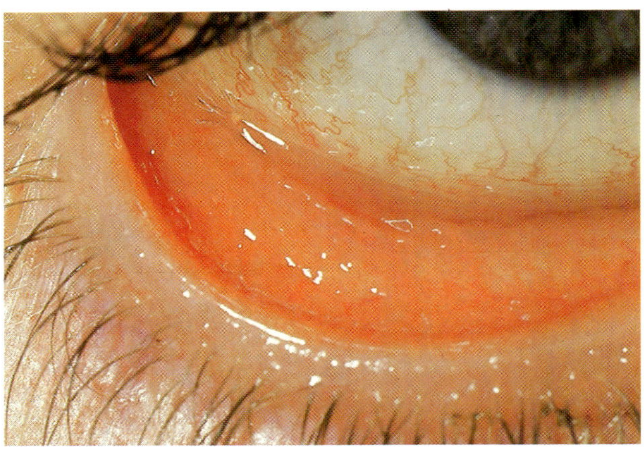

3–32 Follicular conjunctivitis due to molluscum nodule of the lid margin. A chronic follicular conjunctivitis commonly develops in response to a molluscum contagiosum lesion on or near the lid margin. The superior epithelial keratitis and pannus that may form together with the chronic follicular conjunctivitis may simulate trachoma. This 26-year-old female had developed a follicular conjunctivitis with minimal discharge six weeks previously. The edge of the molluscum contagiosum nodule can be seen on the lateral side of the lower eyelid.

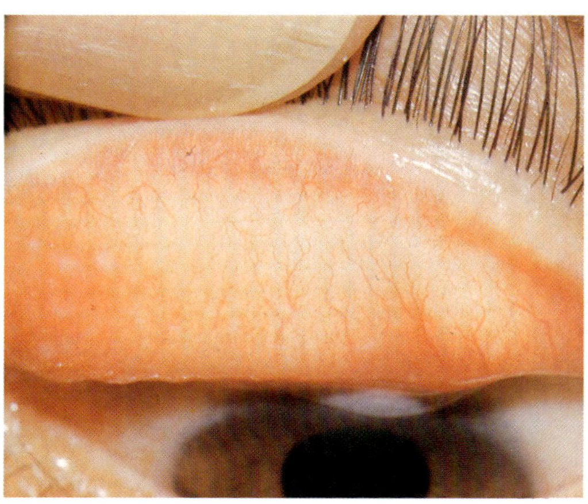

3–33A Herpes simplex conjunctivitis, follicular reaction. A conjunctivitis commonly occurs during primary ocular infections with the herpes simplex virus. The conjunctivitis may be follicular, as seen in this photograph, or may be pseudomembranous. In recurrent ocular herpes simplex infections, however, a conjunctivitis only rarely occurs and is usually follicular in type. A corneal dendrite (Fig. 3–33B) or vesicular lesions on the lid margin (Fig. 3–33C) often suggest the herpetic etiology. This patient developed a primary herpes simplex infection of the conjunctiva and when seen three days later was found to have follicles on the upper and lower tarsus.

3–33B Corneal dendrite in herpes simplex infection. This patient had developed a primary herpes simplex infection of the conjunctiva and cornea 2½ weeks previously. The dendrite, which is evident on the medial aspect of the cornea, is beginning to heal. It is fragmented and is taking up only a small amount of fluorescein. Superficial corneal neovascularization is present.

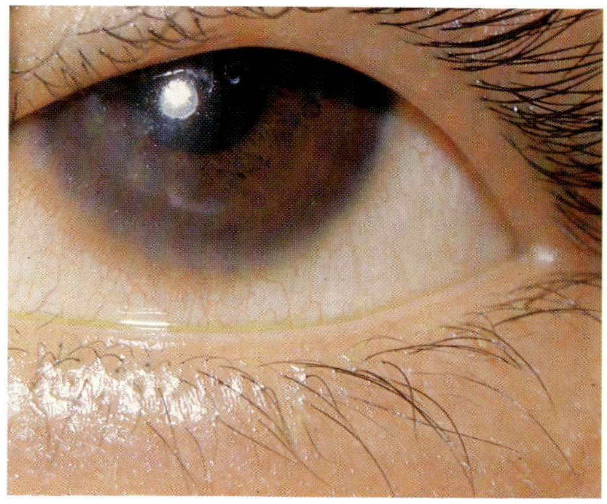

3–33C Herpes simplex vesicles on the eyelid. Vesicles on the lid margin due to herpes simplex infections often furnish a clue to the herpetic etiology of a follicular or pseudomembranous conjunctivitis. The vesicles are multiple and possess an erythematous base. In this patient, the vesicles on the outer aspect of the upper eyelid are beginning to crust and the erythema is subsiding.

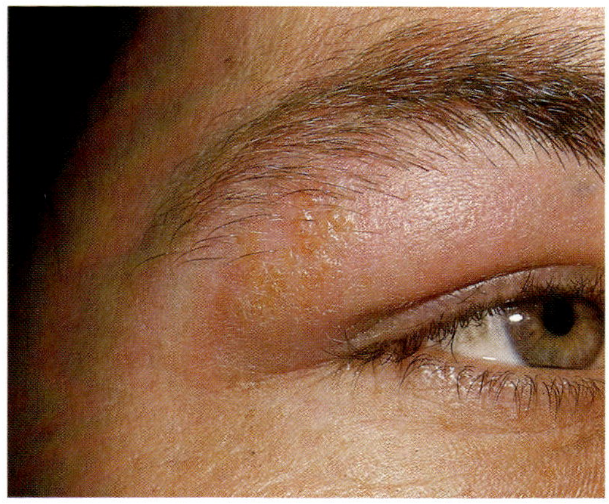

3–33D Scraping from herpes simplex conjunctivitis. Scrapings reveal a predominantly mononuclear reaction, as is evident in this scraping taken from a patient with primary herpes simplex conjunctivitis. Giemsa stain, ×400.

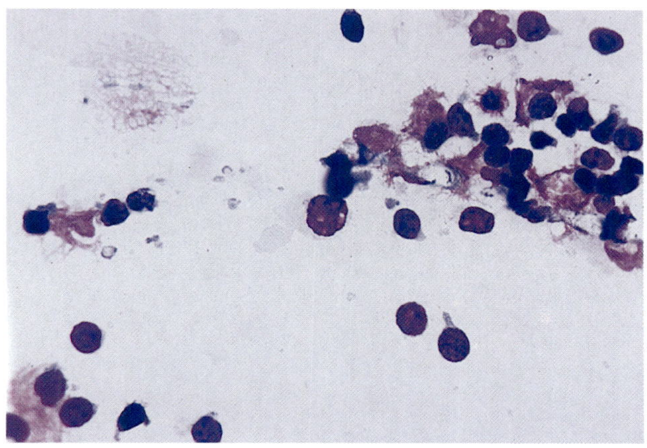

3–34 Herpes zoster conjunctivitis, follicular reaction. Herpes zoster conjunctivitis may be papillary, follicular, or pseudomembranous in character. There are no distinguishing features of the conjunctivitis per se, but when coupled with the ophthalmic distribution of a vesicular skin eruption, herpes zoster ophthalmicus is most likely. The follicular conjunctivitis in this patient was moderate in degree and was present when the patient was first seen one week after onset of his skin lesions.

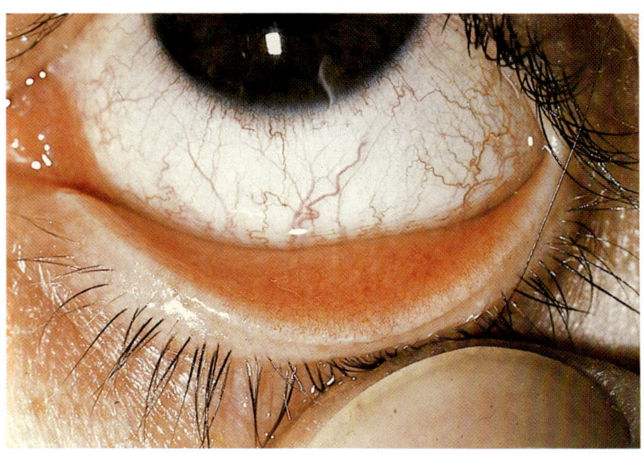

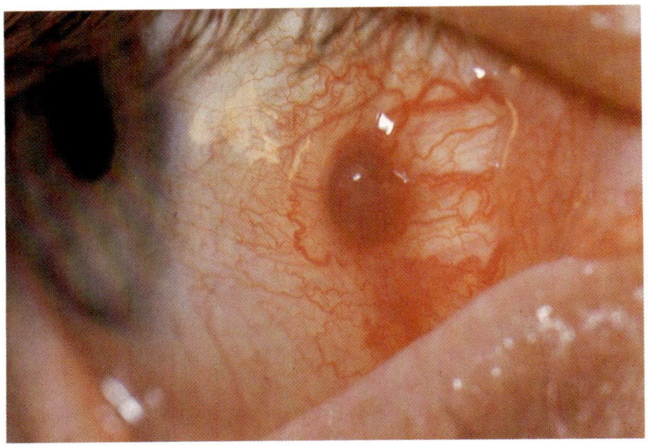

3–35 Kaposi's sarcoma. Kaposi's sarcoma of the conjunctiva may occur in patients with AIDS. In rare instances, the conjunctival injection may be the earliest presentation of infection with the HTLV 3 virus. This patient noted the red spot on his conjunctiva three weeks previously. The lesion persisted with only a slight increase in size until the patient's death eight months later. (Photograph courtesy of Dr. M. Friedlaender.)

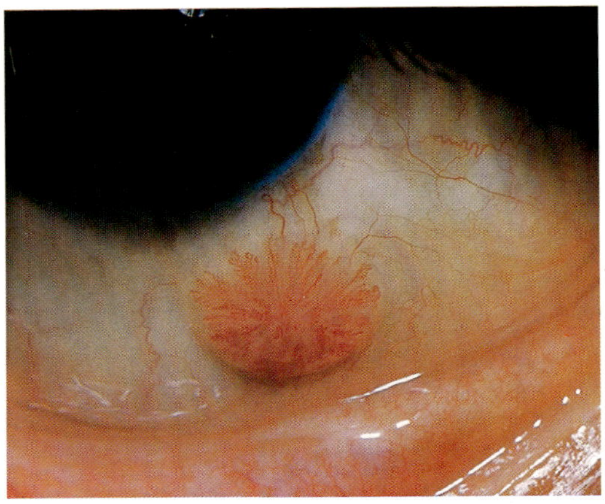

3–36 Verruca of the conjunctiva. Conjunctival verruca is a papillomatous growth containing very delicate frond-like processes. Each of the fronds has a vascular network similar to the veins in a leaf. Conjunctival verrucae tend to be multiple and pedunculated and usually occur in young individuals. This 17-year-old male had a verruca on the bulbar conjunctiva; the fronds are readily visible; the lesion was pedunculated and was noted to have a small base.

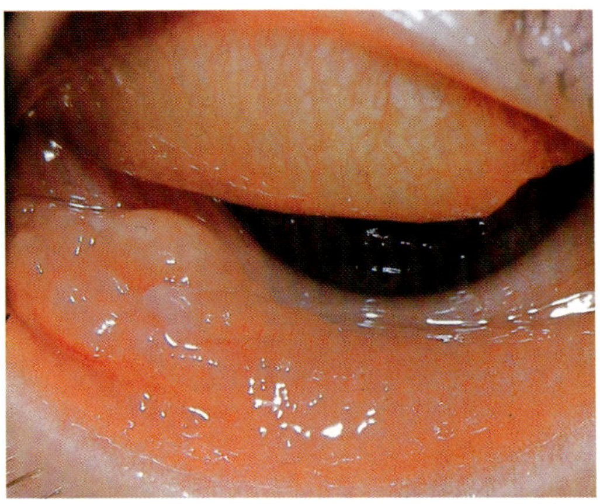

3–37A Conjunctival granuloma in cat scratch fever. Cat scratch fever may cause a focal granulomatous conjunctivitis with an associated grossly visible regional (preauricular) adenopathy (as seen in Fig. 3–37B, Parinaud's oculoglandular syndrome). The granulomatous reaction is usually on the tarsal conjunctiva or within the cul-de sac, but may occur on the bulbar conjunctiva. The granulomas are often associated with some follicular reaction, which arises secondary to the antigenic stimulus, as is evident in this patient. Follicular reactions are unusual in adults who develop Parinaud's oculoglandular syndrome, however.

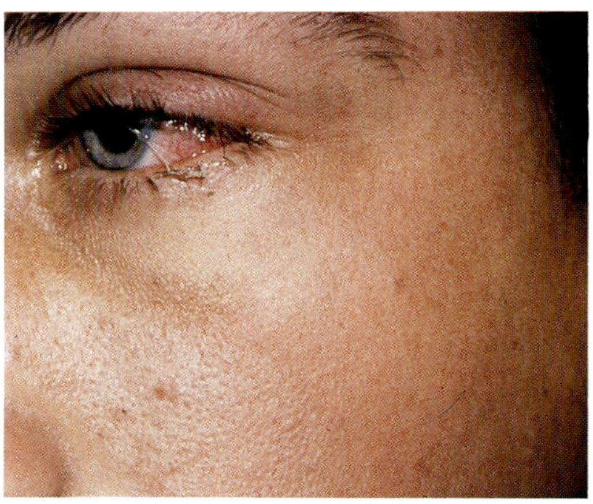

3–37B Grossly visible preauricular node in cat scratch fever. A grossly visible preauricular node may develop in response to many forms of conjunctivitis. When it is associated with conjunctival granulomas (Fig. 3–37A), however, the findings are sufficient to make the diagnosis of Parinaud's oculoglandular syndrome. This 14-year-old male developed a grossly visible preauricular node 1½ weeks prior to examination. The enlarged node and the conjunctivitis are readily visible in this photograph.

3–38 Tuberculosis of the conjunctiva. The granulomas in Parinaud's oculoglandular syndrome may also ulcerate and present as an ulcer of the conjunctiva and/or sclera. This woman was seen by the author in the Philippines. The patient presented with bilateral conjunctival ulcers that had developed from a tuberculous scleritis; she had a small preauricular node. The conjunctivitis and associated preauricular node did not properly fit into the classical Parinaud's oculoglandular syndrome.

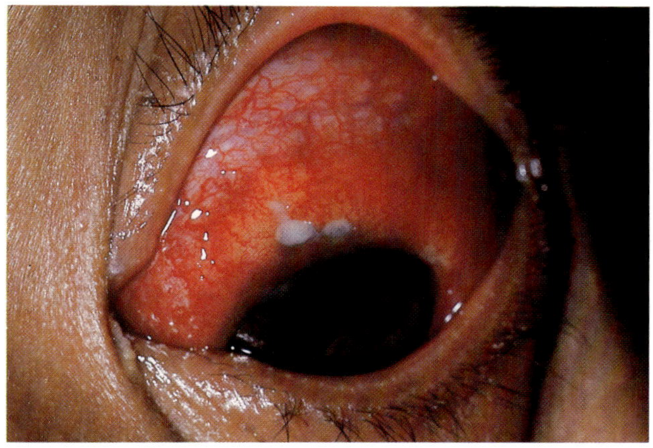

3–39A Tularemia. Infections with *Francisella tularensis* may cause an oculoglandular syndrome. Characteristically, the patient presents with evidence of fever and prostration. This patient developed tularemia after handling an infected rabbit. Note the severe hyperemia of the conjunctiva with a small granuloma on the lateral aspect of the lower tarsal conjunctiva (Anderson 1970). (Reprinted with permission from the *Journal of the Iowa Medical Society.)*

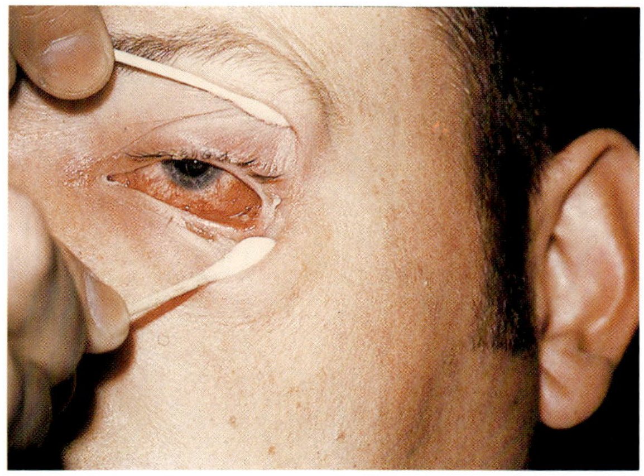

3–39B Grossly enlarged lymph node in tularemia. Tularemia is one of the possible causes of Parinaud's oculoglandular syndrome. This photograph shows the same patient seen in Fig. 3–39A. (Reprinted with permission from the *Journal of the Iowa Medical Society.)*

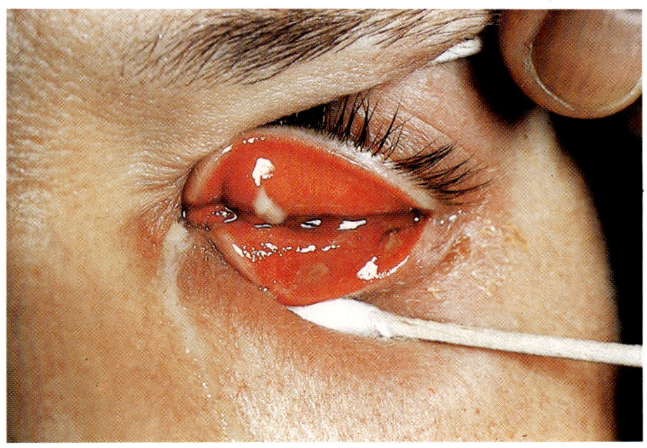

3–40 Infectious mononucleosis. Conjunctival involvement in infectious mononucleosis may be follicular or granulomatous in type. When it is granulomatous and associated with a grossly visible preauricular lymphadenopathy, as seen in this photograph, it is properly classified as Parinaud's oculoglandular syndrome. (Photograph courtesy of Dr. David M. Meisler and reprinted with permission from the *American Journal of Ophthalmology.)*

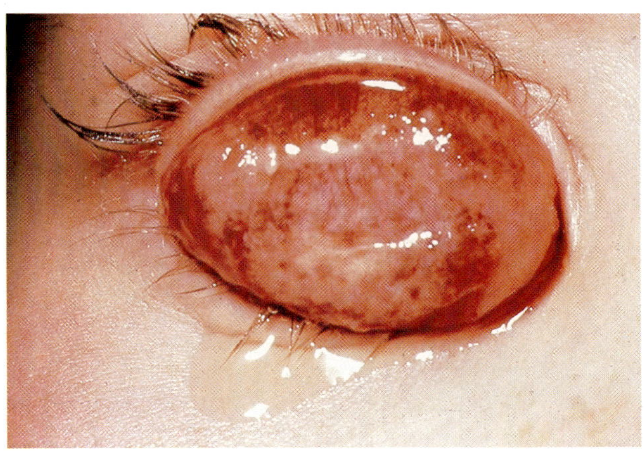

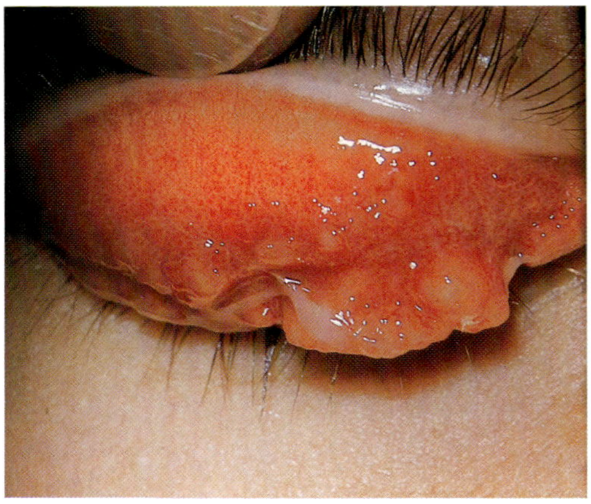

3–41 Coccidioidomycosis granuloma of the conjunctiva. This child developed a granuloma of the conjunctiva together with a grossly enlarged preauricular lymph node. History revealed that he had had a moderate cough and some fever several weeks previously. Biopsy revealed a granuloma due to coccidioidomycosis. There was no other evidence of dissemination. (Photograph courtesy of Dr. Phillips Thygeson and reprinted with permission from the *American Journal of Opththalmology.)*

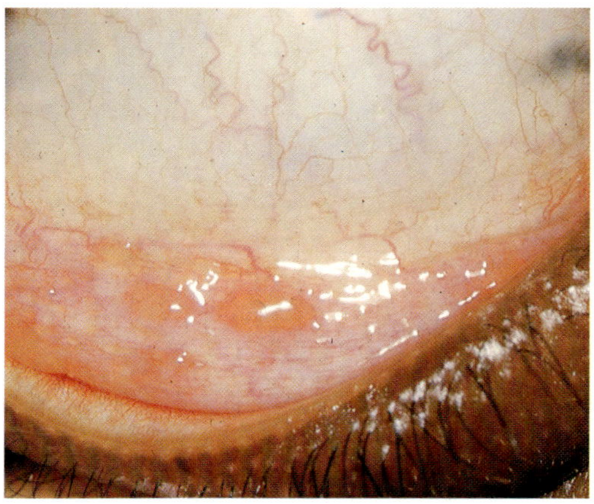

3–42 Sarcoid. In most instances, conjunctival sarcoidosis is characterized by the presence of small multiple granulomas in the inferior cul-de-sac, without involvement of the preauricular lymph nodes. In rare instances, however, a picture of Parinaud's oculoglandular syndrome may develop. This 27-year-old male was seen by the authors, with a request to rule out sarcoid. On biopsy, the nodules in the inferior cul-de-sac were compatible with sarcoid. Since the patient had no preauricular adenopathy, the conjunctival sarcoidosis did not properly fit the diagnosis of Parinaud's oculoglandular syndrome.

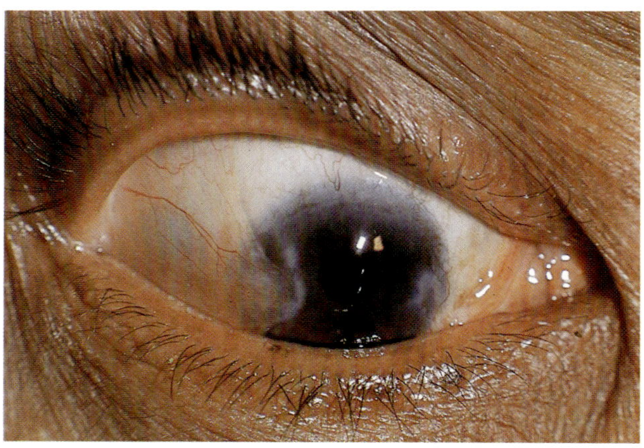

3–43 Pterygium. A pterygium is a fan-shaped or wing-shaped thickening of the conjunctiva that extends onto the limbus and cornea. It is found in the interpalpebral area of the conjunctiva and usually on the medial aspect. The pterygium may be markedly thickened and inflamed or flat and minimally injected, as in this 62-year-old Samoan.

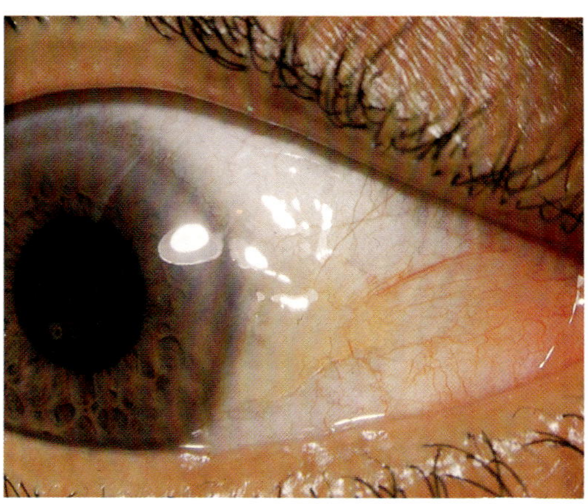

3–44 Pinguecula. A pinguecula occurs in the interpalpebral area of the conjunctiva adjacent to the limbus. It is a yellow triangular patch, and occurs in the aging population. This 64-year-old female had noted a yellow patch in the conjunctiva of each eye for more than 24 years.

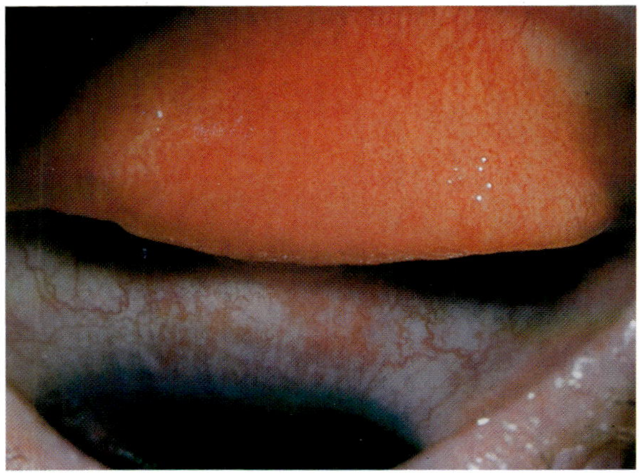

3–45A Superior limbic keratoconjunctivitis (SLK), upper tarsus. A superior limbic keratoconjunctivitis is characterized by a papillary conjunctivitis of the upper tarsus and thickening and keratinization of the superior limbus (Fig. 3–45B). In this 46-year-old female with SLK of eight months duration, marked papillary hypertrophy is evident in the upper tarsal conjunctiva. Thickening and hyperemia of the upper limbus are also visible.

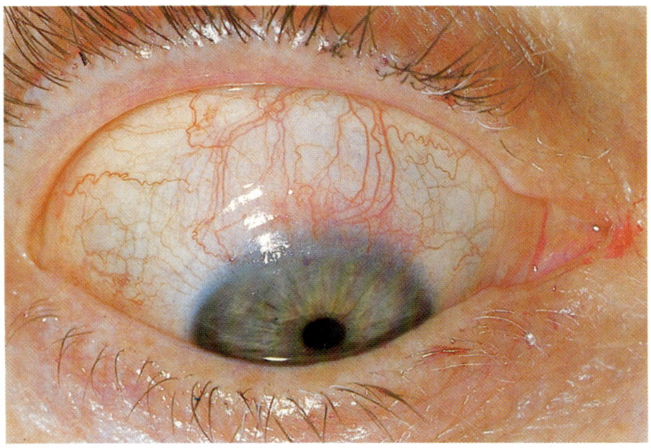

3–45B Superior limbic keratoconjunctivitis, upper limbus. Thickening and hyperemia of the upper limbus are visible in this photograph of a 34-year-old female with SLK. Rose bengal has been instilled into the eye, and the areas that are keratinized or keratinizing have taken up the vital dye.

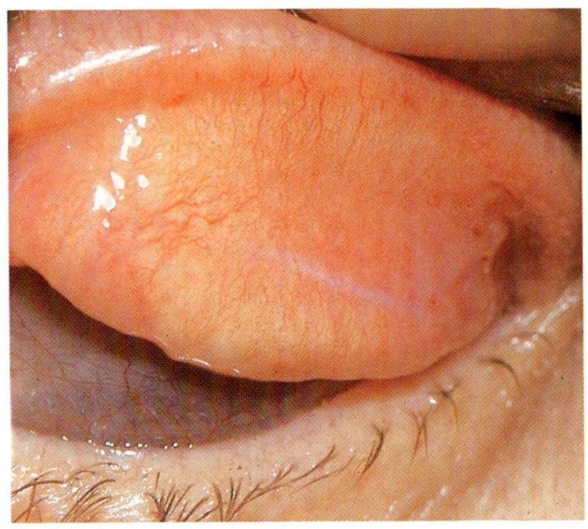

3–46 Toxic follicular conjunctivitis. A follicular conjunctivitis may develop in response to the use of topical medications such as the antivirals (especially idoxuridine), many miotics, and atropine. The reaction is thought to be toxic; the full response takes several weeks to develop, even when the patient is rechallenged with the same topical medication and no eosinophils are found on scrapings of the follicular conjunctivitis. This patient developed a follicular reaction to the topical use of atropine. She had been treated with atropine previously for a herpetic iritis and had developed, follicles; the atropine was discontinued and the follicles subsided. Three weeks after the atropine was reinstituted in her regimen of treatment, conjunctival follicles developed again. The corneal scarring and neovascularization resulted from involvement of her cornea with herpes simplex.

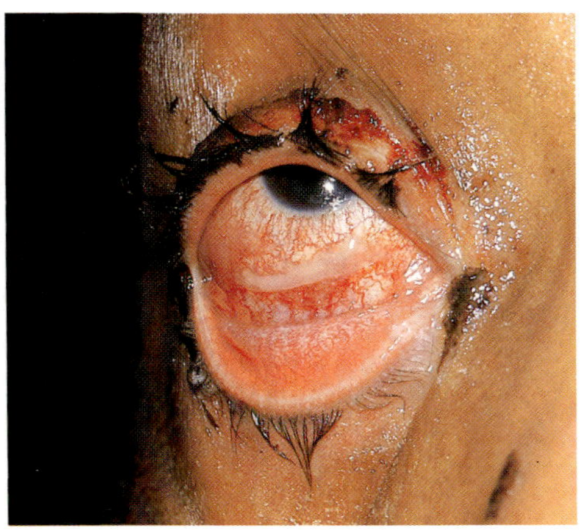

3–47A Erythema multiforme major, early conjunctival changes. In its early phases, the conjunctivitis of erythema multiforme major begins as a papillary conjunctivitis which quickly develops to form vesicles or small bullae. In the presence of moisture, the vesicles and bullae break down to form pseudomembranes which then progress to conjunctival scarring and symblepharon formation. In this 36-year-old male, who developed erythema multiforme major triggered by the use of antibiotics, marked crusting and decadent blood on the eyelids, a pseudomembrane on the bulbar conjunctiva, and a moderate papillary reaction on the tarsal conjunctiva are evident.

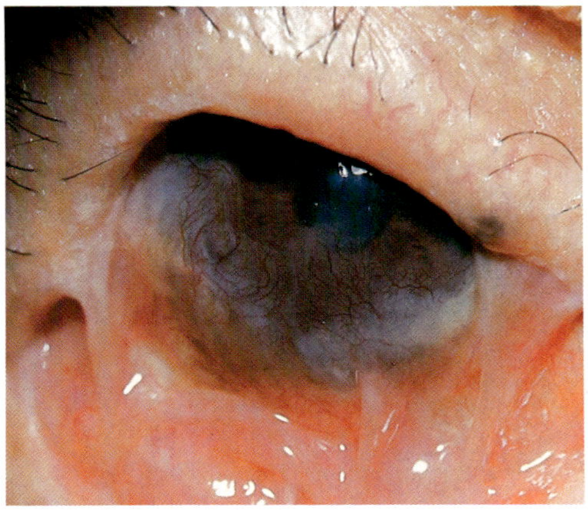

3–47B Erythema multiforme major, late conjunctival changes. In the late phases of erythema multiforme major, symblepharon formation and flat scarring are commonly found.

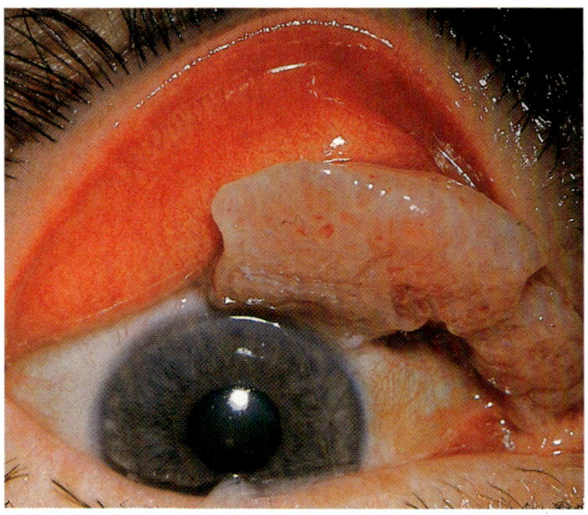

3–48 Ligneous conjunctivitis. This conjunctivitis is of unknown origin and occurs most frequently in young girls. The name ligneous describes the woody, hard feeling of the lid, which is due to the presence of a white membrane covering the palpebral and sometimes the bulbar conjunctiva. This 11-year-old female has had difficulty for more than a year. The membranous lesion was removed many times, and here can be seen overlying the medial aspect of the upper tarsus.

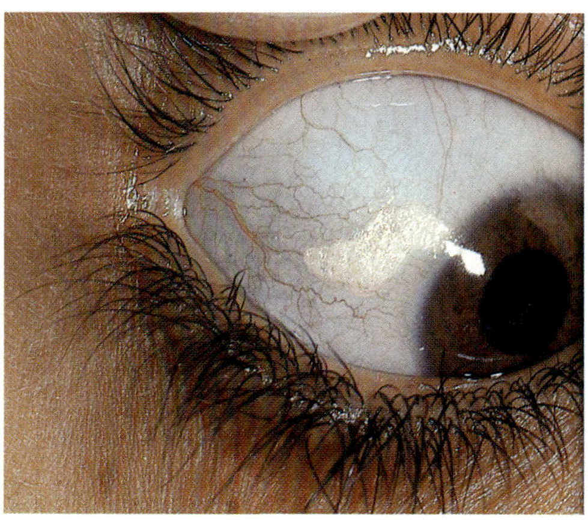

3–49 Bitot's spot. A Bitot's spot is a characteristic of vitamin A deficiency and may persist long after the deficiency has been corrected. It is characteristically found on the interpalpebral conjunctiva and has a dry, thickened, foamy appearance.

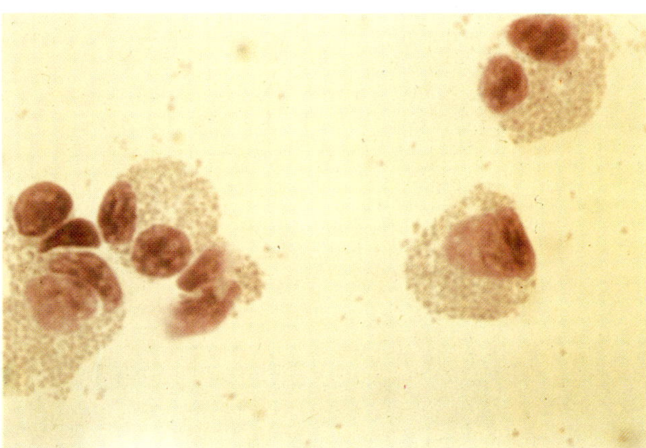

3–50 Eosinophils and free eosinophilic granules in vernal keratoconjunctivitis. Eosinophils and free eosinophilic granules are one of the hallmarks of allergic conjunctivitis, including hay fever conjunctivitis, atopic keratoconjunctivitis, and vernal conjunctivitis.

3–51 Hay fever conjunctivitis. This represents an acute anaphylactic response to an allergen in which the conjunctiva represents the shock organ. The conjunctiva is chemotic and injected, and often the patient is concerned that the cornea is sinking into the socket. The reaction is short lived, unless exposure to the offending antigen continues. This patient developed an acute chemosis and swelling of his lids in reaction to animal dander. The exposure that brought on this attack occurred 30 minutes previously when the patient was exposed to guinea pig dander. Note the marked swelling of the eyelids and conjunctiva, together with tearing.

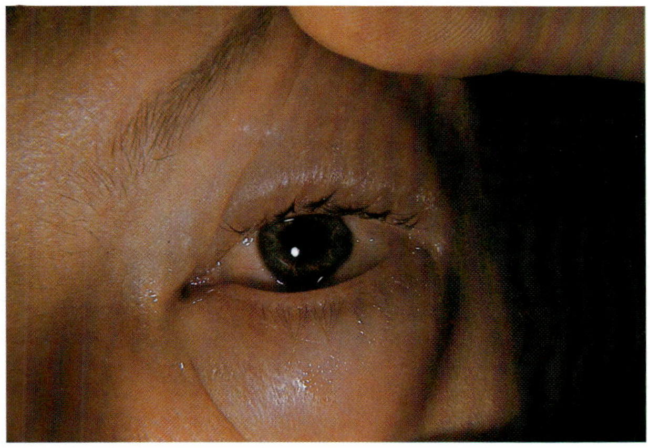

3–52 Atopic keratoconjunctivitis, lower tarsus. The conjunctiva in atopic keratoconjunctivitis appears milky in color because of conjunctival edema. The upper tarsus usually has many small papillae with a few giant papillae, whereas the lower tarsal conjunctiva may have a few or many giant papillae. This 28-year-old male has had atopic keratoconjunctivitis for more than 18 years. A milky appearance of the conjunctiva together with a few giant papillae are seen. The stringy, mucoid discharge is also characteristic.

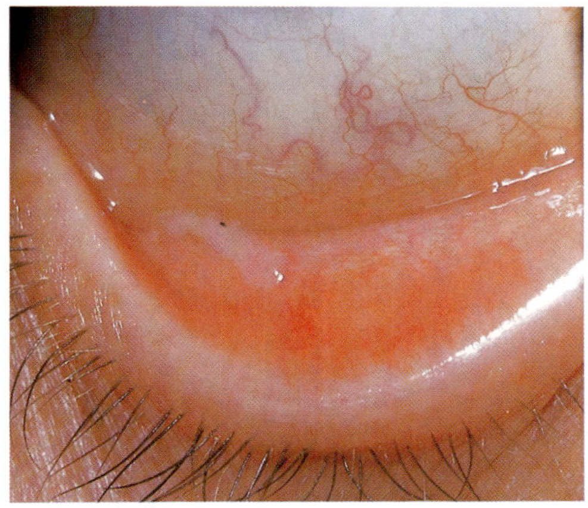

3–53 Atopic keratoconjunctivitis, limbus. Giant papillae may occur at the limbus in atopic conjunctivitis. Because of the edema, the papillae appear somewhat avascular and may appear round since the conjunctiva is more loosely attached to the limbus than to the tarsus. The giant papillae usually occur near the 12:00 area but may occur anywhere on the limbus. Trantas' dots are also frequently seen. (Fig. 3–54). This 18-year-old male has had marked itching and tearing for more than 12 years. The symptoms were more marked during the fall and winter and often occurred with attacks of eczema. Thickening of the upper limbus and many Trantas' dots are evident in the upper limbal area.

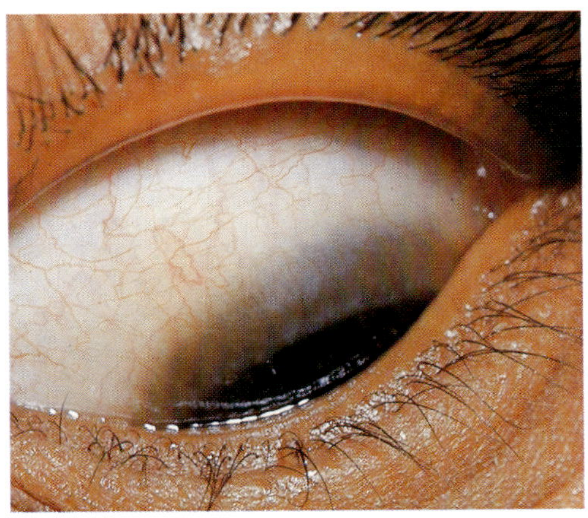

3–54 Trantas' dots. Trantas' dots represent clusters of eosinophils that are gradually working to the surface of the conjunctiva. They are chalky in appearance, and although they are usually found at the limbus may occur on the bulbar or the tarsal conjunctiva. Trantas' dots are usually found in atopic keratoconjunctivitis and in vernal keratoconjunctivitis, as seen in this 19-year-old male.

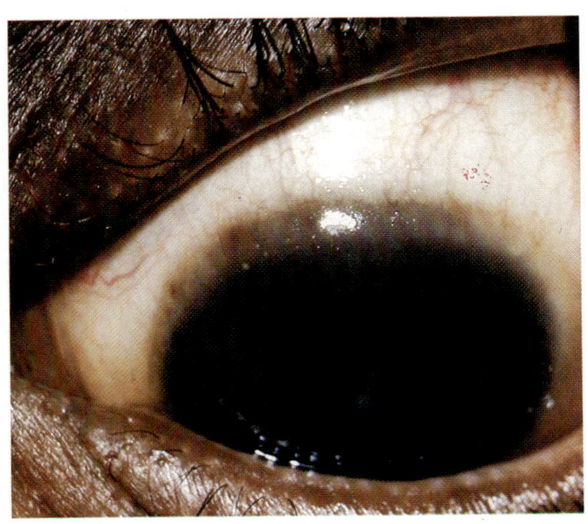

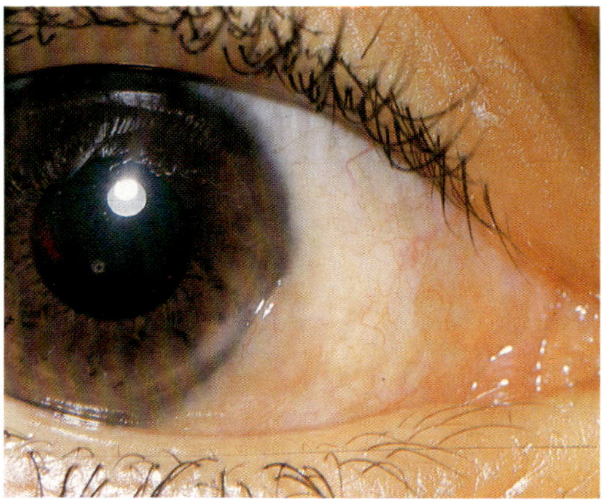

3–55 Pseudogeronotoxin. A pseudogeronotoxin may occur in either limbal vernal keratoconjunctivitis or atopic keratoconjunctivitis. It looks like a small segment of arc of an arcus senilis, and results from prolonged hyperemia at that segment of the limbus due to the presence of giant papillae. After the giant papillae have subsided the pseudogeronotoxin is still evident and is often the only evidence of previous allergic eye disease. In this photograph the pseudogeronotoxin is readily visible adjacent to a large limbal papilla. Note that the arc does not extend superiorly or inferiorly in areas where the limbal papillae are absent.

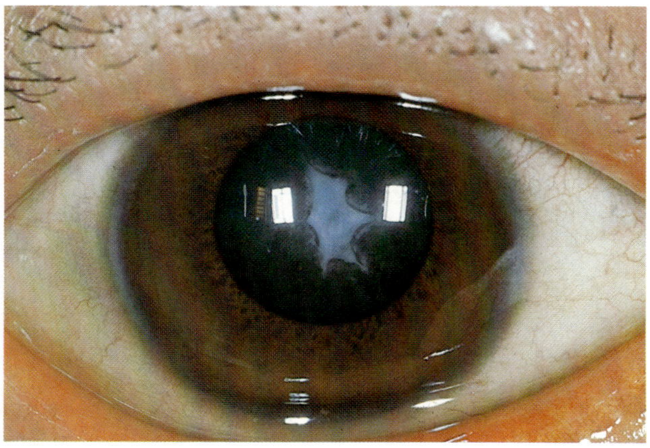

3–56 Anterior shield-like cataract in atopic keratoconjunctivitis. Although a posterior subcapsular cataract occurs more commonly than an anterior shield-like cataract in atopic keratoconjunctivitis, the anterior shield-like cataract is more characteristic of the disease. This patient has had atopic keratoconjunctivitis for more than 24 years and has begun to develop characteristic anterior cataractous changes, as seen in this photograph.

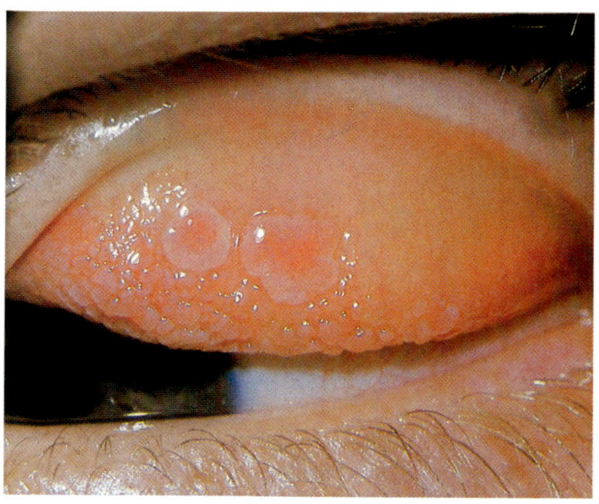

3–57 Palpebral vernal keratoconjunctivitis. This conjunctivitis is manifested by the presence of giant papillae on the upper tarsus; the tarsal conjunctiva appears milky in color. The giant papillae are polygonal and usually flat-topped because of the marked crowding of the papillae and the firm attachment of the conjunctiva to the underlying tarsus. In this 14-year-old male, many medium-sized and two giant papillae are noted on the upper tarsus. The flat-topped papillae and milky color are very characteristic.

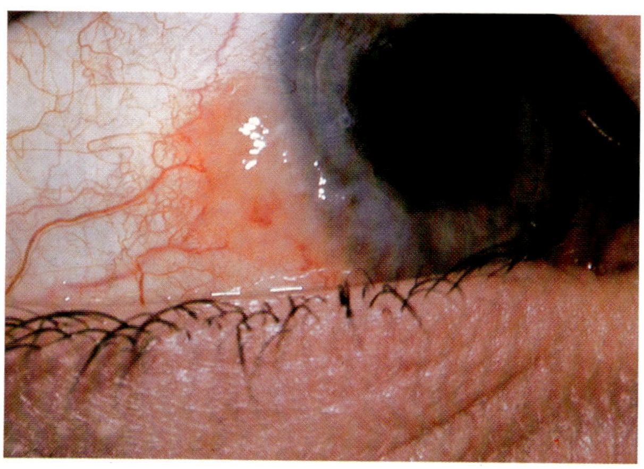

3–58 Limbal vernal keratoconjunctivitis. Giant papillae may occur at the limbus in both limbal vernal keratoconjunctivitis and in the palpebral form of vernal keratoconjunctivitis. The papillae are similar to those seen in atopic keratoconjunctivitis (Fig. 3–52), and although they may occur anywhere on the limbus, are usually found in the interpalpebral area. In this 16-year-old female, the large limbal papillae extend onto the peripheral cornea and onto the bulbar conjunctiva.

3–59 Giant papillae in giant papillary conjunctivitis. The giant papillae that occur in giant papillary conjunctivitis may be confused with follicles because of their avascular appearance. The white appearance arises from a fine superficial scarring, however. The papillae are polygonal in appearance and flat-topped.

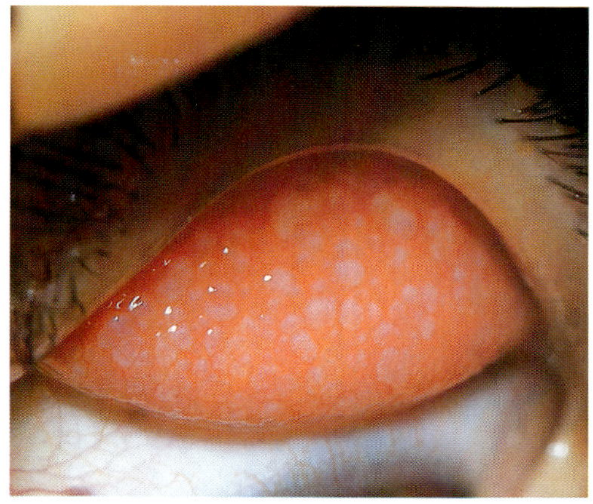

3–60 Scarring following pseudomembranous conjunctivitis. The scarring that develops after a pseudomembranous conjunctivitis is flat and occurs in those areas that were covered by pseudomembrane. In this patient who developed erythema multiforme major, a flat scar is present on the superior aspect of the upper tarsus. Marked erythema of the conjunctiva and loss of keratinization of the medial aspect of the lid margin are also noted, as is some crusting of the lashes.

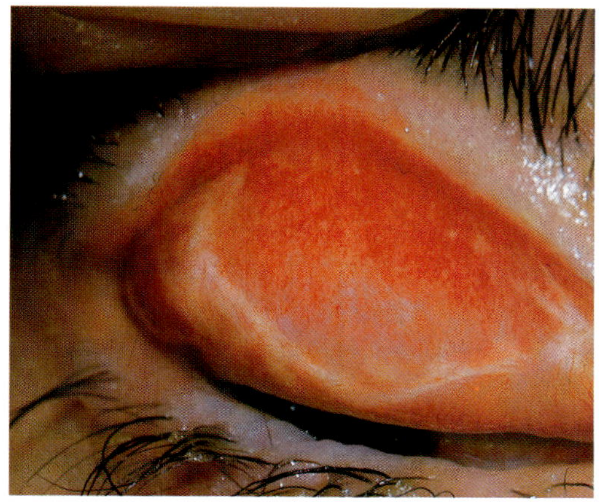

3–61 Cicatricial pemphigoid. The conjunctivitis in cicatricial pemphigoid begins as a nonspecific papillary conjunctivitis and progresses to scarring and obliteration of the inferior fornices, and eventually to total symblepharon formation. The upper cul-de-sac tends to be spared until very late in the disease. In this 64-year-old female total obliteration of the inferior cul-de-sac has occurred, with marked dryness and keratinization of the exposed conjunctiva and cornea. The upper cul-de-sac is still partially spared.

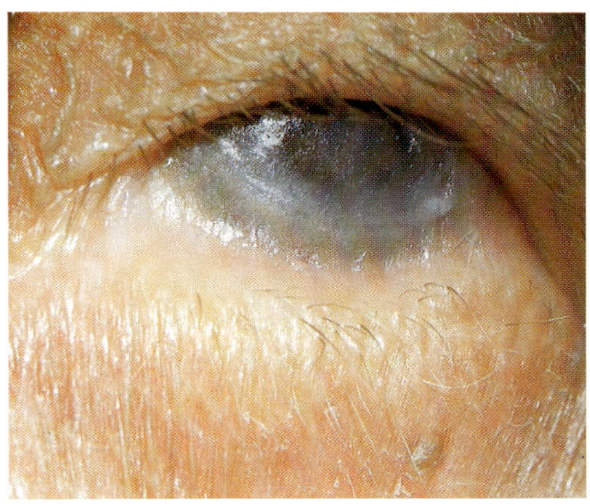

3–62 Conjunctiva in early toxic epidermal necrolysis. The early and late conjunctival changes in toxic epidermal necrolysis are similar to those of erythema multiforme major (Figs. 3–47A, 3–47B). The pseudomembrane formation in this 22-year-old female, who developed toxic epidermal necrolysis from exposure to Gantanol®, is evident on the lower tarsus. Note the marked crusting of the skin of the eyelid.

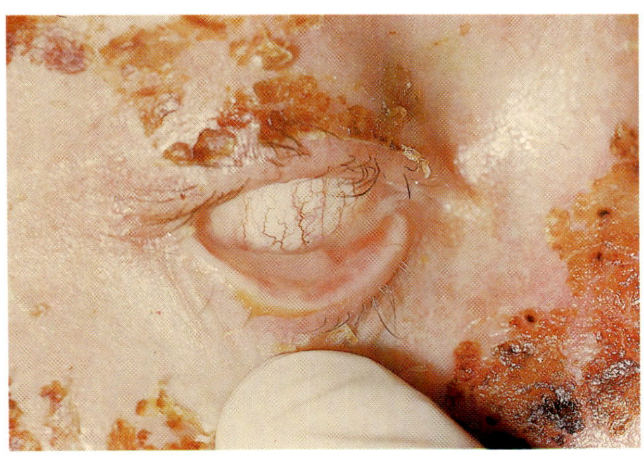

Chapter 4

Infections and Inflammations of the Cornea

Any infection or inflammation that causes irregularity or opacification of the cornea may reduce vision. Although there are many different infectious and inflammatory conditions of the cornea, the types of corneal response are limited and the manifestations of disease are similar in many forms of keratitis.

The advantages of the slit lamp for examination of the cornea and the external eye were appreciated soon after Tullstrand's introduction of the device in 1911. Clinicians should use the full range of techniques available with the modern slit lamp when examining the eye, including diffuse illumination (particularly for the lids and conjunctiva), direct focal illumination, retro-illumination, specular reflection, and indirect lateral illumination (sclerotic scatter). Other instruments designed for examination of the cornea include the specular microscope to examine the endothelium, the keratometer to measure corneal curvature, Placido's disk to examine the cornea for irregular astigmatism, and the pachymeter to measure corneal thickness.

Epithelial Keratitis

The epithelial keratopathies include the entire range of abnormalities of the corneal epithelium that occur during infections and inflammatory diseases of the external eye. Epithelial abnormalities may be classified by their size, morphology, and location. In many instances epithelial changes are not inflammatory in origin, but we include them in the general classification for completeness.

Filamentary Keratitis

A filamentary keratitis may comprise true filaments caused by a curling up of corneal epithelium (Fig. 4–1) or mucous filaments composed of filament-like mucoid threads with a tiny tag of epithelium at the end where the mucous attaches to the cornea. The two types may be differentiated clinically: true epithelial filaments are fewer in number (less than ten) (Fig. 4–2), usually longer in length, twisted in appearance, and more firmly attached to the corneal epithelium; mucoid filaments are more numerous, usually shorter in length, frothy in appearance, and more easily movable (Fig. 4–3). A true epithelial filament arises from a triangular patch of corneal epithelial cells which becomes elevated, while at the same time the surrounding epithelial cells are undergoing degenerative changes. The cells gradually become elongated and undergo torsion, which produces the filament. A filamentary keratopathy is associated with symptoms of photophobia and foreign body sensation; the authors have found them to cause a foreign body sensation even when the corneal sensation is absent. The clinical forms of filamentary keratopathy are listed in Table 4–1.

Epithelial Erosions

Punctate epithelial erosions are depressed areas of the cornea arising from epithelial loss and are usually scattered over the surface of the cornea. The erosions may be fine, i.e., visible only with high magnification such as at the slit lamp (Fig. 4–6), medium (Figs. 4–7, 4–8), or coarse in type (Fig. 4–9). The cornea

Table 4–1 Clinical Forms of Filamentary Keratopathy

Location	*Disease*	*Comments*
	Transitory	
Entire Cornea	Herpes simplex infections (Fig. 4–4)	Small, very evanescent
Area of erosion	Recurrent erosion	Occur at time of erosion
Area of lesion	Ruptured bulla	Occur at time of rupture
	Long lasting	
Superior third of cornea	Superior limbic keratoconjunctivitis (Fig. 4–2)	Presence not constant
	Prolonged ptosis (Fig. 4–5)	Area covered by lid
Entire cornea	Prolonged occlusion	
Inferior cornea	Keratoconjunctivitis sicca (Fig. 4–3)	Usually mucoid

surrounding the erosions appears normal. The loss of superficial epithelial cells results from premature desquamation of the cells, which allows vital dyes such as fluorescein to stain the immature epithelial cells developing within the deficient area and to stain the underlying corneal stroma. The clinical forms of epithelial erosions are listed in Table 4–2.

Recurrent Epithelial Erosions

Recurrent epithelial erosions are macroscopic epithelial defects usually occurring inferior to the visual axis. The epithelial defects are readily seen with the aid of a vital dye such as fluorescein, and characteristically produce recurrent pain, photophobia, redness, and tearing. Symptoms usually begin during sleep or as the patient first awakens. Unless the erosion is of long standing, the underlying corneal stroma and Bowman's layer are clear (Shoch et al., 1985). Recurrent epithelial erosions commonly occur in lattice, macular, and anterior membrane (map-dot-fingerprint) dystrophies, and also commonly follow trauma (Weene, 1985). Fuchs' endothelial-epithelial dystrophy may also cause a recurrent erosion, but the other

Table 4–2 Clinical Forms of Epithelial Erosions

Type/Location	*Disease**	*Comments*
Linear/Any location	Conjunctival foreign body or misdirected lash	Actual abrasion of cornea
Fine/Diffuse	Staphylococcal blepharitis (Fig. 4–6)	Due to dermatonecrotoxin
	Chemicals	
	Molluscum contagiosum	Toxic effect, usually grouped in appearance
	Verruca of lid margin	Toxic effect, usually grouped in appearance
	Viral exanthemas	Usually grouped
	Adenoviral conjunctivitis	Probably actual infection
	Chlamydia	Associated micropannus or pannus
Fine/Superior cornea	Molluscum contagiosum	Toxic effect, associated pannus
	Verruca of lid margin	Toxic effect, usually grouped in appearance
	Trachoma	Associated pannus formation
Fine/Inferior cornea	Chemicals	
	Staphylococcal blepharitis	Due to dermatonecrotoxin
	Seborrhea of lid margin	
Fine/Exposure area	Seborrhea of lid margin	
	Familial corneal hypes thesia	Bilateral
Fine/Any location	HSV keratitis	Quickly forms dendrite
	VZ keratitis	May form pseudodendrite
Medium/Diffuse	Staphylococcal blepharitis	
	Molluscum contagiosum (Fig. 4–8)	Toxic effect
	Verruca of lid margin	Toxic effect, usually grouped
	Chlamydia	Associated micropannus or pannus
Medium/Superior cornea	Molluscum contagiosum	Toxic effect
	Verruca of lid margin	Toxic effect, usually grouped
	Trachoma	Associated pannus
Medium/Inferior cornea	Staphylococcal blepharitis	Due to dermatonecrotoxin
	Medicamentosa	Toxic effect (antivirals, antibiotics)

Type/Location	*Disease**	*Comments*
Medium/Exposure area	Medicamentosa	Toxic effect (antivirals, antibiotics)
	Familial corneal hypesthesia (Fig. 4–7)	Bilateral
Medium/Any location	HSV keratitis	Quickly forms dendrite
	VZ keratitis	May form pseudodendrite
	Viral exanthemas	Usually grouped
Coarse/Diffuse	Chemicals	Usually grouped
Coarse/Inferior cornea	Medicamentosa	Toxic effect (antivirals, antibiotics)
Coarse/Exposure area	Medicamentosa	Toxic effect (antivirals, antibiotics)
	Keratoconjunctivitis sicca (Fig. 4–9)	
Coarse/Peripheral	Reiter's syndrome	Associated with conjunctivitis
Coarse/Central	Erythema multiforme major	Large erosions
	Toxic epidermal necrolysis	Large erosions
Coarse/Any location	HSV keratitis	Quickly forms dendrite
	VZ keratitis	May form pseudodendrite
	Viral exanthemas	Usually grouped
	Keratoconjunctivitis sicca	
	Epidemic keratoconjunctivitis (Fig. 4–10)	May form large erosion

* Abbreviations used: HSV, herpes simplex virus; VZ, varicella/zoster ophthalmicus

findings of corneal edema and endothelial cell loss usually overshadow those of the recurrent erosion. The dystrophic forms of epithelial erosions are bilateral but initially present unilaterally.

Several theories have been suggested to explain the cause of recurrent erosion. These include a tendency for the corneal epithelium to adhere to the lid margin or to the palpebral conjunctiva and then to be pulled off from the cornea when the eyelids are first opened, or a tendency for the eyelids to exert suction on the corneal epithelium as they are first opened. Histologically, absence of hemidesmosomes, loss of the basement membrane and alteration in the basal cells of the epithelium, and changes within the corneal stroma have been documented (Messer et al., 1983).

Epithelial Keratopathy (Keratitis)

An epithelial keratopathy presents as fine, medium, or coarse opaque areas within the corneal epithelium. It differs from epithelial erosions by the presence of opaque areas and the tendency for the lesions to stain readily with rose bengal and only poorly with fluorescein. The epithelial keratopathy results from the loss of vitality of epithelial cells. Pathophysiologically, edema of the epithelial basal cells and the spaces between the epithelial cells develops together with loss of the hemidesmosomes. These changes lead to loss of individual epithelial cells. The clinical forms of epithelial keratopathy (keratitis) are listed in Table 4–3.

Table 4–3 Clinical Forms of Epithelial Keratopathy (Keratitis)

Type/Location	*Disease**	*Comments*
Fine/Diffuse	Viral exanthemas	
	Adenoviral conjunctivitis	Represents actual infection
	Acute hemorrhagic conjunctivitis	Probably from actual infection
	Seborrheic blepharitis	

Type/Location	*Disease**	*Comments*
Fine/Superior	Superior limbic keratoconjunctivitis	Associated micropannus
	Chlamydial infections	Associated micropannus or pannus
	Molluscum contagiosum	Toxic effect
	Vernal keratoconjunctivitis	Syncytium (Fig. 4–11)
Fine/Inferior	Staphylococcal blepharitis	Due to dermatonecrotoxin
	Medicamentosa	Toxic effect (antivirals, antibiotics)
	Keratoconjunctivitis sicca	
Fine/Exposure area	Keratoconjunctivitis sicca	
	Exposure keratitis (neuroparalytic and neurotrophic)	
	Medicamentosa	Toxic effect (antivirals, antibiotics)
Fine/Any location	HSV keratitis	Quickly forms dendrite
	VZ keratitis	May form pseudodendrite
	Superficial punctate keratitis (Thygeson)	Oval may be elevated
Medium/Superior	Superior limbic keratoconjunctivitis	Associated micropannus
	Chlamydial infections	Micropannus or pannus
	Molluscum contagiosum	Toxic effect
	Vernal keratoconjunctivitis	Syncytium (Fig. 4–11)
Medium/Exposure	Keratoconjunctivitis sicca (Fig. 4–12)	
	Exposure keratitis (neuroparalytic and neurotrophic)	
	Medicamentosa	Toxic effect (antivirals, antibiotics)
Medium/Any location	HSV keratitis	Quickly forms dendrite
	VZ keratitis	May form pseudodendrite
	Superficial punctate keratitis (Thygeson)	Oval may be elevated
Coarse/Superior	Vernal keratoconjunctivitis	Syncytium or oval ulcer
	Chlamydial infections	Associated micropannus or pannus
	Molluscum contagiosum	Associated pannus
	Superior limbic keratoconjunctivitis	
Coarse/Exposure area	Keratoconjunctivitis sicca (Fig. 4–13)	
	Exposure (neuroparalytic, neurotrophic)	
	Dystrophic lesions of recurrent erosion	e.g., Anterior membrane dystrophy
	Medicamentosa (Fig. 4–14)	Toxic effect (antivirals, antibiotics)
Coarse/Any location	Superficial punctate keratitis (Thygeson) (Figs. 4–15 A and B)	Oval may be elevated
	HSV keratitis	Blotchy, stellate, dendritic (Fig. 4–16)
		Geographic (Fig. 4–17)
	VZ keratitis	Blotchy, pseudodendrite (Figs. 4–18 A and B)
	Chemical injury	
	Hypovitaminosis A (Pham, 1985)	Cornea lusterless, Bitot's spot

* Abbreviations used: HSV, herpes simplex virus; VZ, varicella/zoster ophthalmicus.

Subepithelial Keratitis

Disciform Keratitis

Disciform keratitis, a disk-shaped opacity, may occur in the center of the cornea in viral corneal infections (Liesegang, 1985) and especially herpes simplex keratitis (Fig. 4–19). The lesion appears to be mediated by immune mechanisms, or in some instances by infection within the cornea (Tullo et al., 1985). The opacity primarily represents corneal edema.

Round Superficial Subepithelial Opacities

Round superficial subepithelial opacities (focal avascular superficial keratitis) (Fig. 4–20) may occur in the cornea. In herpes simplex infections they develop in areas underlying an epithelial keratitis or within the area of a disciform keratitis as it begins to clear, especially if it has been treated with glucocorticoids.

In epidemic keratoconjunctivitis, the round subepithelial opacities are grossly visible (Figs. 4–21 A and B) and are more prominent in the central cornea. In rare instances the opacities become confluent.

Dimmer's nummular or padi keratitis is usually unilateral and is associated with round subepithelial opacities (Fig. 4–22) which may become faceted as the lesions heal (Valenton, 1974). The opacities may be irregularly shaped because of confluence of several lesions. The lesions occur in one or several levels of the corneal stroma. Neovascularization of the cornea may also occur.

Round, often irregular superficial infiltrates also occur in varicella-zoster keratitis, phlyctenulosis, and Reiter's syndrome (Mark and McCulley, 1982). Round subepithelial corneal opacities may develop early in the course of Hansen's disease; as the disease progresses, the opacities also involve the midstromal and deep stromal layers. At onset, they occur in the superior temporal region, but eventually involve the entire circumference of the cornea.

During the parasitemia of onchocerciasis, round irregular snowflake–like subepithelial opacities may develop in both the exposure and the inferior areas of the peripheral cornea. As the disease progresses, the lesions gradually involve the central cornea.

Limbal-based Triangular Corneal Opacities

Triangular, limbal-based opacities result from phlyctenulosis (Fig. 4–23). Vascularization of the cornea may also develop in phlyctenulosis and lead to a fascicular keratitis (see below).

Fascicular Keratitis

A fascicular keratitis is defined as a superficial corneal inflammatory lesion accompanied by a "bundle" of superficial blood vessels. The inflammatory lesion seemingly wanders aimlessly across the cornea as the infection progresses. A fascicular keratitis may be produced by herpes simplex infections (Fig. 4–24), or by the progressive development of new phlyctenules central to the ends of new vessels (a wandering phlyctenule) (Fig. 4–25) during a delayed hypersensitivity reaction to tubercular protein or staphylococcal products.

Marginal Keratitis

A marginal keratitis is characterized by an inflammatory focal lesion in the peripheral cornea, which has a tendency to remain near or associated with the limbal vessels as the inflammation progresses. Marginal infiltrates usually progress to produce epithelial and occasionally superficial stromal necrosis. As a general rule, these lesions are more benign than central corneal are lesions, especially central corneal ulcers, although neovascularization of the cornea often occurs.

A marginal keratitis may begin as an infiltrate of the superficial stroma which proceeds to ulceration, as occurs in staphyloccocal marginal ulcers (Fig. 4–26). Alternatively, the lesion may begin in the epithelium and involve the superficial stroma secondarily, as occurs in herpes simplex infections of the cornea (Fig. 4–27).

Simultaneously with the development of the marginal keratitis, the adjacent limbal conjunctiva becomes hyperemic, edematous, and infiltrated, but a hypopyon does not occur unless there is severe stromal necrosis. Except for marginal herpes simplex keratitis, which is usually quite asymptomatic, a marginal keratitis usually causes severe pain, tearing, and photophobia.

Catarrhal Corneal Infiltrates and Ulcers

In staphylococcal blepharokeratitis, *Haemophilus aegyptius* keratoconjunctivitis, and probably other types of keratoconjunctivitis, the catarrhal corneal infiltrate or ulcer (Fig. 4–28) is mediated by immune complexes.

Catarrhal corneal infiltrates or ulcers may also occur in gonorrheal conjunctivitis, coliform bacterial infections of the conjunctiva or lid margin, and actinomycotic and beta-hemolytic streptococcal infections of the canaliculus or lacrimal sac. The catarrhal corneal ulcer occurring with *Moraxella lacunata* conjunctivitis is probably due to a hypersensitivity reaction to the staphylococcus.

A catarral corneal infiltrate begins as a subepithelial infiltrate that runs concentric to the limbus; a small area of clear cornea (a lucid interval) usually separates the infiltrate from the limbus (Fig. 4–29). If the infiltrate progresses, it enlarges concentrically forming a bow-shaped infiltrate that is readily visible with the naked eye. The epithelium overlying the infiltrate usually breaks down during the disease process to form a marginal corneal ulcer with a gray base. Because of necrosis, new vessels are usually attracted to the area. As the corneal ulcer heals, a permanent, gray, arc-shaped opacity remains, which may later become infiltrated with fat or hematogenous pigmentation. Corneal thinning is uncommon unless the catarrhal infiltrates recur, but in such cases may develop into a mild corneal ectasia.

Recurrent catarrhal corneal infiltrates may occur in front of the newly formed blood vessels, producing a picture of a wandering phlyctenule (fascicle) (see above) (Fig. 4–25).

A catarrhal infiltrate and ulceration occasionally develops during a lowgrade gonorrheal conjunctivitis, especially with inadequate antibiotic therapy. The infiltrate is similar to the staphylococcal variety. On the other hand, peripheral corneal ulcers are commonly found in a hyperacute gonorrheal conjunctivitis with copious discharge. In such instances, there is massive inflammatory infiltration of the peripheral cornea, which subsequently breaks down to form the peripheral ulcer. These ulcers are frequently infected (see below).

The catarrhal corneal ulcers resulting from coliform bacterial infections of the conjunctiva or lid margin probably arise from a hypersensitivity to the endotoxin produced by the infecting organism (Belmont et al., 1982). The infiltrate or ulcer is usually large and may extend circumferentially to form a ring-shaped infiltrate. In some instances the infiltrate occurs in the midperipheral cornea (Fig. 4–30).

Catarrhal corneal ulcers occur rarely with lymphogranuloma venereum conjunctivitis. The ulcer is narrow and is associated with an epaulet (a heavily vascularized thickened limbus). A catarrhal corneal infiltrate with regular pannus formation occurs rarely during actinomycotic infection of the canaliculus or conjunctiva. The canaliculitis is usually relatively silent.

Marginal Corneal Ulcers Arising from Direct Infection

Marginal corneal ulcers may result from direct bacterial, chlamydial, or viral infection of the corneal epithelium or stroma. These ulcers are less benign than catarrhal corneal ulcers and may lead to perforation. Corneal thinning is also more common. In such instances, the causative organisms are found on scrapings and cultures of the marginal ulcer.

Infected marginal corneal ulcers may occur during an episode of conjunctivitis of Morax, in which beta-hemolytic streptococci invade the peripheral cornea at the same time that they are producing a hyperacute conjunctivitis (see Chapter 6).

In the hyperacute conjunctivitis due to *Neisseria gonorrhoeae, N. meningitidis,* and *Corynebacterium diphtheriae,* the conjunctiva may become so chemotic as to overhang the corneal margin, thus entrapping polymorphonuclear leukocytes between the conjunctiva and the corneal epithelium. A breach in the corneal epithelium then occurs from the action of leukocytic enzymes. This allows the infecting organism to gain access to the stroma producing an infectious marginal corneal ulcer.

In trachoma, gray marginal infiltrates or yellow pustules occasionally develop central to an active pannus. The infiltrates are at first elevated but soon become flat and later may ulcerate. The infecting organism is found in the corneal epithelium but not in the stroma or the subepithelial infiltrate. Rarely, a ring-like gutter and eventually a ring ulcer are produced in trachoma. The ring-like ulcer extends circumferentially, attracting superficial vessels, but it is otherwise benign and indolent.

Vesicles of primary varicella occasionally involve the limbus, causing a marginal infiltrate or phlyctenule-like picture, often associated with an underlying sectoral iris atrophy (Fig. 4–31). In some instances the vesicular lesion develops in the peripheral cornea and then progresses to pustulation, descemetocele formation, and finally corneal perforation. Primary varicella may also produce a ring ulcer and disciform keratitis.

In herpes zoster ophthalmicus, marginal corneal infiltration and ulceration may develop in association with herpes zoster scleritis; in such an event, infiltration and ulceration occur (Fig. 4–32). In addition, the pseudodendrite of herpes zoster may occur in the peripheral corneal epithelium (see the section on central corneal ulcers).

Herpes simplex keratitis occasionally produces a peripheral corneal ulcer. In this case, the epithelial ulceration precedes corneal infiltration (Fig. 4–27), whereas in catarrhal corneal ulcers, the infiltration of the corneal stroma precedes epithelial ulceration. The herpetic epithelial lesion is linear or dendritic in character, or may appear as a small defect with irregular borders. Unlike herpes simplex infections of the central cornea, marginal herpes simplex corneal infections may not affect the corneal sensation. As in the central herpetic lesions, however, the patient notes minimal symptoms of foreign-body sensation and photophobia. The combination of slightly reduced corneal sensation and minimal photophobia in the presence of a peripheral ulcer or infiltrate is highly suggestive of marginal herpes simplex keratitis.

Phlyctenules

Phlyctenulosis represents a delayed hypersensitivity reaction in response to an endogenous (tubercular or coccidioidal) or an exogenous (tubercular or staphylococcal) antigen. It occurs most frequently in children 3 to 15 years of age and is most common in areas where malnutrition, crowding, and poor hygiene prevail.

Phlyctenules usually occur at the limbus, but may develop anywhere on the conjunctiva or cornea. The marginal phlyctenule does not have a lucid interval and produces neovascularization of the local peripheral cornea. In many instances it produces severe scarring of the cornea and decreased vision. The pannus that is produced is irregular (Fig. 4–33) and is readily differentiated from the pannus of trachoma. When the phlyctenule involves the cornea, and especially if it arises from a hypersensitivity to tuberculoprotein, severe photophobia, tearing, blepharospasm, and pain occur. Phlyctenules that arise from a hypersensitivity reaction to staphylococcal antigen are less symptomatic.

Conjunctival phlyctenules begin as erythematous infiltrated areas, which after 2 to 3 days develop a gray-white center (Fig. 4–34) representing early necrosis, and, if untreated, ulcerate and heal within 10 to 14 days. When the cornea is involved a scar is produced, whereas if the conjunctiva alone is involved no scarring occurs. Limbal phlyctenules characteristically straddle the limbus, affecting both cornea and conjunctiva (Figs. 4–35 A and B). As a limbal phlyctenule heals, a limbal-based triangular scar is produced from scarring of the corneal portion and complete resolution of the conjunctival portion. Recurrent corneal phlyctenules are uncommon.

Phlyctenules associated with tuberculosis respond very rapidly to treatment with topical glucocorticoids. Those associated with staphylococcal lid infections resolve only slowly with glucocorticoids, however, unless the bacterial infection is also treated.

Mooren's Ulcer (Chronic Serpiginous Ulcer)

Mooren's corneal ulcer is a chronic, progressive, relentlessly destructive ulceration that begins at the margin of the cornea and advances irregularly and progressively to involve the entire cornea. The ulcers are probably autoimmune in origin, and about one-third of them occur bilaterally (Fig. 4–36 A). The lesions begin as multiple gray or white infiltrates near the limbus which then spread, coalesce, and break down to form a shallow ulcer extending to about half of the depth of the stroma. Characteristically, there is no clear interval between the sclera and the ulcer, and the sclera is involved in the same necrotizing process. Centrally, there is a steep overhanging edge, and the edge gradually slopes upward peripherally to the scleral rim. The peripheral edge heals slowly and new vessel formation occurs (Fig. 4–36 B), whereas the central edge actively ulcerates. Iritis may accompany the ulceration. In older persons, corneal perforation is rare, while in younger patients, more than one-third of the cases perforate. The painful and relentless course is characteristic of Mooren's ulcer.

Peripheral Corneal Furrows or Ulcers Associated with Collagen-Vascular Diseases

A peripheral corneal furrow or ulcer may arise in association with a vasculitis and is therefore associated with collagen-vascular diseases such as rheumatoid arthritis (Fig. 4–37) (Pham, 1985), polyarteritis nodosa (Fig. 4–38), Wegener's midline granuloma, systemic lupus erythematosus and ulcerative colitis (Fig. 4–39). Except for polyarteritis nodosa, in which inflammation of the limbal area may be intense, minimal inflammatory signs are usually associated with the marginal thinning. In midline granuloma and Wegener's granulomatosis, a limbal granuloma usually occurs before the marginal furrow. A furrow frequently develops in an area contiguous to a necrotizing scleritis or episcleritis resulting from collagen diseases.

Marginal Furrows and Ring Furrows or Ring Ulcers

Ring ulcers may develop from a hypersensitivity reaction or a vasculitis and are therefore usually associated with an infection or a systemic disease. Ring ulcers and ring infiltrates may also arise when multiple marginal catarrhal ulcers or corneal infiltrates become confluent.

A ring abscess, beginning as a ring infiltrate or from confluence of discrete marginal infiltrates, may occur in endophthalmitis or panophthalmitis. A lucid interval frequently separates the limbus from the yellow-appearing ring abscess. In the early course of ring abscess development the central cornea is clear, but as it progresses the central cornea becomes cloudy and the corneal epithelium is lost. The epithelium over the ring abscess breaks down producing a ring ulcer as the endophthalmitis progresses into frank panophthalmitis. In some instances, late in the disease process, the cornea sloughs en bloc.

Ring ulcers may also result from direct bacterial invasion of the cornea, such as by *Neisseria gonorrhoeae, N. meningitidis,* and *Corynebacterium diphtheriae* (see the section on marginal corneal ulcers).

Marginal Corneal Changes Associated with Scleritis

Peripheral corneal changes frequently develop in areas contiguous to a scleritis (Fig. 4–40). The corneal changes are therefore usually much more extensive in cases of diffuse scleritis than in nodular scleritis (see Chapter 5).

Terrien's Marginal Degeneration

Terrien's marginal degeneration is relatively rare and occurs bilaterally, although one eye may be involved earlier and be much more advanced than the other. It occurs most frequently in males and appears to have a bimodal onset. In the younger age groups (10 to 40 years) the patient frequently notes irritation, foreign-body sensation, redness and tearing during stages of activity, whereas in the older age group (over 40 years) the condition is usually asymptomatic.

Terrien's marginal degeneration begins superiorly (Fig. 4–41), then progresses to involve the superior temporal area. The degeneration gradually extends circumferentially over a period of 10 to 20 years to involve the entire peripheral cornea (Fig. 4–42). The degenerative process may deepen, and in about one-third of cases a traumatic or spontaneous perforation occurs. The prognosis in spite of perforation is usually good. Terrien's marginal degeneration is manifested by opacification, vascularization, and thinning of the peripheral cornea. As the condition progresses, vascularization and ectasia may occur along with increasing astigmatism resulting from corneal flattening.

Keratitis Marginalis Superficialis (Fuchs')

Keratitis marginalis superficialis is a rare disease occurring during the middle years of life. The ulceration begins peripherally and remains superficial; it spreads circumferentially and toward the central cornea (but does not reach the center of the cornea) as the disease progresses. The edge of the ulcer is not undermined, and the lesion is demarcated from the central cornea by a sinuous gray line. As the ulcer heals, the conjunctiva is drawn over the cornea to form a pseudopterygium (Fig. 4–43). The peripheral ulcer does not advance uniformly, and periods of remissions and relapses occur during the many years of progression. The patient experiences no pain but notes moderate symptoms of irritation.

Senile Marginal Atrophy of the Cornea (Senile Marginal Ectasia)

In rare instances, an arcus senilis may become quite wide and be associated with a gutter-shaped depression. Later, the remaining cornea within the depression may become ectatic. The disease is usually benign and asymptomatic, except for producing changes in the refractive error.

Pellucid Degeneration

Pellucid degeneration is characterized by thinning of the inferior peripheral cornea, without limbal involvement. There is no neovascularization or deposition of lipid.

Dellen

Dellen are peripheral, saucer-shaped excavations of the cornea usually occuring in association with elevation of the adjacent conjunctiva, such as occurs following muscle, glaucoma, or cataract surgery. A dellen may also be associated with a pterygium, pinguecula, limbal tumor, or nodular episcleritis, or may develop after the use of an anesthetic.

Dellen result from desiccation of the corneal epithelium resulting from improper lid surfacing. The eyelid's normal movement over the surface of the cornea is blocked by the elevated conjunctiva, which prevents the mixing of the mucous and aqueous in the tear film and allows desiccation to occur in the area adjacent to the elevation. Obliteration of the limbal capillaries has also been suggested as a cause of dellen.

Interstitial Keratitis

Interstitial keratitis is defined as an inflammation of the corneal stroma without evidence of primary involvement of the epithelial or endothelial surfaces. In most instances, it represents an immune complex phenomenon from antigens associated with *Treponema pallidum, Mycobacterium tuberculosis,* and *M. leprae.* Interstitial keratitis also occurs in Cogan's syndrome, the etiology of which is unknown.

Syphilitic Interstitial Keratitis

Syphilitic interstitial keratitis causes an intense inflammatory reaction, most marked in the posterior stroma. It usually involves the entire cornea, although in rare cases it is sectoral in type. The interstitial keratitis is of sudden onset, becoming "full-blown" within one to three weeks; the symptoms of photophobia, pain, tearing, and pericorneal injection, suggesting early ciliary body involvement, are severe. Early in the course of the inflammation, the corneal endothelium appears hazy and there are a few keratic precipitates (KPs). Grayish maculae (more marked in the peripheral cornea but distributed irregularly throughout the cornea) develop, increase in size, and coalesce. Large folds in Descemet's membrane serve as evidence of marked corneal edema. The corneal epithelium becomes markedly cloudy, and an iritis of variable intensity invariably occurs.

As the syphilitic interstitial keratitis progresses, neovascularization of the deep corneal stroma develops and advances toward the gray maculae (Fig. 4–44). As the vessels approach the maculae, the infiltrates extend further toward the center of the cornea. Epaulets, which appear as crescent-shaped swellings of engorged vessels at the edges of the cornea, and salmon patches, the color of which is produced by the advancing vessels and the overlying corneal infiltrate, are commonly seen in syphilitic interstitial keratitis. As the inflammation resolves, the symptoms abate rapidly and the inflammatory process clears first at the periphery. The maculae may completely disappear, but the newly formed blood vessels are permanent and appear as "ghost vessels" lying at the level of Descemet's membrane.

Syphilitic interstitial keratitis is seen most frequently in congenital syphilis, but occasionally occurs in acquired syphilis. Other stigmata of congenital syphilis include frontal bossing, saddle nose, high arched palate, dacryocystitis, semilunar notching of the incisors (Hutchinson's teeth), a nerve-type deafness, and synovitis of the knee joints (Clutton's joints).

Tuberculous Interstitial Keratitis

The interstitial keratitis from tuberculosis is less severe in intensity than syphilitic interstitial keratitis and is usually sectoral in type (Fig. 4–45). Moreover, the neovascularization usually occurs in mid to deep stroma instead of at the level of Descement's membrane.

Interstitial Keratitis Due to Hansen's Disease

Interstitial keratitis due to Hansen's disease may occur in the deep cornea, as in syphilitic interstitial keratitis, or may be more superficial. The deep interstitial keratitis begins in the temporal quadrant and may be associated with a mild neovascularization, although this is not a prominent feature of the disease. The superficial keratitis causes corneal neovascularization only late in the disease (Fig. 4–46), and begins as fine white dots surrounded by grayish maculae.

Interstitial Keratitis Due to Cogan's Syndrome

Cogan's syndrome represents a nonsyphilitic interstitial keratitis with many of the features of syphilitic interstitial keratitis; its etiology is unknown. Moreover, it is commonly associated with vestibuloauditory symptoms (McDonald et al., 1985). The corneal changes begin as faint subepithelial nummular lesions at the periphery of the cornea, which progress to involve the deep stromal areas (Cobo and Haynes, 1984).

Endotheliitis

Endotheliitis (inflammation of the endothelium) occurs in herpes simplex and herpes zoster infections of the cornea (Maudgal et al., 1980; Reijo et al., 1983). It represents an immune reaction against viral-infected endothelial cells. The inflammation can be recognized by the presence of keratic precipitates which are confined to the area of endothelial damage (Sundmacher, 1983); on specular microscopy, nonreflecting black areas are seen within the endothelium (Vannas and Ahonen, 1981; Reijo et al., 1983).

Central Corneal Ulcers

Regardless of the site of inoculation of organisms into the central stroma, most central corneal ulcers progress toward the center of the cornea, away from the vascularized limbus. The infection usually causes loss of epithelium and destruction of stroma and may cause marked loss of vision. Central corneal ulcers were formerly called hypopyon corneal ulcers because of a tendency for inflammatory cells to settle out as a layer of pus in the anterior chamber during the suppurative process in the corneal stroma.

As a general rule, a thorough laboratory study of scrapings and cultures of all central corneal ulcers should be made prior to treatment, unless the ulcer is obviously viral in nature.

Viral Corneal Ulcers

Herpes Simplex Keratitis

Herpes simplex viruses are the major cause of corneal ulcers in the United States. Because of their epithelial tropism, herpes simplex viruses produce mainly epithelial ulcers, unless the patient's defense mechanisms have been compromised (as with the use of topical glucocorticoids), in which case the infection may involve the stroma. Herpes simplex keratitis usually causes minimal symptoms of pain, irritation, and photophobia because of the loss of corneal sensation.

A dendritic epithelial lesion (a linear branching lesion, like the branches in a tree) that has terminal bulbs (Fig. 4–47) should be considered almost pathognomonic for herpes simplex infection, especially when corneal sensation is absent or markedly reduced. Scrapings of the edge of the epithelial lesion reveal multinucleated giant cells (Fig. 4–48), which further substantiates the diagnosis.

Geographic or ameboid ulcers (large angulated epithelial defects) (Fig. 4–49) are also characteristic of herpes simplex infections, especially if the corneal sensation is absent. Other corneal manifestations of herpes simplex keratitis include a disciform keratitis (a round opacity in the superficial corneal stroma) (Fig. 4–50), focal avascular interstitial keratitis (coin-shaped stromal opacities without evidence of corneal neovascularization), an indolent hypopyon corneal ulcer (often distinguished by the presence of a small hemorrhage within the hypopyon) (Fig. 4–51), and medium white keratic precipitates located underneath the area of infiltration in the cornea.

Herpes Zoster Ophthalmicus

The cornea is frequently involved in ophthalmic zoster. The epithelial lesions may be fine or blotchy, or may appear as a pseudodendrite (an elevated linear epithelial defect with minimal branching and no terminal bulbs). As in herpes simplex keratitis, the corneal sensation is absent, and scraping of the epithelial defect reveals multinucleated giant cells (Fig. 4–48).

Stromal involvement in herpes zoster often produces nummular opacities, in which multiple round, slightly irregular opacities develop within the stroma, or it may produce a disciform keratitis similar to that seen in herpes simplex keratitis (Figs. 4–52 A and B). Marked neovascularization with deposition of lipid-like material in the corneal stroma (Fig. 4–53) may also occur in herpes zoster. Epithelial lesions are also frequently seen in other viral infections such as adenoviral conjunctivitis, acute hemorrhagic conjunctivitis, and the viral exanthema (see the sections on epithelial keratitis and keratopathy).

Bacterial Corneal Ulcers

Although *Streptococcus pneumoniae* (Fig. 4–54 A) was formerly the major cause of bacterial corneal ulcers, opportunistic organisms such as *Streptococcus viridans* (Fig. 4–55 A) and *Staphylococcus epidermidis* (Fig. 4–56 A) are now the most frequent causes of bacterial corneal ulcers (Ostler et al., 1976). The organisms are usually readily found on scraping of the corneal ulcer (Figs. 4–54 B, 4–55 B, 4–56 B), unless treatment has already been initiated. Other common bacterial organisms found in central corneal ulcers include *Pseudomonas aeruginosa* (Figs. 4–57 A and B), *Moraxella* spp., *Staphylococcus aureus* (Figs. 4–58 A and B), and *Nocardia* spp. (Figs. 4–59 A and B). Mixed bacterial corneal ulcers also occur, and there is a group of bacterial corneal ulcers caused by organisms such as the *Mycobacterium fortuitum/cheloni* complex (Meisler et al., 1982; Newman et al., 1984). As a general rule, bacterial corneal ulcers caused by the more virulent organisms progress rapidly and provoke greater inflammatory reactions, including hypopyon formation, whereas corneal ulcers caused by opportunistic organisms tend to be more indolent and spread superficially. Although a few bacterial corneal ulcers have some distinguishing clinical features, a clinical impression should not be relied upon to determine treatment of a central corneal ulcer.

Pneumococcal Corneal Ulcers

Pneumococcal corneal ulcers may be quite distinctive: a grayish infiltrate develops rapidly at the area of inoculation of the pneumococcal organism into the stroma (Fig. 4–54A), whereas the surrounding cornea is usually clear. The infiltrate rapidly "breaks down" into an ulcer and at the same time spreads rapidly and irregularly toward the center of the cornea. The advancing border is active while the trailing edge shows signs of healing. This phenomenon has led to the term serpiginous corneal ulcer. A scraping of the advancing edge reveals Gram-positive diplococci, which are usually lancet-shaped and may show evidence of capsule formation (Fig. 4–54B).

Moraxella Corneal Ulcers

Moraxella corneal ulcers occur most frequently in alcoholics, diabetics, or patients who are otherwise immunosuppressed (Fedukowicz and Horwich, 1953). They are usually indolent and progress toward the deep stroma. The ulcer is usually found in the inferior cornea (Fig. 4–60A), and in only about one-half of the cases is a hypopyon noted. Scraping reveals very large, square-ended, Gram-negative diplobacilli (Fig. 4–60B).

Pseudomonas Corneal Ulcers

The proteolytic enzymes produced by *Pseudomonas* usually cause the corneal ulcer to be superficial and round in shape (Fig. 4–57A). The corneal infection develops and progresses rapidly, and early in the course of the infection, severe pain is a common symptom.

Nocardial Corneal Ulcers

Nocardial corneal ulcers are indolent ulcers in which the base of the ulcer frequently has a "cracked windshield" appearance (Fig. 4–59A). A hypopyon is produced in about one-half of cases. Scraping of the ulcer reveals Gram-positive filamentous organisms (Fig. 4–59B).

Fungal Corneal Ulcers

Most fungi that infect the cornea are opportunistic and cause corneal ulcers as a result of previous suppression of the cornea's defense mechanisms (Thygeson and Okumoto, 1974), or because the number of organisms inoculated is so large that defense mechanisms of the cornea are overwhelmed. The principal causes of fungal corneal infections include *Candida* spp. (Figs. 4–61 A and B), *Aspergillus* spp. (Figs. 4–62 A and B), and *Fusarium* spp. (Figs. 4–63 A and B). Other fungi, including *Penicillium* spp., *Acremonium (Cephalosporium)* spp., *Helminthosporium* (Figs. 4–64 A and B), and *Alternaria* spp., are occasional causes of fungal corneal ulcers.

The filamentous fungi usually produce indolent corneal ulcers with features suggesting a fungal etiology. These include severe inflammation, satellite lesions (infiltrates in the cornea that are separate from the major focus of infiltration), fuzzy or hyphate edges of the infiltrates, a tendency for the infiltrate to be elevated above the surface of the surrounding cornea because of stromal edema, the presence of an endothelial plaque underlying the infiltrate or ulcer, and an immune ring (Fig. 4–65).

Candidal corneal ulcers may resemble either opportunistic bacterial corneal ulcers or fungal corneal ulcers caused by the filamentous fungi (see above).

Parasitic Corneal Ulcers

Parasitic corneal ulcers are uncommon and occur from the free-living opportunistic parasitic *Acanthamoeba* spp. (Samples et al., 1984). The corneal ulcer is indolent and has many of the features of a corneal ulcer caused by the filamentous fungi.

Elevated Corneal Lesions

Except for pterygia (see Chapter 3), elevated corneal lesions are uncommon and usually represent leukoplakia or Salzmann's nodular degeneration of the cornea.

Leukoplakia (Conjunctival Intraepithelial Neoplasia)

Conjunctival intraepithelial and conjunctival squamous cell carcinomas may affect the contiguous area of the cornea. The lesions usually develop in the interpalpebral area of the conjunctiva at or near the limbus. They appear thickened, white, or gelatinous, and typically have fronds of blood vessels that appear to grow perpendicular to the surface of the lesions (Fig. 4–66) (Waring et al., 1984). Leukoplakia occurs more frequently in older patients.

Salzmann's Nodular Degeneration

Salzmann's nodules appear as elevated bluish-gray

nodules (Fig. 4–67) (Vannas et al., 1975). They usually develop near corneal scars and are more commonly found in women. Conditions with which they are associated include pterygia, trachoma, phlyctenulosis, vernal keratoconjunctivitis, and other diseases that cause corneal scarring.

Corneal Granulomas

A corneal granuloma is exceedingly rare, although the authors have seen several following penetrating corneal lacerations (Fig. 4–68) and one following contact lens wear. The lesion is elevated, vascularized, and "fleshy" in appearance.

Miscellaneous Corneal Involvement

Other forms of corneal involvement include corneal dystrophies and corneal degenerations. Corneal dystrophies differ from corneal degenerations by the presence of a hereditary pattern, a tendency to be bilateral, the absence of corneal neovascularization, preferential involvement of the central cornea, and a symmetrical appearance.

Corneal Dystrophies

The corneal dystrophies discussed here are anterior membrane, Reis-Buckler's, granular, lattice, macular, posterior polymorphic, and Fuchs' endothelial dystrophies.

Anterior Membrane Dystrophies

Many names are used for anterior membrane dystrophy; these include Cogan's microcystic epithelial dystrophy, map-dot-fingerprint dystrophy, and dystrophic recurrent erosion.

Anterior membrane dystrophy is commonly associated with recurrent erosions, in which the patient complains of a sudden onset of pain, tearing, and photophobia (see the section on recurrent epithelial erosions). It occurs most commonly in women over the age of 30 years. The lesions occur in various forms (maps, dots, and fingerprints) in the subepithelial area of the central or paracentral area of the cornea. The lesions consist of fine blebs or gray dots, flat opacities that are variable in size and gray in color (maps), grossly visible cysts, and refractile lines (fingerprints) (Fig. 4–69). The lesions usually occur in combination and it is thought that dots do not occur without the presence of maps.

Reis-Buckler's Dystrophy

Reis-Buckler's dystrophy arises during the first decade of life and is associated with recurrent painful corneal erosions that persist until about the fourth decade of life, at which time the recurrent erosions are less frequent and are accompanied by less pain. In this dystrophy, lesions in the central cornea appear as reticular blue-white opacities which may be grouped or isolated and have a ring, crescentic, or geographic shape. The cornea appears like frosted glass. The lesions spare the peripheral cornea, and the most dense opacities are located in the midperiphery.

Stromal Dystrophies

The major stromal dystrophies are granular dystrophy, with an autosomal dominant hereditary pattern; lattice dystrophy, with an autosomal dominant hereditary pattern but a low level of penetrance; and macular dystrophy, with an autosomal recessive hereditary pattern.

Granular Dystrophy. Granular dystrophy occurs in young people, often beginning during the first decade of life. The lesions are white and have a bread-crumb appearance (Fig. 4–70); the peripheral cornea remains clear, although the central lesions enlarge and gradually coalesce.

Lattice Dystrophy. Lattice dystrophy is characterized by the presence of small refractile lines (Fig. 4–71), white dots, and a faint central haze in the anterior stroma. The refractile lines slowly enlarge, thicken, and become radially oriented. In some instances the refractile lines may be seen only by retro-illumination (Sturrock, 1983), and often resemble ropes. As the dystrophy progresses, the stroma between the lesions becomes hazy, which causes a marked decrease in vision. Frequently, recurrent erosions occur during the first decades of life.

Macular Dystrophy. Macular dystrophy affects the anterior layers of the central cornea. Diffuse gray-white spots with indistinct edges develop, and, by the third decade of life, diffuse stromal opacities are found which extend to the deep stroma and eventually to the endothelium, where guttate changes are noted. Descement's membrane eventually becomes opacified.

Posterior Corneal Dystrophies

The major dystrophies that primarily involve the posterior cornea are posterior polymorphous dystrophy and Fuchs' epithelial-endothelial dystrophy.

Posterior Polymorphous Dystrophy. Posterior polymorphous dystrophy is inherited as an autosomal dominant trait. The lesions are subtle and easily missed; they appear as small, discrete, round vesicles surrounded by a gray opacity. They occur in the posterior stroma, usually immediately anterior to Descemet's membrane. Gray opacities with minimal or no evidence of vesicle formation may also be found.

Fuchs' Epithelial-Endothelial Dystrophy. Although Fuchs' epithelial-endothelial dystrophy occurs bilaterally, it is often asymmetric, much more advanced in one eye than the other. The endothelial cell loss resembles corneal guttata. Pigment dusting of the corneal endothelium can usually be seen. Descemet's membrane appears thickened and somewhat opaque. Stromal edema followed by epithelial edema gradually develops and appears at first like epithelial bedewing, but large bullae later develop (Fig. 4–72).

Corneal Edema Due to Damaged Endothelium

Although this type of corneal change is usually not dystrophic in nature, it is included here because the corneal changes are due to endothelial damage such as occurs in endothelial dystrophies. The corneal opacity usually involves the entire cornea. It may be found in hereditary corneal edema, infantile glaucoma, or congenital rubella (de Luise et al., 1983), or following endothelial trauma such as from intraocular surgery.

Corneal Degenerations

Corneal degenerations are usually bilateral but may be unilateral. There is no definite inheritance pattern, and corneal neovascularization commonly occurs. The corneal degenerations include band keratopathy, climatic droplet degeneration, keratoconus, keratoglobus, and pellucid marginal degeneration.

Band Keratopathy

Calcific band keratopathy typically involves the interpalpebral area of the cornea. It appears as a superficial grayish opacity interspersed with numerous round, clear zones of varying diameter. At onset the band keratopathy involves the peripheral cornea and is separated from the limbus by a thin clear zone (Fig. 4–73). Later, as the condition progresses, the band keratopathy spreads to the central cornea. The lesion is superficial, involving Bowman's layer and the basement membrane of the corneal epithelium. Its location helps to distinguish it from calcareous degeneration of the cornea, which involves both superficial and deep layers of the cornea.

Climatic Droplet (Spheroidal) Degeneration

Climatic droplet degeneration preferentially involves the interpalpebral fissure area of the cornea. It consists of whitish to yellow almost oil-like droplets that develop subepithelially and later coalesce to form a yellowish-gray subepithelial band (Fig. 4–74). The yellow droplets may enlarge and even cause the corneal epithelium to be elevated. The lesion usually begins peripherally and progresses to involve the central corneal area. The conditions probably results from excessive exposure to ultraviolet light (Johnson, 1981; Johnson et al., 1984; Taylor, 1980).

Keratoconus

Keratoconus is often classified as a corneal dystrophy, especially because it may have a dominant or recessive inheritance pattern. It is characterized by thinning of the cornea and the development of a cone with its apex immediately inferior and lateral to the center of the cornea (Fig. 4–75). Vertical striae in the deep stroma, increased prominence of corneal nerves, and an iron ring at the base of the cone are also commonly found. Ruptures of Descemet's membrane and Bowman's membrane may occur (Krachmer et al., 1984).

Keratoglobus

Keratoglobus is similar to keratoconus, except that the ectasia is more extensive and involves the entire cornea (Krachmer et al., 1984).

Pellucid Marginal Degeneration

Pellucid marginal degeneration is a degenerative change in which corneal thinning is a prominent feature. The thinning occurs in the inferior cornea and extends almost to the limbus, but a narrow strip of normal cornea separates the thinned area from the limbus. It is not associated with neovascularization or lipid deposition, and the corneal sensation remains normal. In rare instances, pellucid marginal degeneration may be associated with a keratoconus.

References

Ahmad, A, Hogan, M, Wood, I, and Ostler, HB: Climatic droplet keratopathy in a 16-year-old boy. *Arch. Ophthalmol.* 95: 149–151, 1977.

Belmont, JB, Ostler, HB, Dawson, CR, Schwab, I, and Dulay, D: Noninfectious ring-shaped keratitis associated with *Pseudomonas aeruginosa. Am. J. Ophthalmol.* 93: 338–341, 1982.

Cobo, LM, and Haynes, BF: Early corneal findings in Cogan's syndrome. *Ophthalmology* 91: 903–907, 1984.

de Luise, VP, Cobo, LM, and Chandler, D: Persistent corneal edema in the congenital rubella syndrome. *Ophthalmology* 90: 835–839, 1983.

Fedukowicz, H, and Horwich, H: The Gram-negative diplobacillus in hypopyon keratitis. *Arch. Ophthalmol.* 49: 202–205, 1953.

Johnson, GJ: Aetiology of spheroidal degeneration of the cornea in Labrador. *Br. J. Ophthalmol.* 65: 270–283, 1981.

Johnson, GJ, Green, JS, Paterson, GD, and Perkins, ES: Survey of ophthalmic conditions in a Labrador community. II. Ocular disease. *Can. J. Ophthalmol.* 19: 224–233, 1984.

Krachmer, JH, Feder, RS, and Belin, MW: Keratoconus and related noninflammatory corneal thinning disorders. *Surv. Ophthalmol.* 28: 293–322, 1984.

Lemp, MA, and Gold, JB: An in vivo study of the corneal surface in keratoconjunctivitis sicca. *Trans. Ophthalmol. Soc. UK* 104: 436–438, 1985.

Liesegang, TJ: Corneal complications from herpes zoster ophthalmicus. *Ophthalmology* 92: 316–324, 1985.

Mark, DB, and McCulley, JB: Reiter's keratitis. *Arch. Ophthalmol.* 100: 781–784, 1982.

Maudgal, PC, Misotten, L, DeClergq, E, and Descamps, J: Varicella-zoster virus in the human corneal endothelium: A case report. *Bull. Soc. Belge Ophtalmol.* 190: 71–86, 1980.

McDonald, TJ, Volertsen, RS, and Younge, BR: Cogan's syndrome: Audiovestibular involvement and prognosis in 18 patients. *Laryngoscope* 95: 650–654, 1985.

Meisler, DM, Friedlaender, MH, and Okumoto, M: *Mycobacterium chelonei* keratitis. *Am. J. Ophthalmol.* 94: 398–401, 1982.

Messer, G, Isakow, I, Dabush, S, and Romem, M: Posttraumatic recurrent epithelial erosion. 2. Ultrastructural findings in epithelium and stroma. *Metab. Pediatr. Syst. Ophthalmol.* 7: 59–66, 1983.

Newman, PE, Goodman, RA, Waring, GO III, Finton, RJ, Wilson, LA, Wright, J, and Cavanagh, HD: A cluster of cases of *Mycobacterium chelonei* keratitis associated with outpatient office procedures. *Am. J. Ophthalmol.* 97: 344–348, 1984.

Ostler, HB, Okumoto, M, and Wilkey, C: The changing pattern of the etiology of central bacterial corneal (hypopyon) ulcers. *Trans. Pac. Coast Ophthalmol. Soc.* 57: 235–241, 1976.

Pham, DT: Keratomalacia perforans, klinische und pathohistologische befunde. *Klin. Monatsbl. Augenheilkd.* 187: 290–292, 1985.

Reijo, A, Antti, V, and Jukka, M: Endothelial cell loss in herpes zoster keratoiritis. *Br. J. Ophthalmol.* 67: 751–754, 1983.

Samples, JR, Binder, PS, Luibel, FS, Font, RL, Visvesvara, GS, and Peter, CR: Acanthamoeba keratitis possibly acquired from a hot tub. *Arch. Ophthalmol.* 102: 707–710, 1984.

Shoch, DE, Stock, EL, and Schwartz, AE: Stromal keratitis complicating anterior membrane dystrophy. *Am. J. Ophthalmol.* 100: 199–201, 1985.

Sturrock, GD: Lattice corneal dystrophy: A source of confusion. *Br. J. Ophthalmol.* 67: 629–634, 1983.

Sundmacher, R: Endotheliitis cornea. Begriffsbestimmung und klinisch abgrenzung. *Klin. Monatsbl. Augenheilkd.* 184: 163–167, 1983.

Taylor, HR: Aetiology of climatic droplet keratopathy and pterygium. *Br. J. Ophthalmol.* 64: 154–163, 1980.

Thygeson, P, and Okumoto, M: Keratomycosis, a preventable disease. *Trans. Am. Acad. Ophthalmol. Otolaryngol.* 78: 433–439, 1974.

Tullo, AB, Easty, DL, Shimeld, C, Stirling, PE, and Darville, JM: Isolation of herpes simplex virus from corneal discs of patients with chronic stromal keratitis. *Trans. Ophthalmol. Soc. UK* 104: 159–165, 1985.

Valenton, MJ: Deep stromal involvement in Dimmer's nummular keratitis. *Am. J. Ophthalmol.* 78: 897–902, 1974.

Vannas, A, and Ahonen, R: Herpetic endothelial keratitis. A case report. *Acta Ophthalmol.* 59: 296–301, 1981.

Vannas, A, Hogan, MJ, and Wood, I: Salzmann's nodular degeneration of the cornea. *Am. J. Ophthalmol.* 79: 211–219, 1975.

Waring, GO III, Roth, AM, and Ekins, MB: Clinical and pathologic description of 17 cases of corneal intraepithelial neoplasia. *Am. J. Ophthalmol.* 97: 547–559, 1984.

Weene, LE: Recurrent corneal erosion after trauma: A statistical study. *Ann. Ophthalmol.* 17: 521–522, 1985.

Zaidman, GW, Geeraets, R, Paylor, RR, and Ferry, AP: The histopathology of filamentary keratitis. *Arch. Ophthalmol.* 103: 1178–1181, 1985.

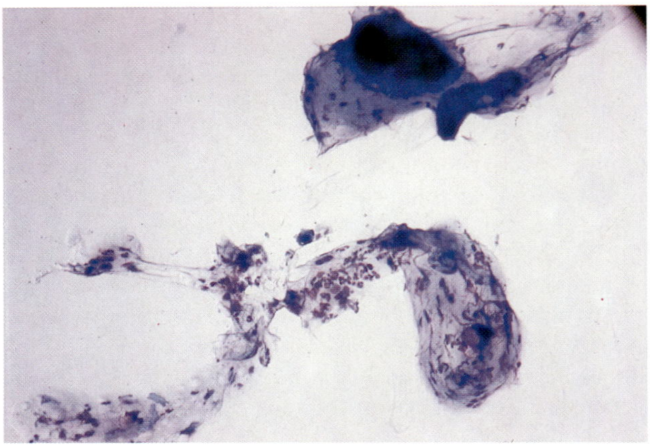

4–1 Biopsy of corneal epithelial filament. Corneal filaments may be made up of epithelium or mucus. An epithelial filament, such as is seen in this scraping, represents a scroll of epithelium that is attached to the corneal epithelium at one end and is rolled up like a scroll at the other end. It is usually quite long. Mucoid filaments, on the other hand, tend to be shorter and more numerous. In mucoid filaments, epithelial cells are found only at the area where the filament was attached to the epithelium. Giemsa stain, × 100.

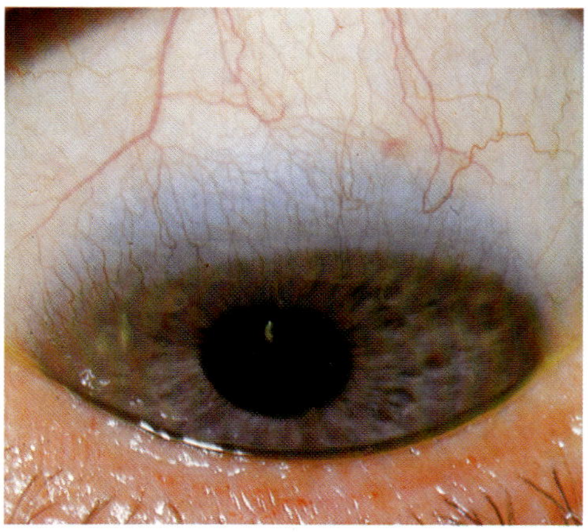

4–2 Epithelial filaments in superior limbic keratoconjunctivitis. The epithelial filaments found in superior limbic keratoconjunctivitis occur in the superior third of the cornea. The cornea had been stained with fluorescein in this patient, and minimal injection was present in the superior limbal area.

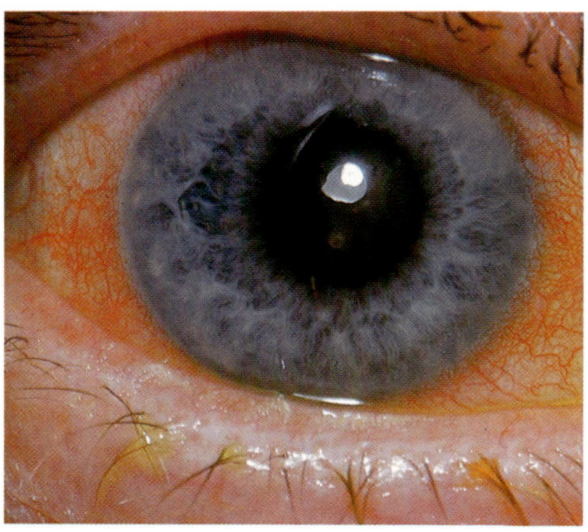

4–3 Mucoid filaments in keratoconjunctivitis sicca. Mucoid filaments are only loosely attached to the corneal epithelium. The filaments in this patient are visible immediately adjacent to and over the pupillary area. Injection of the conjunctiva is also evident. An accelerated cell loss may be the cause of the filaments in keratoconjunctivitis sicca (Lemp and Gold, 1985). Histologically, scattered groups of inflammatory cells and fibroblasts can be found immediately beneath the basal epithelium; these cells may damage the epithelium, thus giving rise to the filaments (Zaidman et al., 1985).

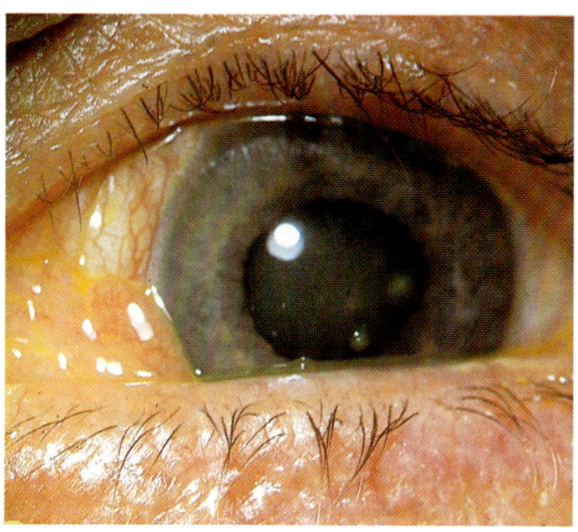

4–4 Filaments in herpes simplex keratitis. Transitory filaments as noted in this patient may occur in herpes simplex keratitis. They are short and quite firmly attached to the cornea. Within days, stellate or dendritic figures usually develop in the same location. This man had been followed for several years for herpes simplex keratitis, and complained of a foreign-body sensation at the time this photograph was taken, although the corneal sensation was absent.

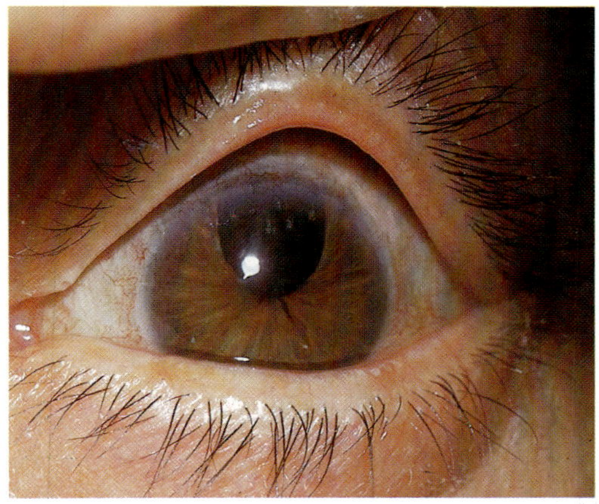

4–5 Filamentary keratitis from prolonged ptosis which developed following cataract extraction. A filamentary keratitis may occur in ptosis or following prolonged occlusion of the eye. The filaments occur in the area covered by the eyelid, such as in this patient who developed ptosis following a cataract extraction six weeks previously. Multiple filaments are present in the superior cornea. Filaments in such cases may develop from failure of the lid to properly wipe the corneal surface like a knife blade, which in turn allows the corneal epithelial cells to mature at different rates of growth, thus allowing scrolls of epithelial tags to develop.

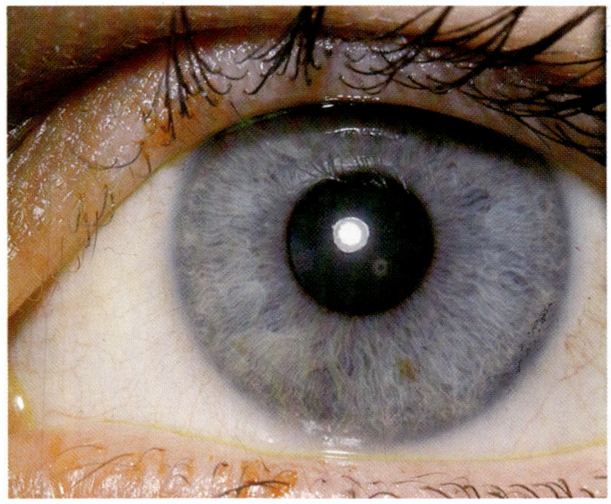

4–6 Fine punctate epithelial erosions occurring over most of the cornea in staphylococcal blepharitis. Fine or punctate epithelial erosions are slightly depressed areas in the surface of the cornea that represent areas of premature epithelial desquamation. These areas stain readily with vital dyes such as fluorescein. The epithelial erosions shown in this photograph are most readily visible in the central area of the cornea because of the black background of the pupil. The erosions are due to the toxic action of the staphylococcal dermatonecrotoxin. The patient usually complains of a foreign-body sensation and/or pain upon awakening.

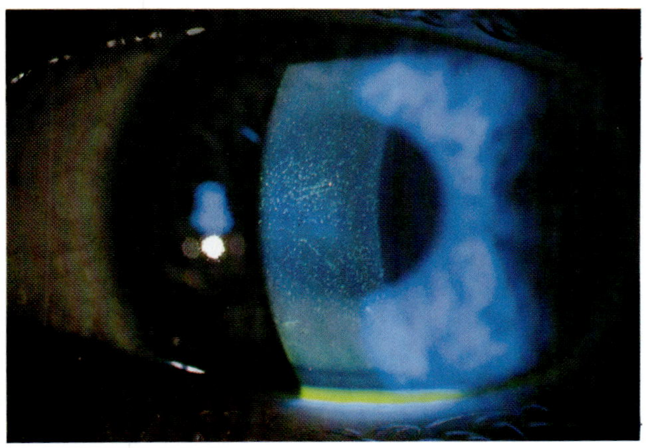

4–7 Fine to medium-sized corneal erosions occurring in familial hypesthesia. This patient was seen for persistent bilateral medium-sized corneal erosions, most marked in the exposure area but involving most of the cornea. Both he and his mother had bilateral corneal hypesthesia.

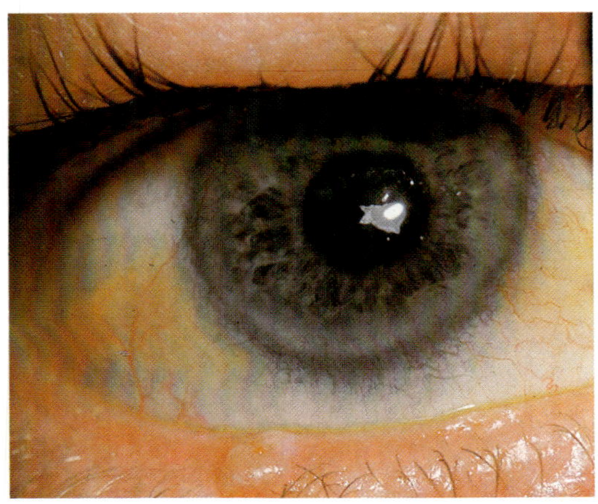

4–8 Medium-sized epithelial erosions due to a molluscum contagiosum nodule of the lid margin. A molluscum contagiosum nodule of the lid margin may produce epithelial erosions involving either the superior third of the cornea or the entire cornea, such as is evident in this 38-year-old female. The erosions are probably due to a toxic action of the products produced by the virus within the epithelium of the skin. The molluscum nodule is evident on the margin of the lower eyelid. A corneal pannus extending from the 9:00 to 4:00 area is also evident and resulted from the toxic action of the molluscum.

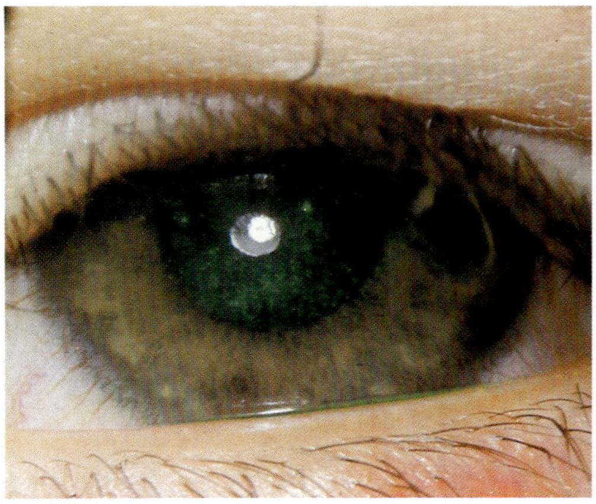

4–9 Coarse epithelial erosions due to keratoconjunctivitis sicca. This 57-year-old female had medium to coarse epithelial erosions from keratoconjunctivitis sicca. The erosions are evident over the pupil. The corneal epithelium is particularly susceptible to drying in keratoconjunctivitis sicca because it normally derives part of its nutritional and oxygen requirements from the tear film.

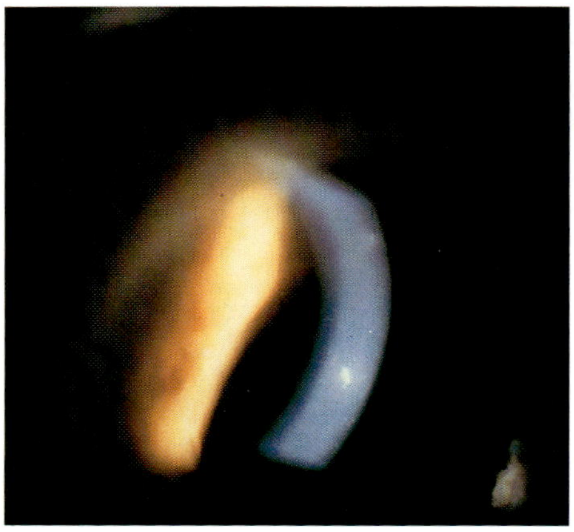

4–10 Macropunctate medium to coarse epithelial erosions in epidemic keratoconjunctivitis. An epithelial keratitis develops early during an infection of epidemic keratoconjunctivitis. The epithelial involvement is medium to coarse, as is evident in this patient who had developed epidemic keratoconjunctivitis seven days earlier.

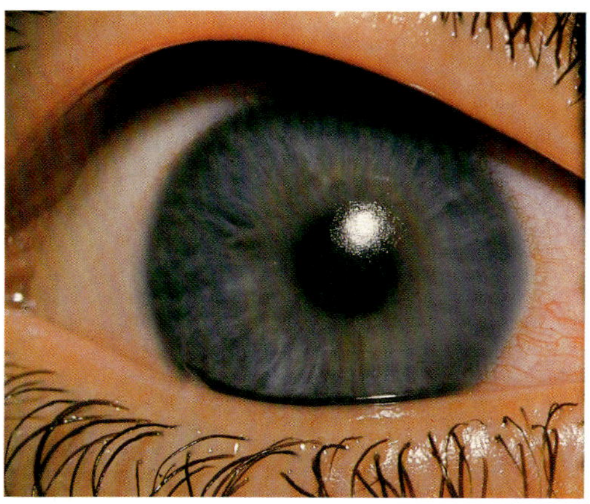

4–11 Syncytium due to vernal keratoconjunctivitis. The superior third of the corneal epithelium is frequently involved in vernal keratoconjunctivitis. When the corneal epithelium is first involved, a syncytium of epithelial cells becomes evident and resembles flour dusted on the surface of the cornea. Later, the same epithelial cells slough, producing an oval ulcer. In this 14-year-old male, a syncytium can be seen in the area of the pupil. Two days later an oval ulcer developed that involved the central cornea. Hyperemia of the bulbar conjunctiva and some mucoid discharge are evident.

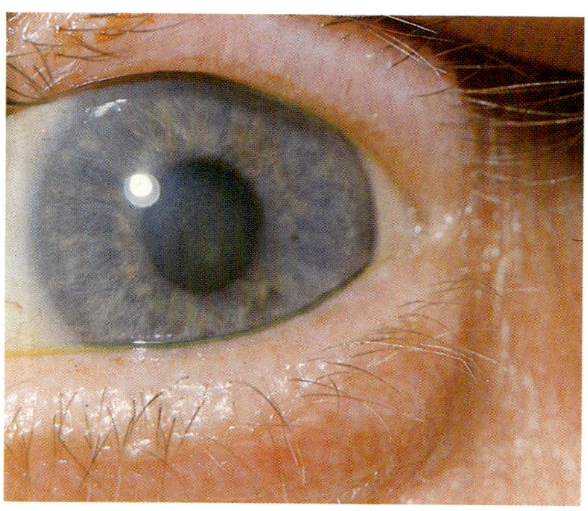

4–12 Medium-sized epithelial keratopathy of the exposure area of the cornea due to keratoconjunctivitis sicca. An epithelial keratopathy (keratitis) is characterized by the presence of tiny white opaque areas, which represent degenerating epithelial cells. The tiny opaque areas take up rose bengal in preference to fluorescein, although fluorescein staining may also be prominent since epithelial erosions are present. In this 59-year-old female with keratoconjunctivitis sicca, medium-sized epithelial changes are evident in the exposure area of the cornea.

4–13 Coarse epithelial keratopathy in keratoconjunctivitis sicca. In this patient, the coarse (grossly visible) epithelial keratopathy is visible in the pupillary area and inferior portion of the cornea. A prominent arcus senilis can also be seen.

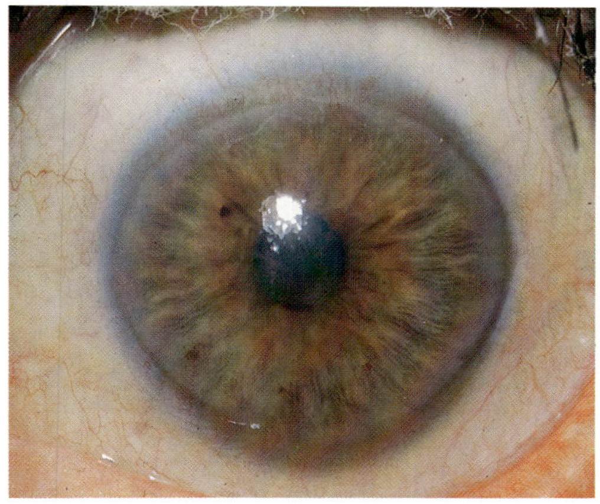

4–14 Coarse epithelial keratopathy resulting from the toxic effects of antivirals (idoxuridine). A common cause of a coarse epithelial keratopathy is the chronic administration of antivirals. This 28-year-old female had used idoxuridine for several months. The bright-staining areas of epithelial erosions and the gray opacities of the keratopathy are readily visible. Meibomian froth and conjunctival hyperemia are also evident, together with a disciform keratitis superior to the epithelial keratopathy.

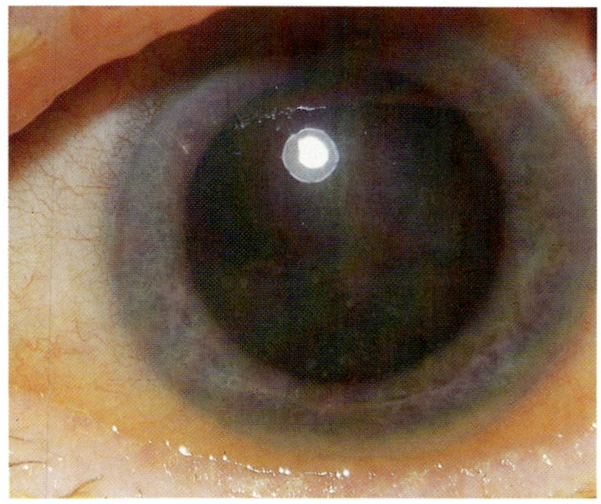

4–15 A Superficial punctate keratitis of Thygeson. Superficial punctate keratitis (SPK) occurs in all age groups. It is a bilateral recurrent epithelial keratopathy of unknown etiology, which characteristically has periods of remission and exacerbation. During periods of remission, the lesions disappear completely or become flat and fail to take up stain. During exacerbations, the lesions, which are composed of fine dots grouped together to make up the coarse lesion, often take up stain. The lesions are oval in shape and the areas in between the lesions are clear.

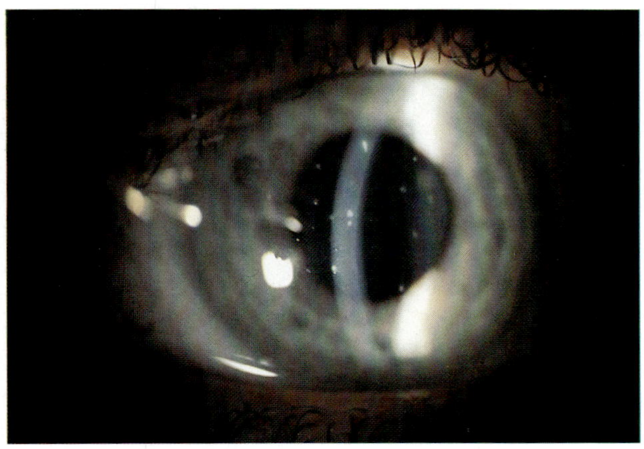

4–15 B Superficial punctate keratitis of Thygeson, demonstrating epithelial involvement. The epithelial nature of SPK is evident in this photograph. In almost all instances in which subepithelial changes occur, antivirals have been used.

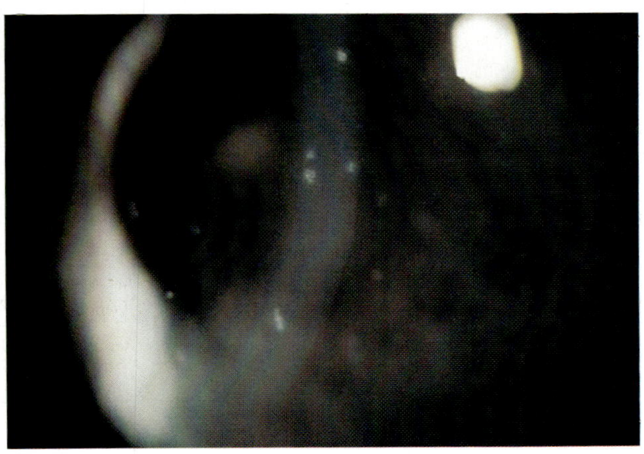

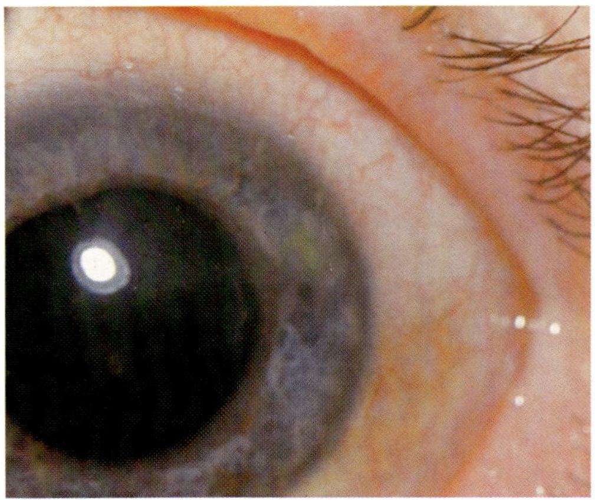

4–16 Herpes simplex dendritic keratitis. Characteristically, a dendritic keratitis is a linear, branching epithelial ulcer. The appearance is almost pathognomonic for herpes simplex keratitis, especially if terminal knobs are also present. In this 24-year-old male, the dendritic ulcer is associated with an underlying opacity suggesting that the keratitis is recurrent. The dendrite is fragmenting, and the terminal knobs are small, suggesting that the lesion is responding to therapy. Note the small posterior synechiae at the 11:00 position.

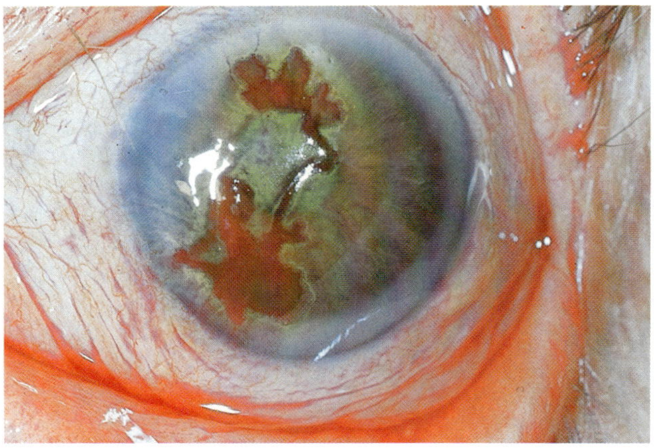

4–17 Herpes simplex geographic (ameboid) ulcer. A geographic ulcer is a large angulated ulcer that often looks like a map. In this 31-year-old male, the angulated outline and fuzzy edges of the ulcer suggest that there is virus still present in the epithelium. The ulcer was stained with both rose bengal and fluorescein. The fluorescein has leaked into the surrounding (diseased) epithelium, while the rose bengal has stained the area of epithelial cell loss.

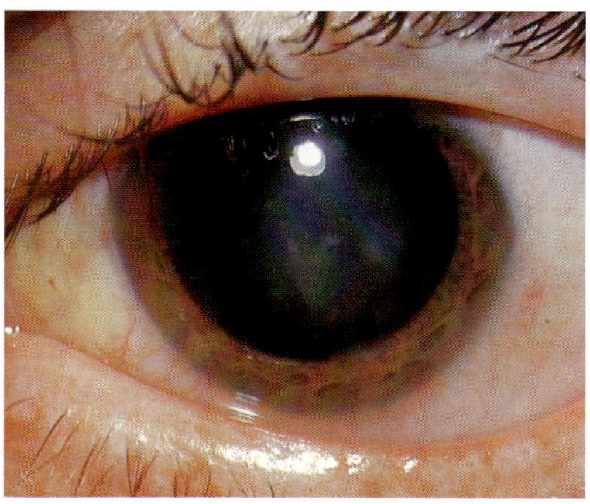

4–18A Pseudodendrite of herpes zoster ophthalmicus. Herpes zoster ophthalmicus may produce linear lesions or "medusa head" types of lesions which resemble a rope or branch of a tree lying on the cornea. There are no terminal knobs. This type of lesion is often called a pseudodendrite because of its similarity to a dendrite. Its surface stains poorly and appears elevated above the surrounding epithelium. In this 67-year-old male with herpes zoster, a pseudodendrite is present along with a disciform keratitis. Many pigmented keratic precipitates are also evident, and the globe is moderately injected.

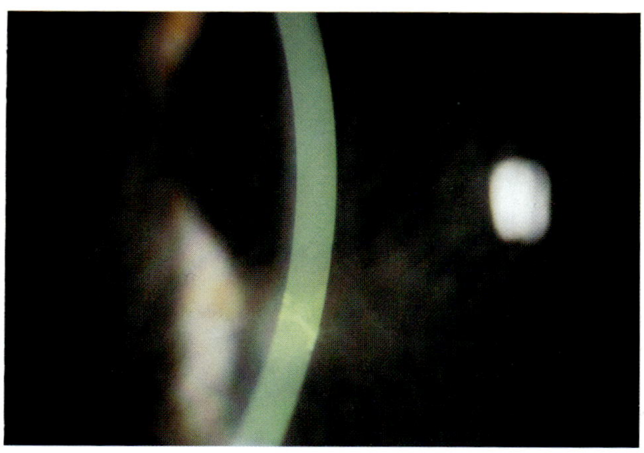

4–18B Pseudodendrite of herpes zoster ophthalmicus, demonstrating epithelial involvement. The epithelial nature of the pseudodendrite can be seen in the parallelepiped of the slit lamp in this photograph.

4–19 Disciform keratitis due to herpes simplex infection. Disciform keratitis is a term used to describe the disk-shaped opacities that may occur in viral infections, especially in herpes simplex keratitis. The opacity occurs because of stromal edema. The lesion usually occurs within the center of the cornea, as noted in this 23-year-old female with recurrent herpes simplex keratitis. Circumcorneal injection is also evident.

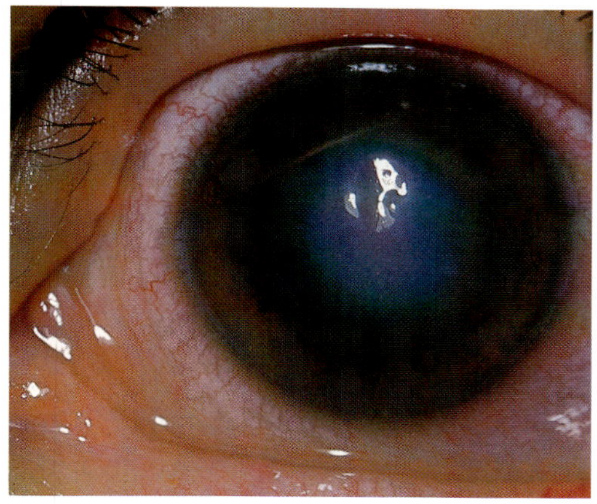

4–20 Focal avascular interstitial keratitis due to herpes simplex infection of the cornea. Focal avascular interstitial keratitis may occur in herpes simplex keratitis. The individual lesions appear as round avascular inflammatory areas in the superficial cornea and are usually seen in an area of disciform keratitis as it is subsiding. In this patient, the focal avascular areas became readily visible when the disciform of herpes simplex keratitis was disappearing and the patient's use of glucocorticoids was being tapered.

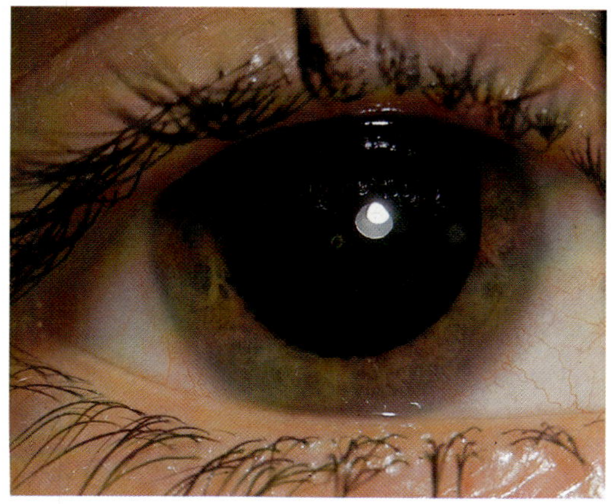

4–21A Subepithelial opacities of epidemic keratoconjunctivitis. The round subepithelial opacities that develop in epidemic keratoconjunctivitis (EKC) occur more prominently in the central cornea. They are grossly visible and occur in the superficial stroma, as can be seen in the pupillary area of this 28-year-old female who developed EKC four weeks previously.

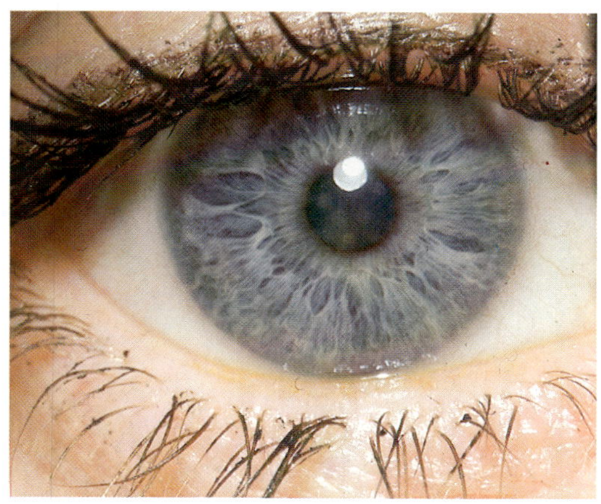

4–21B Opacities of epidemic keratoconjunctivitis, demonstrating their subepithelial location. The subepithelial nature of the opacities in epidemic keratoconjunctivitis is readily visible in the parallelapiped of the slit lamp in this photograph.

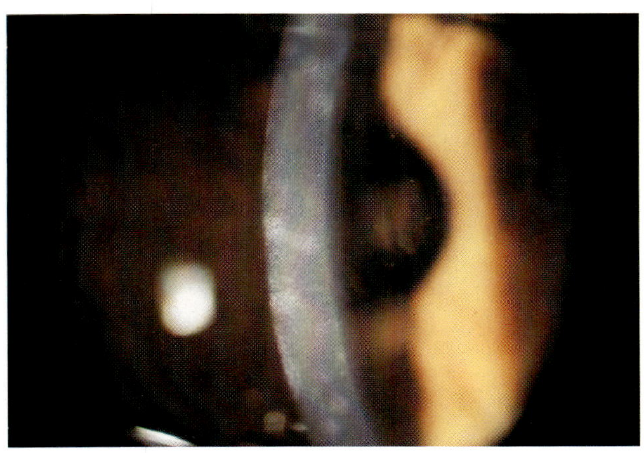

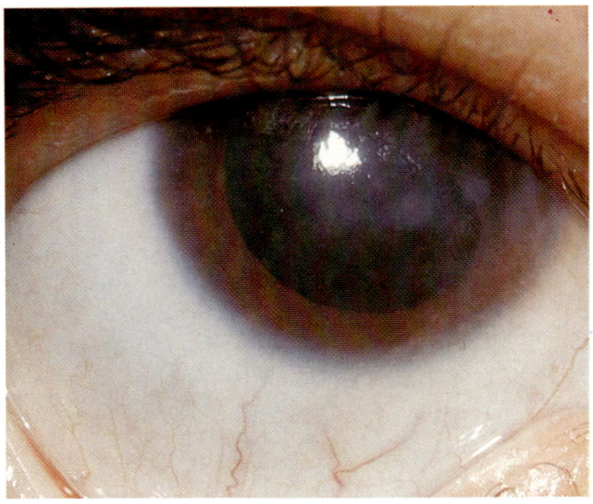

4–22 Nummular keratitis. A nummular keratitis is usually unilateral and is not associated with or preceded by a conjunctivitis. The opacities usually occur in one plane of the cornea, but occasionally occur at various levels. The opacities are usually round, but may appear irregular because of confluence of several lesions, as in this 37-year-old male.

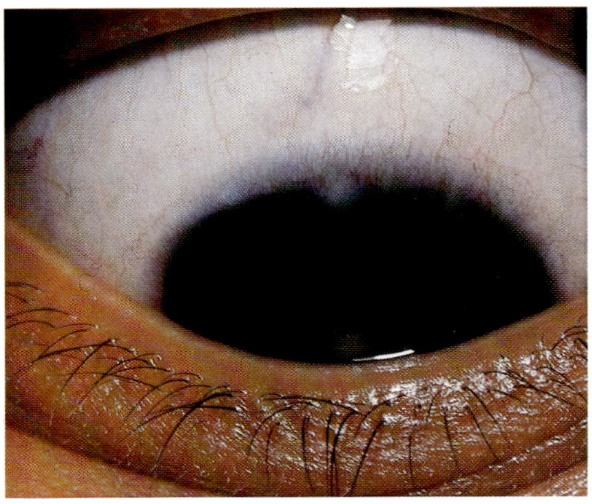

4–23 Limbal scars from phlyctenulosis. Limbal-based triangular opacities, as seen in this 14-year-old male, are highly suggestive of phlyctenulosis. Phlyctenules have a predeliction for straddling the limbus, affecting both cornea and conjunctiva. As healing occurs, the conjunctival portion of the phlyctenule heals without producing scarring, whereas the corneal portion heals to give the characteristic triangular scar.

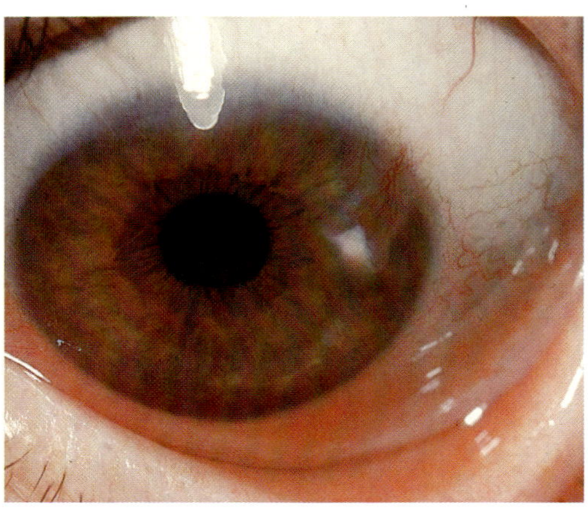

4–24 Fascicular keratitis due to herpes simplex. The major cause of fascicular keratitis in the United States is herpes simplex keratitis. The lesion begins as an inflammatory focus in the superficial cornea, which attracts vessels as it progresses across the cornea in a seemingly aimless fashion. The focus of inflammation and the vessels can be seen in this 17-year-old female. Hyperemia of the globe is also evident.

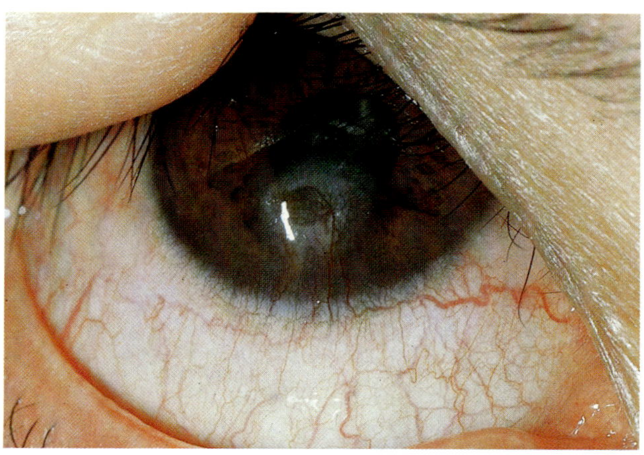

4–25 Fascicular keratitis arising from a delayed hypersensitivity to staphylococci. A fascicular keratitis may develop in recurrent phlyctenulosis in which phlyctenules progressively develop, one in front of the other, as seen in this 7-year-old female with staphylococcal blepharitis. The leash of superficial vessels that was attracted to the area of inflammation is readily seen.

4–26 Staphylococcal marginal infiltrate. A staphylococcal marginal (catarrhal) infiltrate begins in the superficial stroma and involves the overlying epithelium secondarily. There is usually a lucid interval separating the infiltrate from the limbus, as seen in this 17-year-old female who developed a catarrhal ulcer extending from the 5:30 to 7:30 positions.

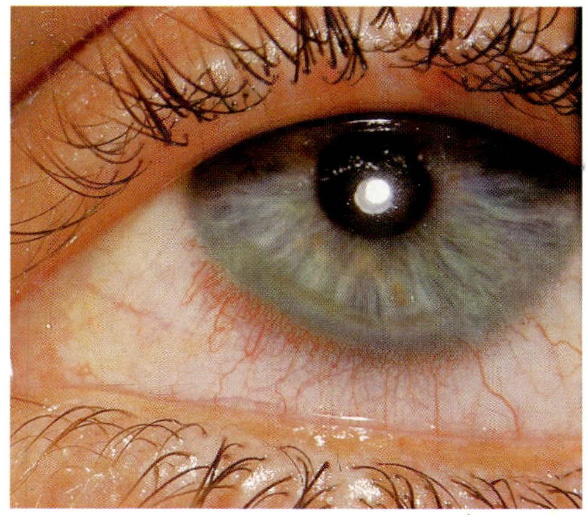

4–27 Marginal herpes simplex keratitis. Characteristically, herpes simplex corneal infections cause epithelial ulceration before causing a subepithelial infiltrate, as seen in this very early marginal dendrite. Branching of the dendrite and terminal knobs are beginning to develop.

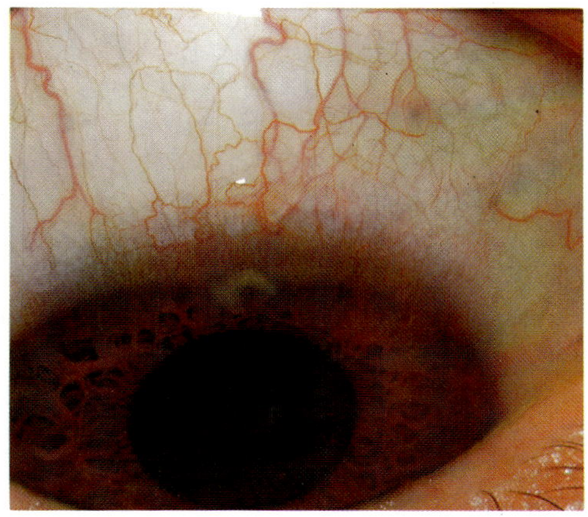

4–28 Catarrhal infiltrate due to staphylococcal blepharokeratitis. The catarrhal infiltrate from staphylococcal blepharokeratitis is mediated by immune complexes. The staphylococcal antigen and the patient's antibodies combine and fix complement, which attracts polymorphonuclear leukocytes. The combination of these factors causes visible infiltration, as seen in this 26-year-old male. The infiltrate extends from the 3:30 to the 6:30 positions. Tiny twigs of new vessels are developing in the cornea in response to the necrosis occurring within the infiltrate. Marked injection of the globe is evident.

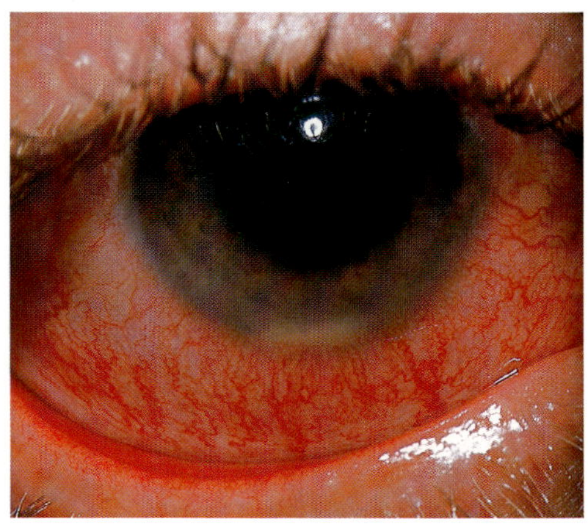

4–29 Early catarrhal corneal infiltrate central to corneal vessels. A catarrhal corneal infiltrate often develops central to corneal vessels. This 32-year-old male has had recurrent catarrhal infiltrates, which have caused superficial corneal neovascularization at the 7:00 region of the limbus. A new infiltrate has developed central to the vessels and subsequently caused the vessels to grow even further into the cornea (Fig. 4–25). Catarrhal infiltrates frequently develop at the 2:00, 4:00, 8:00, or 10:00 positions (areas where the lid margin crosses the limbus).

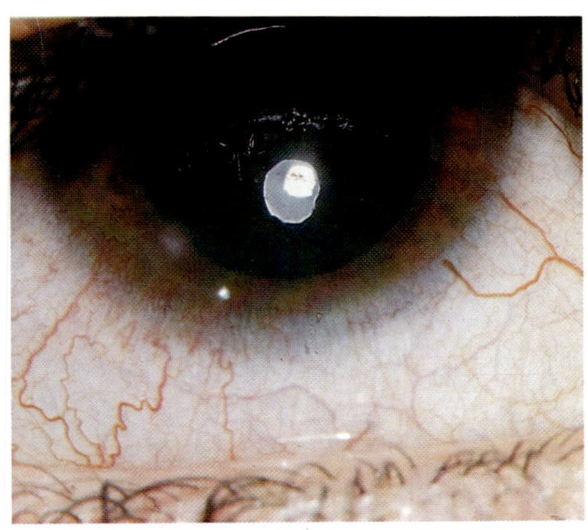

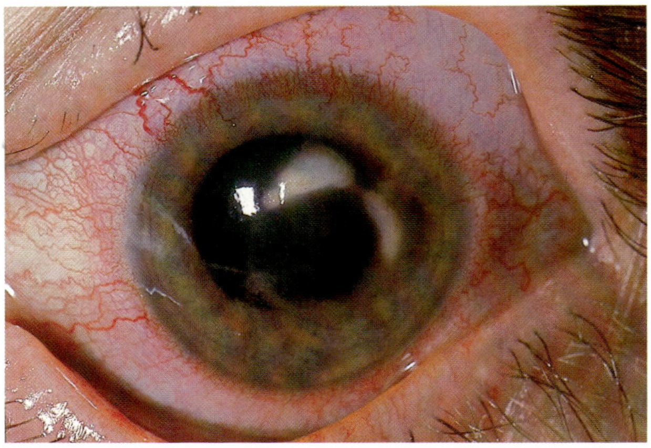

4–30 Midperipheral stromal infiltrate associated with contact lenses. In this patient, a midperipheral corneal infiltrate developed following the use of a continuous-wear soft contact lens. The corneal epithelium was intact. The authors believe that the infiltrate had occurred as a reaction to endotoxin from *Pseudomonas aeruginosa.* (Reprinted with permission from *The American Journal of Ophthalmology.*)

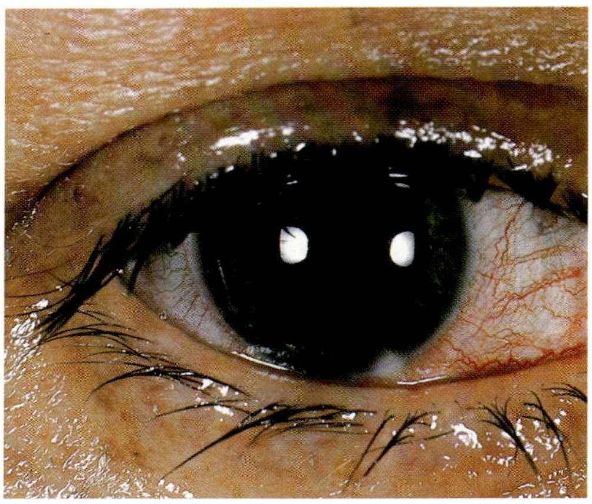

4–31 Marginal infiltrate due to primary varicella. The eruption of chicken pox may involve the limbus, as is evident in this patient with primary varicella. Corneal involvement may lead to sector atrophy of the iris. (Photograph courtesy of Dr. Phillips Thygeson.)

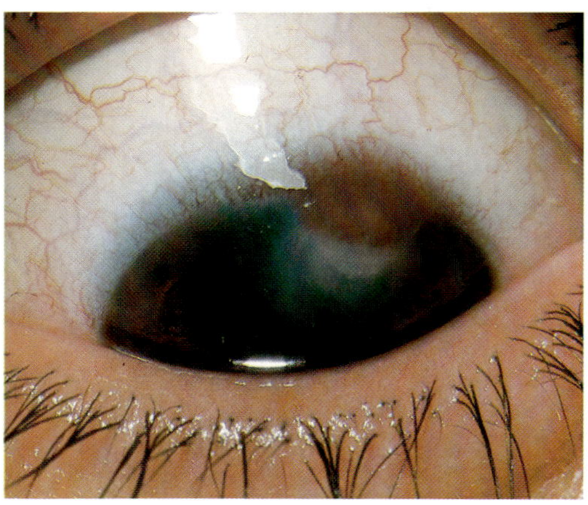

4–32 Marginal herpes zoster keratitis with epaulet-like vascularization of the cornea. This 61-year-old male developed a marginal infiltrate due to herpes zoster four weeks after onset of his skin lesions. Intense neovascularization of the cornea is developing in the same area. (The shiny irregular opacity extending onto the limbus is an artifact.)

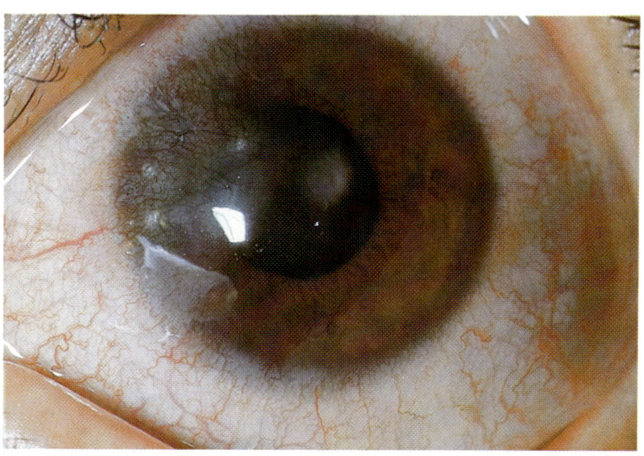

4–33 Irregular pannus caused by staphylococcal phlyctenulosis. This 15-year-old female developed multiple, recurrent phlyctenules with subsequent thinning, scarring, and vascularization of the cornea. In contrast to the pannus of trachoma, the pannus is very irregular. A resolving corneal infiltrate is evident near the center of the cornea. (The irregular opacity near the 7:00 limbus is an artifact.)

4–34 Conjunctival phlyctenules. Although phlyctenules develop most frequently at the limbus, a conjunctival phlyctenule may occur anywhere in the conjunctiva. In this patient, the phlyctenules at the 11 : 30 position developed as a result of a hypersensitivity reaction to staphylococci. The gray-white center of the phlyctenule ulcerated after eight days and the phlyctenule healed without evidence of scarring. Thickening, hyperemia, and crusting of the lid margin are evident.

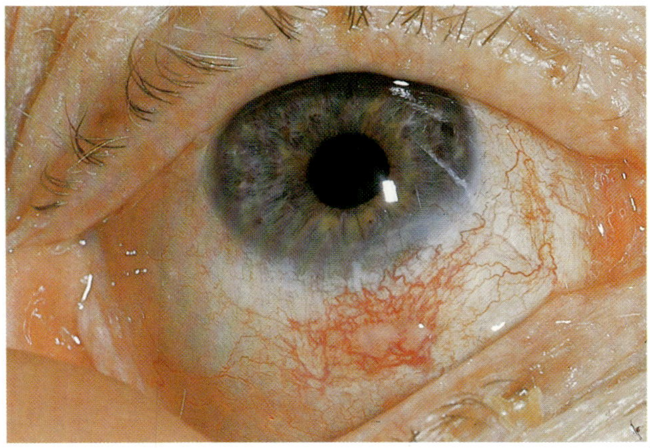

4–35A Limbal phlyctenules. Phlyctenules occur most frequently at the limbus. In this patient, two tiny limbal phlyctenules are evident. They subsided rapidly with the use of topical glucocorticoids.

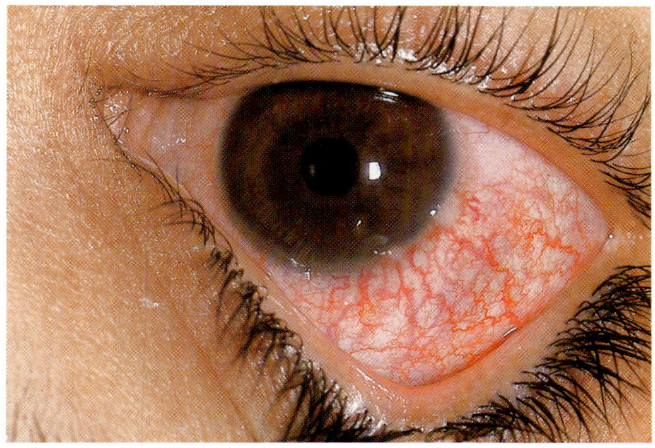

4–35B Resolving limbal phlyctenule. This 18-year-old female noted redness and tearing with minimal pain and photophobia. She had a staphylococcal blepharitis as evidenced by the erythema and pustule formation. (Reprinted with permission from *Transactions of the Pacific Coast Ophthalmology and Otolaryngology Society.)*

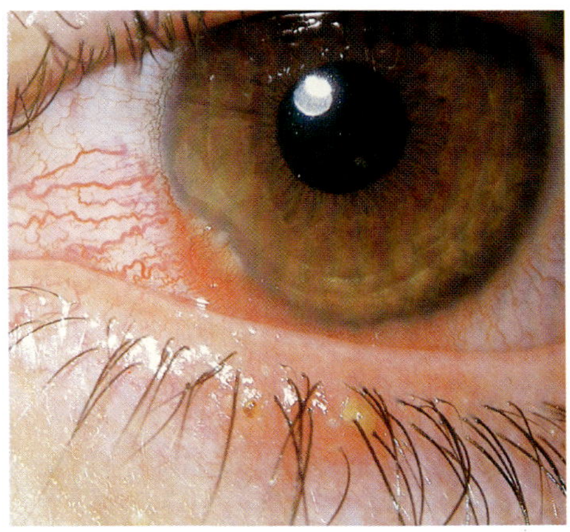

4–36A Bilateral Mooren's ulcer. About one-quarter to one-third of Mooren's ulcers are bilateral, as seen in this 27-year-old male. Peripheral ulceration and injection are evident; it is obvious that the patient is in pain and has photophobia. (Photograph courtesy of Dr. Phillips Thygeson.)

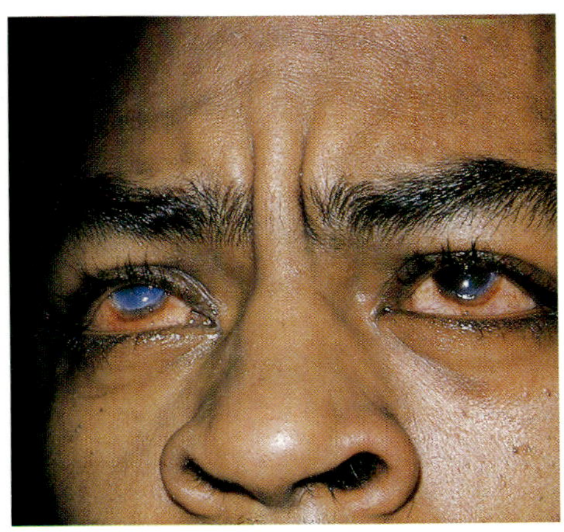

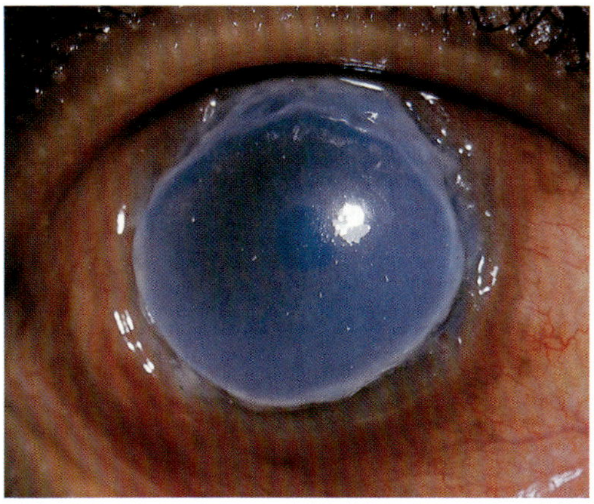

4–36B Closeup of the right cornea of patient with Mooren's ulcer. This photograph of the same patient shown in Fig. 4–36A demonstrates the central steep overhanging edge and limbal involvement that are characteristic of Mooren's ulcer. (Photograph courtesy of Dr. Phillips Thygeson.)

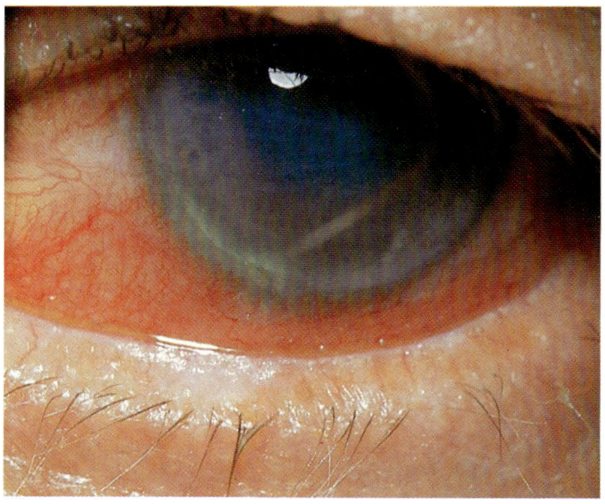

4–37 Peripheral corneal ulcer associated with rheumatoid arthritis. This 61-year-old male presented with symptoms of photophobia, blurred vision, and discomfort. He had severe deformity of the hands and feet and gave a history of having rheumatoid arthritis for more than 18 years. He was noted to have a peripheral corneal ulcer extending from the 6:30 to the 8:30 position and a moderate to severe iritis. Injection of the globe and edema and haziness of the central cornea are evident.

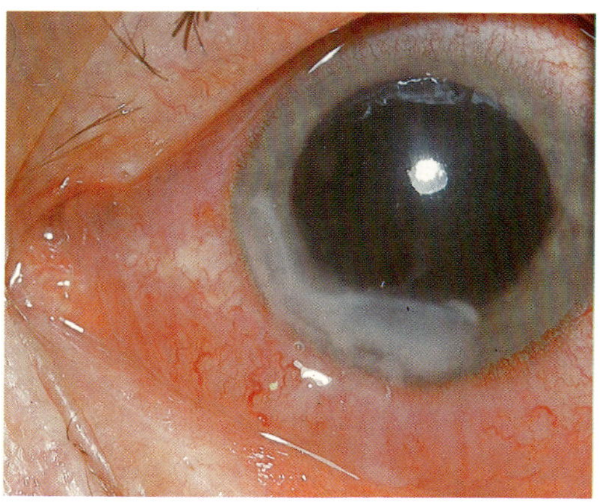

4–38 Peripheral corneal ulcer occurring in polyarteritis nodosa. The peripheral corneal ulcer that occurs with polyarteritis is usually extensive and may encircle the cornea. In this 46-year-old male, edema and hyperemia of the conjunctiva are evident, together with an extensive corneal ulcer and infiltrate.

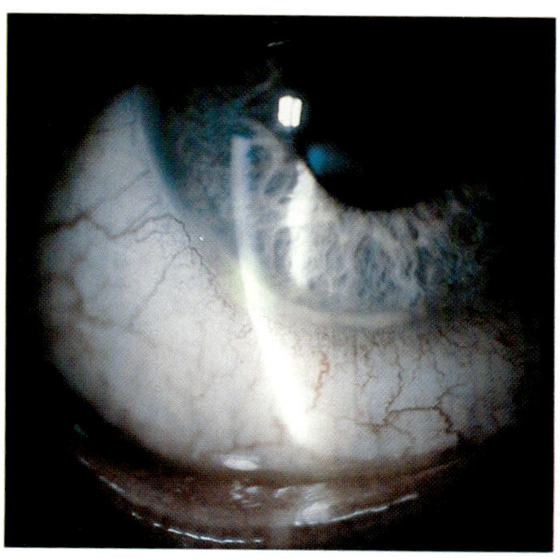

4–39 Peripheral corneal infiltrate associated with granulomatous colitis. This patient had a granulomatous colitis and later developed peripheral corneal infiltration and ulceration. The corneal involvement usually occurred synchronously with the flareup of colitis.

4–40 Peripheral corneal changes occurring in scleritis. Peripheral corneal changes frequently occur in areas contiguous to scleritis, as can be seen in this 45-year-old male with sclerokeratitis. Extensive superficial neovascularization is evident, along with conjunctival edema in the area nearest to the cornea. (Photograph courtesy of Dr. Phillips Thygeson.)

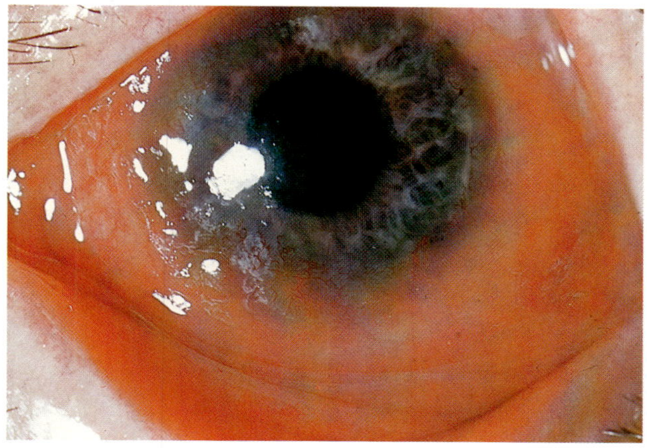

4–41 Terrien's marginal degeneration. This type of degeneration usually begins in the superior nasal quadrant and over a period of many years extends circumferentially to involve the entire peripheral cornea (Fig. 4–42). Corneal thinning of the superior nasal quadrant together with neovascularization of the cornea in the bed of corneal thinning are evident in this 61-year-old male.

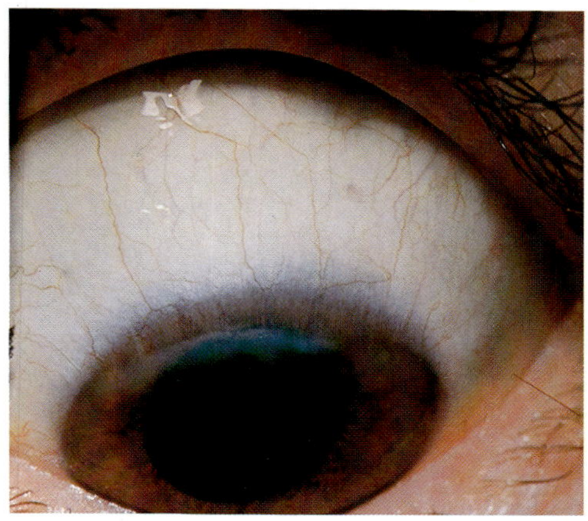

4–42 Advanced Terrien's marginal degeneration. Terrien's marginal degeneration progresses over a 10 to 20 year period to eventually involve the entire circumference of the cornea. This patient has had very few symptoms and was unable to state when he first had difficulty. Compare the marginal, corneal changes to those seen in Fig. 4–38 (polyarteritis), in which much inflammation is evident.

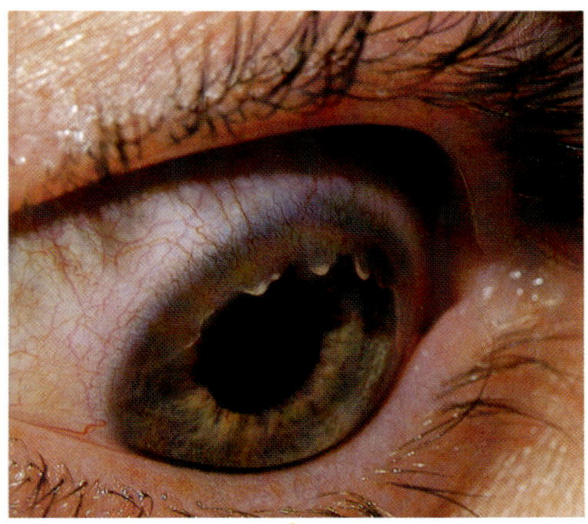

4–43 Fuchs' keratitis marginalis superficialis. Many consider Fuchs' keratitis marginalis superficialis to be a variant of Terrien's marginal degeneration. In Fuchs' keratitis marginalis superficialis, however, the process may extend centrally and a pseudopterygium develops to fill the corneal defect, as seen in this 27-year-old male.

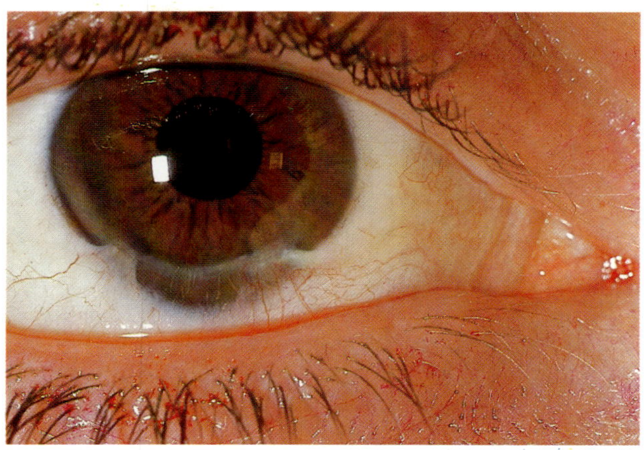

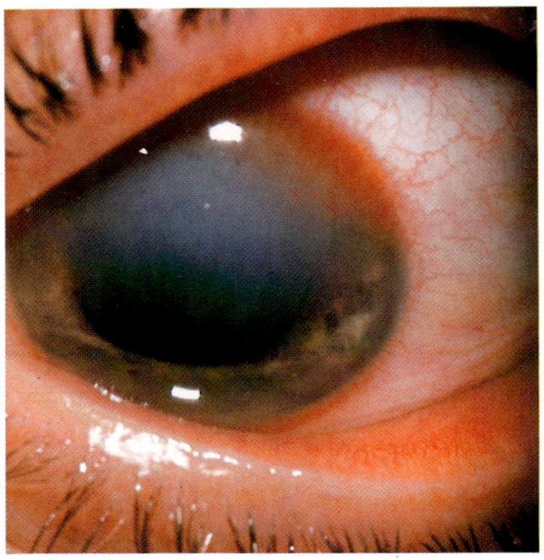

4–44 Syphilitic interstitial keratitis. In this 8-year-old female, early corneal infiltration has developed in the deep and superficial stroma. Neovascularization of the cornea is also developing. Within four days, the infiltration that preceded the vessels had begun to encroach upon the visual axis of the cornea.

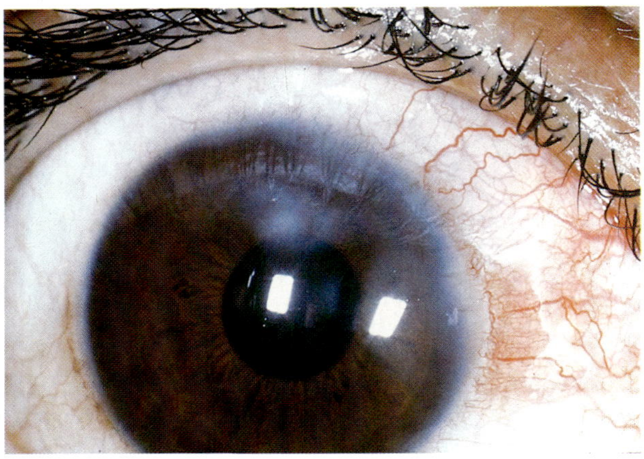

4–45 Inactive sectoral tuberculous interstitial keratitis. The interstitial keratitis occurring in tuberculosis is usually sectoral; the vessels and scarring develop in the mid and superficial stroma, in contrast to the deep stromal involvement in syphilis.

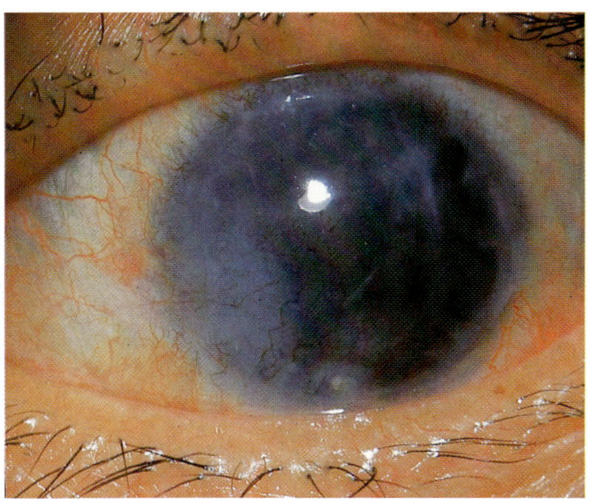

4–46 Deep interstitial keratitis of Hansen's disease. The deep interstitial keratitis that occurs in Hansen's disease begins in the superior temporal quadrant. Corneal neovascularization occurs late in the infection, is moderate in amount, and is not a prominent part of the picture. Both deep and superficial vascularization are evident in this 43-year-old female with lepromatous leprosy. Marked corneal infiltration is evident.

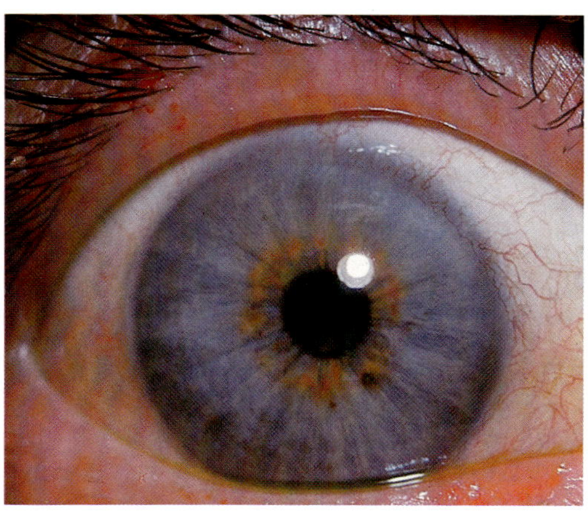

4–47 Dendritic corneal ulcer due to herpes simplex infection. Dendritic corneal ulcers are quite distinctive. They appear as linear branching ulcers with terminal knobs. This patient has three small dendrites which later coalesced to form a large dendrite. Note the terminal knobs.

4–48 Multinucleated giant cell in scraping from herpes simplex keratitis. The herpetic giant cell is a product of nuclear fusion from a number of adjacent epithelial cells; characteristically, the individual nuclei appear to be tightly molded against each other. Giemsa stain, ×1000.

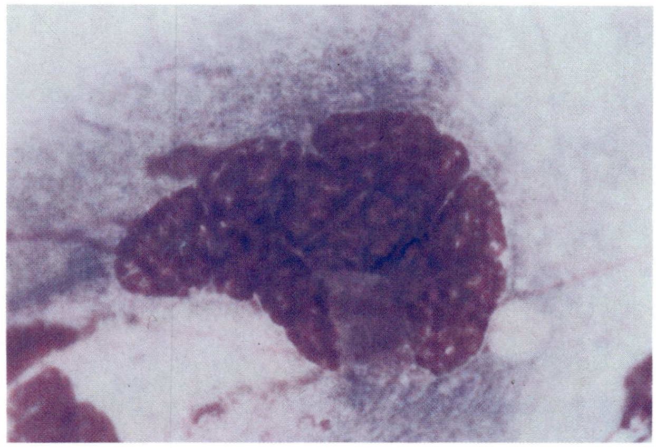

4–49 Geographic corneal ulcer. A geographic or ameboid corneal ulcer is a large ulcer with angulated edges. The finding of such an ulcer, especially when the corneal sensation is reduced or absent, is highly suggestive of herpes simplex keratitis. In this patient, a large geographic ulcer together with central corneal edema, folds in Descemet's membrane, superficial corneal neovascularization, and hyperemia of the conjunctiva are evident. The irregular contour and fuzzy margins of the ulcer suggest that there is still active virus present in the epithelium.

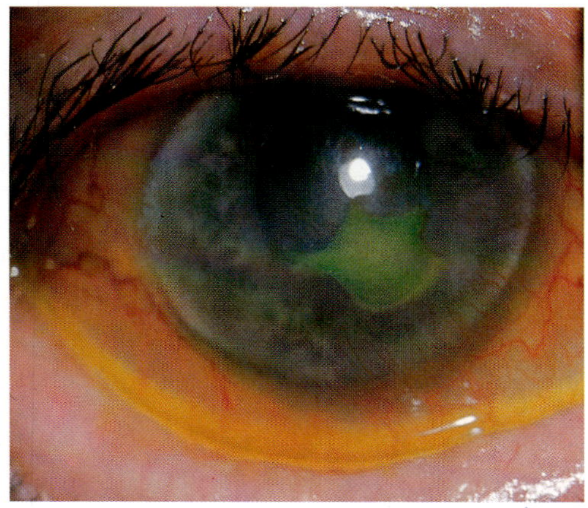

4–50 Disciform keratitis (herpes simplex infection). A disciform keratitis frequently occurs in herpes simplex infections of the cornea. The lesion is round, usually occurs centrally, and involves the superficial stroma. It represents an immune complex reaction in which the antigen is absorbed into the stroma from the overlying infected corneal epithelium, similar to a blotter absorbing fluid. Several small foci of intense inflammation can be seen at the 2:00 region of the disciform keratitis.

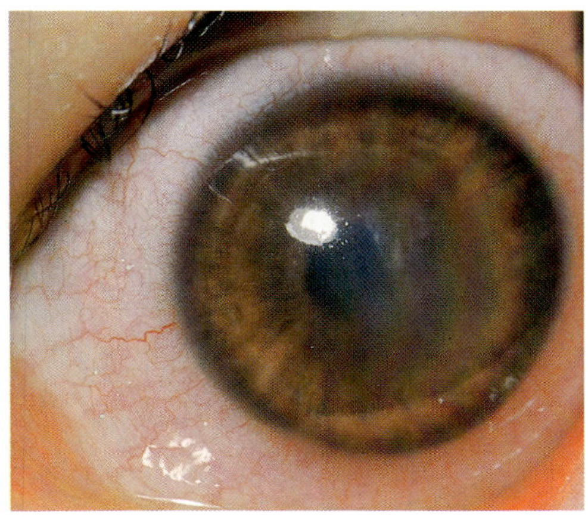

4–51 Herpes simplex geographic corneal ulcer with a hypopyon. An indolent hypopyon ulcer may occur in herpes simplex keratitis as a result of necrosis in the cornea. Smears and cultures for bacterial, fungal, and parasitic organisms must be made to ensure that the ulcer has not become secondarily infected. In this 46-year-old female the large central geographic ulcer has been stained with fluorescein. A corneal infiltrate is present in the bed of the ulcer, and a small hypopyon and superficial corneal novascularization are all visible. Scrapings and cultures were negative for bacteria, fungi, and parasites.

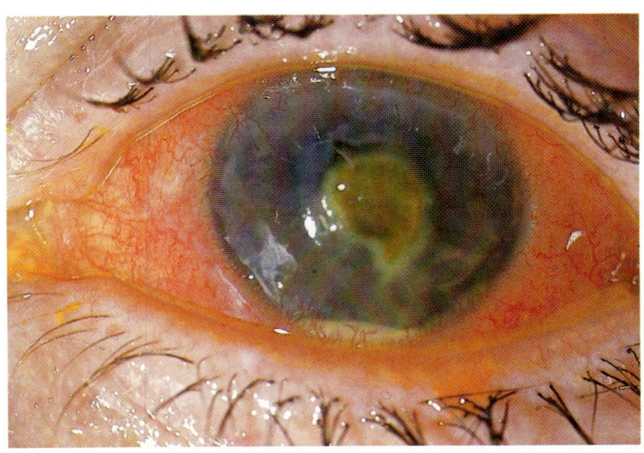

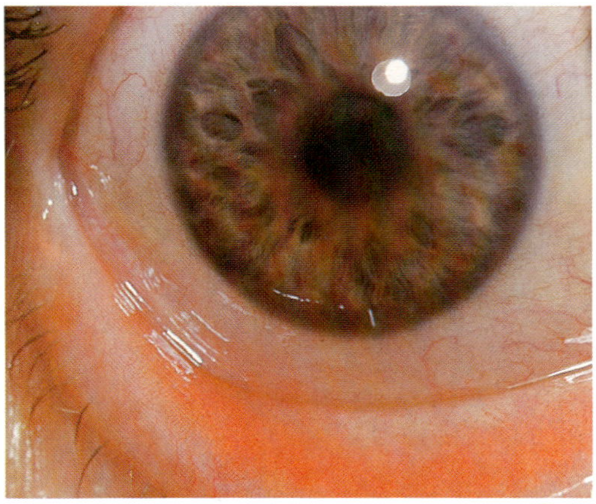

4–52 A Disciform keratitis in herpes zoster ophthalmicus. A disciform keratitis similar to that seen in herpes simplex infections of the cornea (Fig. 4–50) may occur in herpes zoster ophthalmicus. The central disk-like lesion in this patient developed during the third week of illness.

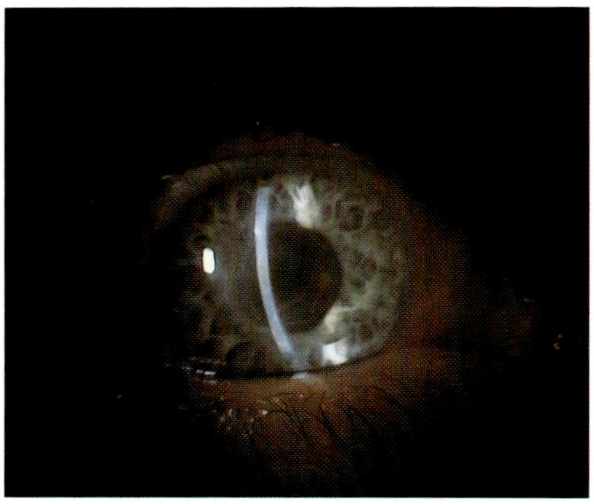

4–52 B Disciform keratitis in herpes zoster ophthalmicus, demonstrating edema and corneal opacity. The edema and corneal opacity of the corneal stroma in disciform keratitis are evident in this slitlamp photograph of a patient with herpes zoster ophthalmicus.

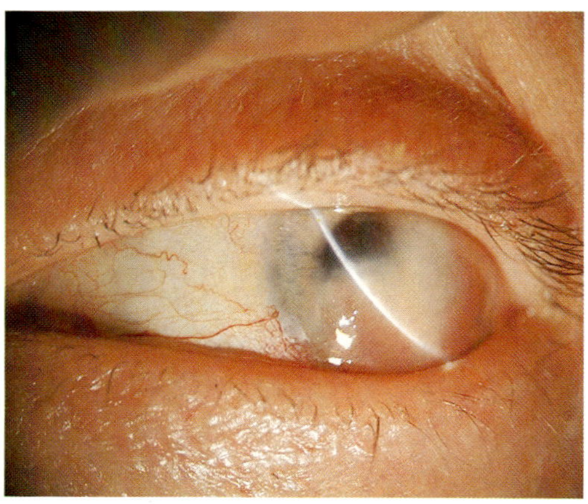

4–53 Marked neovascularization of the cornea with lipid-like deposition in the corneal stroma in herpes zoster ophthalmicus. Lipoidal material commonly occurs when the cornea is involved in herpes zoster ophthalmicus. The material is associated with corneal neovascularization and probably arises from leakage of the lipoidal material through the walls of the newly formed blood vessels. In this patient, deep vascularization of the cornea has occurred together with deposition of lipoidal material into the cornea.

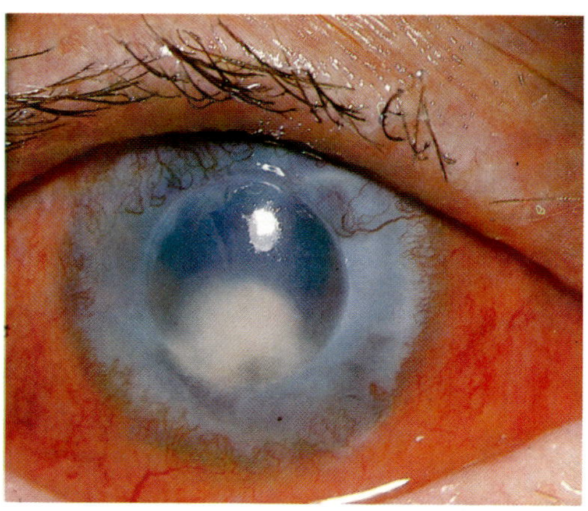

4–54 A *Streptococcus pneumoniae* corneal ulcer. Formerly, *S. pneumoniae* was a very frequent cause of central corneal ulcers. In this atopic patient, the infection has occurred in the donor portion of his corneal graft. The large infiltrate extends into the recipient bed in the 7:00 to 8:00 area. Corneal edema is present superiorly, and corneal vessels approach but do not cross the margin of the graft. A hypopyon did not develop in this patient.

4–54B Scraping taken from pneumococcal corneal ulcer. Typically, untreated pneumococcal corneal ulcers show numerous Gram-positive diplococci, as seen here. Note the prominent capsules. A few pneumococci demonstrate the "classic" lancet morphology. Gram's stain, ×1000.

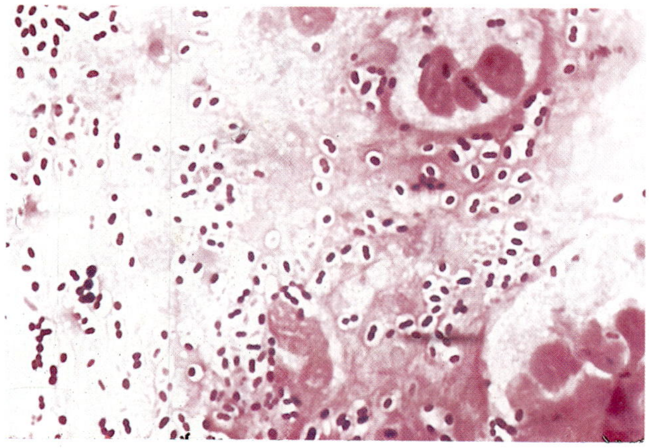

4–55A Viridans streptococcal corneal ulcer. A major cause of central corneal ulcers is the opportunistic viridans streptococcus. This infection frequently occurs in patients who are being treated with topical glucocorticoids for prolonged periods of time. This patient was being treated with glucocorticoids for a mild graft rejection when the infection occurred.

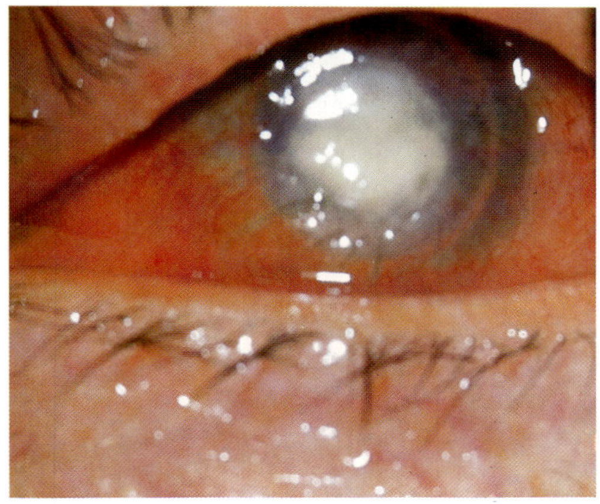

4–55B Scraping from a viridans streptococcal corneal ulcer. In scrapings from viridans streptococcal corneal ulcers, numerous cocci are seen but chain formation is usually lacking. Inflammatory cells are generally absent. Giemsa stain, ×1000.

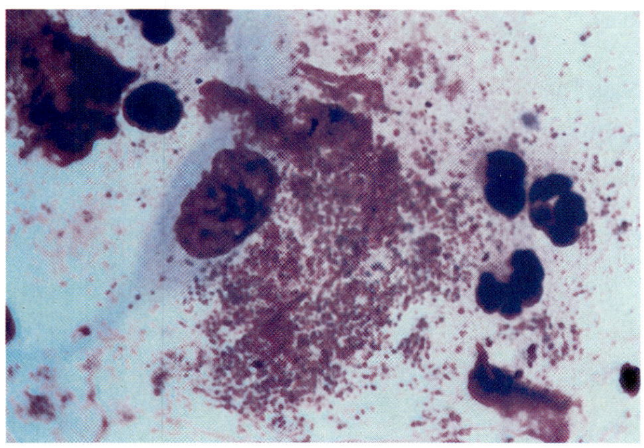

4–56A *Staphylococcus epidermidis* corneal ulcer. Like viridans streptococcus (Fig. 4–55A), *S. epidermidis* is a frequent cause of central corneal ulcers. The ulcer is usually indolent in character.

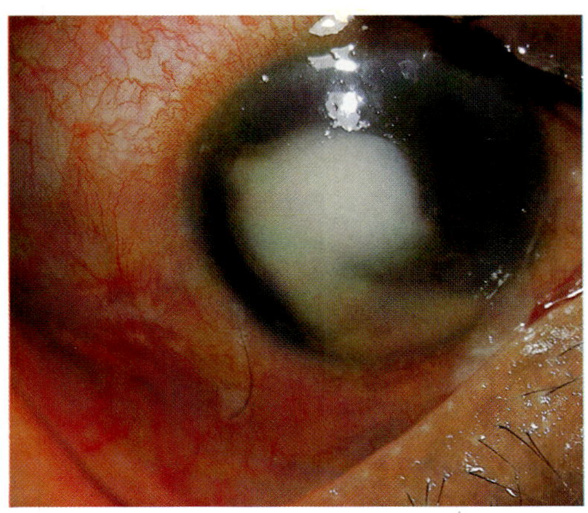

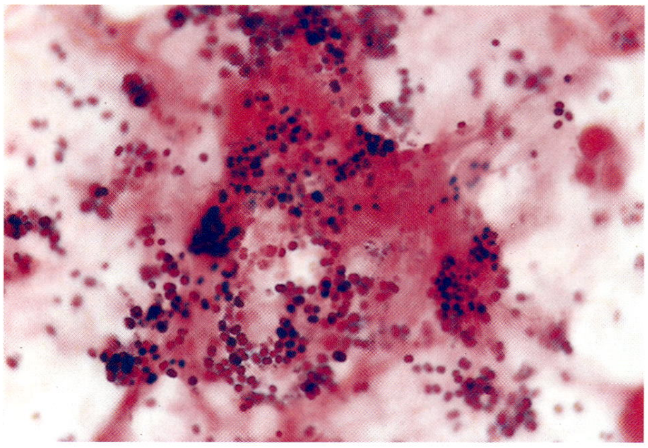

4–56B Scraping from *Staphylococcus epidermidis* corneal ulcer showing many Gram-positive cocci. In this scraping taken from the cornea of the patient in Fig. 4–56A, many Gram-positive cocci and few inflammatory cells are evident. Gram's stain, × 1000.

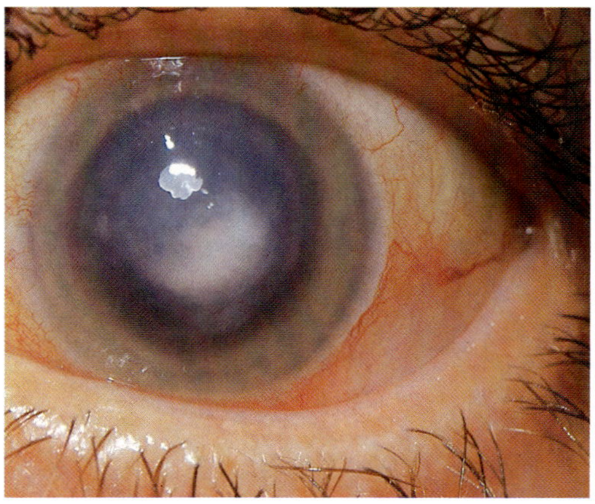

4–57A *Pseudomonas* corneal ulcer. *Pseudomonas* infections of the cornea are common causes of bacterial corneal ulcers. They are round and have a "soupy appearance". This patient abraded her cornea with a mascara brush one day previously. The immune-like ring suggests a reaction to endotoxins.

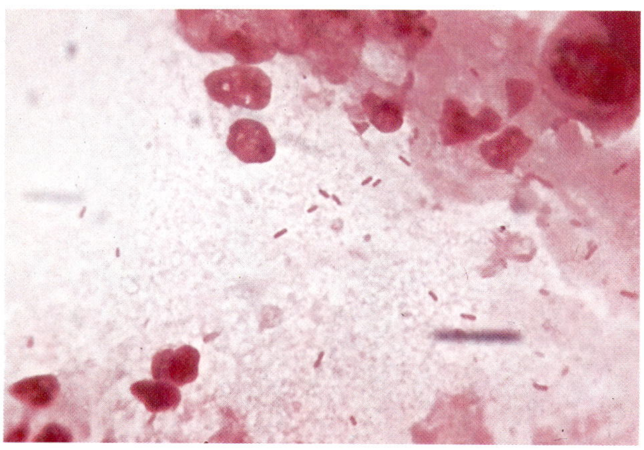

4–57B Scraping from *Pseudomonas* corneal ulcer. A moderate number of slender Gram-negative rods of varying length are seen. Polymorphonuclear granulocytes are usually abundant. Gram's stain, × 1000.

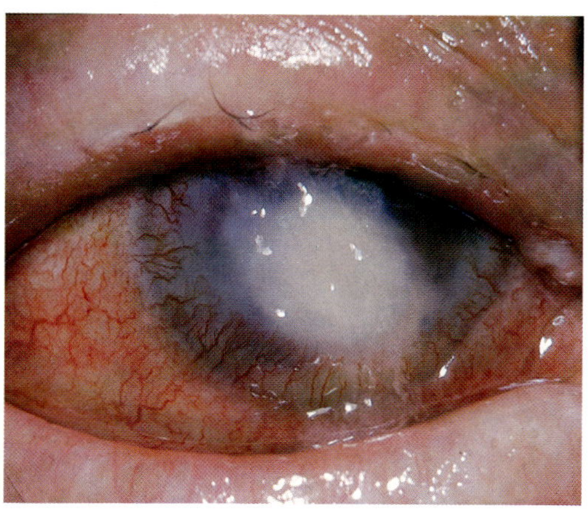

4–58A *Staphylococcus aureus* central corneal ulcer. A *S. aureus* corneal ulcer has no distinguishing features. In this patient with atopy, the ulcer developed as a secondary infection during prolonged treatment with antivirals for herpes simplex keratitis. The central infiltrate extends past the overlying epithelial defect, and a moderate-sized hypopyon is evident. The superficial corneal neovascularization occurred prior to the development of the bacterial infection in response to the herpes simplex infection.

4–58B Scraping of staphylococcal corneal ulcer. A corneal scraping from a *Staphylococcus aureus* corneal ulcer usually reveals many Gram-positive cocci together with a moderate number of inflammatory cells. Gram's stain, × 1000.

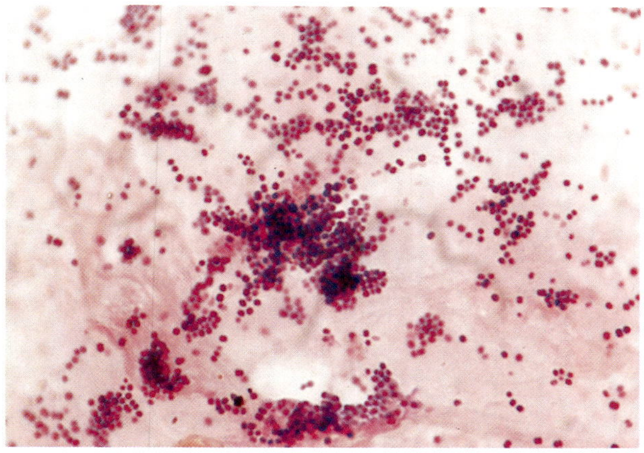

4–59A *Nocardia* spp. central corneal ulcer. Nocardia is a frequent inhabitant of soil and should be suspected as a possible cause of a corneal ulcer when there is contamination with soil. An indolent corneal ulcer that has a "cracked windshield" appearance is suggestive of a nocardial corneal ulcer. This patient, who received a corneal abrasion while working on a tractor, developed a corneal ulcer that was unresponsive to a combination of antibiotics and glucocorticoids. The ulcer is superficial and extends over most of the cornea. Near the edge of the dense infiltrate, dense linear opacities interspersed with clear areas suggest a cracked windshield. A small hypopyon is also evident.

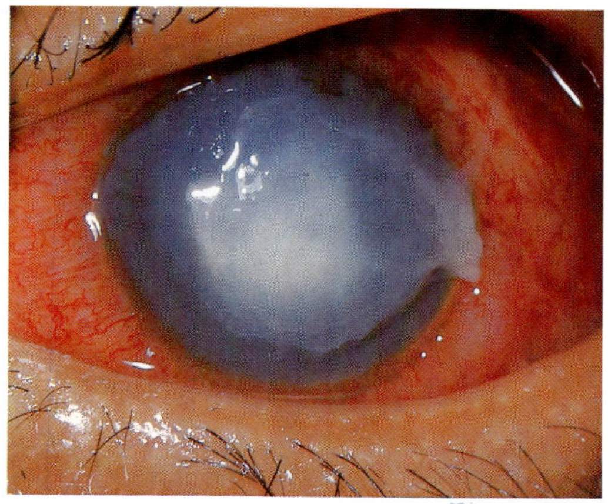

4–59B Scraping from nocardial corneal ulcer. Many Gram-positive branching filaments can be seen. They resemble fungal hyphae, but can be differentiated on the basis of their width: *Nocardia* filaments measure one micron or less in diameter, whereas true fungi are many times thicker. Note the beaded staining of the organism, which is quite characteristic. Gram's stain, × 1000.

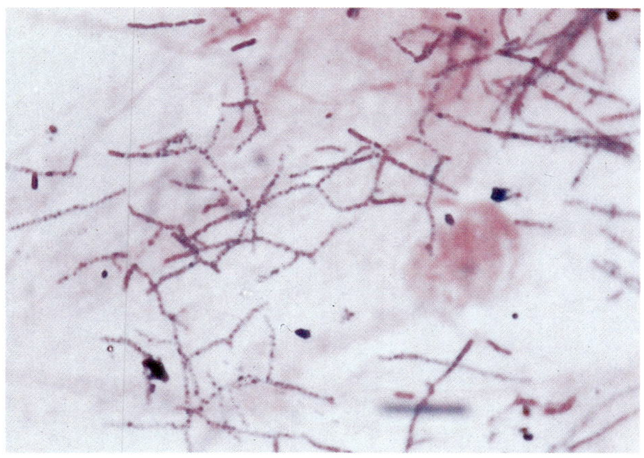

4–60A *Moraxella* corneal ulcer. *Moraxella* corneal ulcers tend to be indolent and are seen most frequently in alcoholics. The ulcer usually occurs in the lower third of the cornea. In this aphakic patient, the corneal ulcer had developed one week previously.

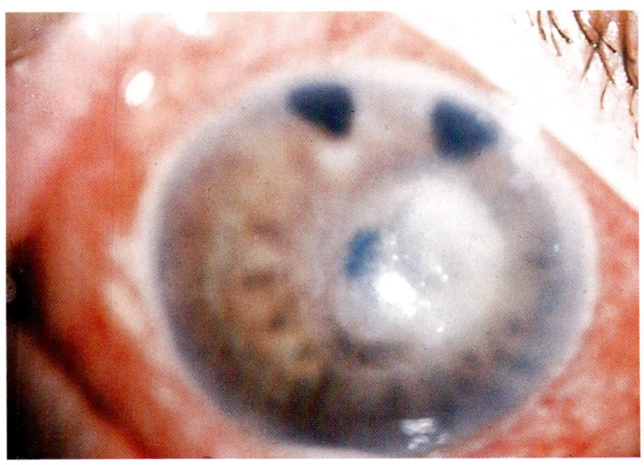

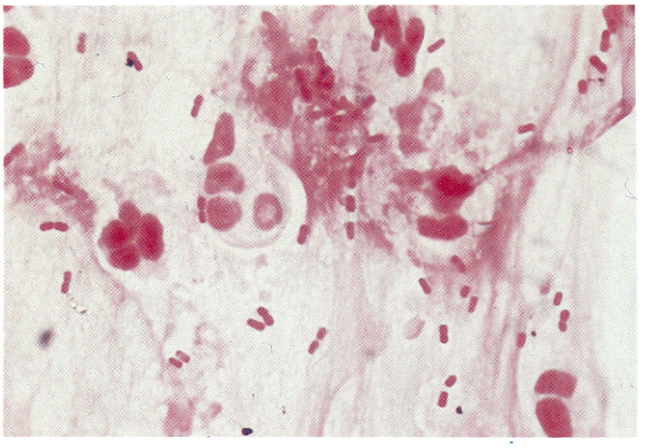

4–60B Scraping of *Moraxella* corneal ulcer. *Moraxella* organisms are large, square-ended, Gram-negative diplobacilli. The organisms can be readily seen in this scraping taken from a patient with a *Moraxella* corneal ulcer. Gram's stain, × 1000.

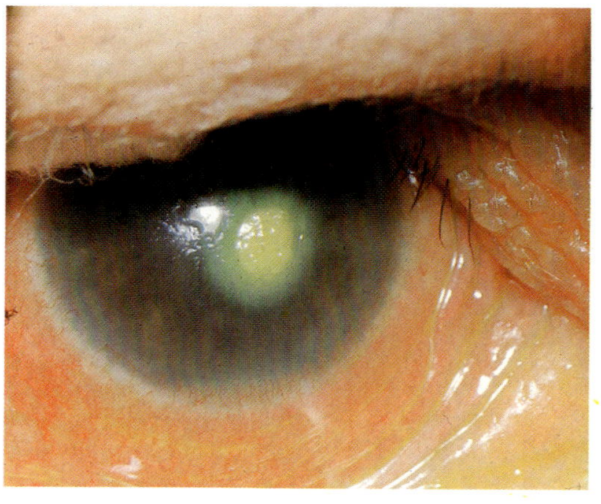

4–61A *Candida* corneal ulcer. A candidal corneal ulcer may resemble an indolent central bacterial corneal ulcer, lacking the characteristics often ascribed to fungal corneal ulcers. This 74-year-old male with keratoconjunctivitis sicca developed a corneal ulcer that suggested a bacterial corneal ulcer, but scraping showed yeast-like organisms. Note the central corneal ulcer with a dry-appearing infiltrate and early corneal neovascularization.

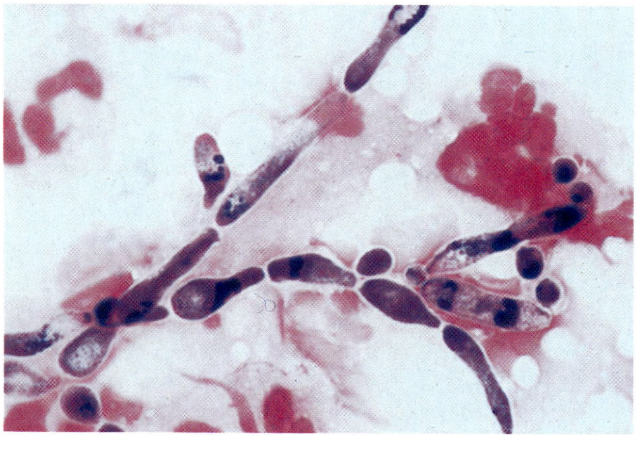

4–61B Scraping from candidal corneal ulcer. This photograph shows *Candida* in its pseudohyphal form as well as a few yeast-forms. The pseudohyphae are formed from successive budding in which the "daughter" cells remain attached to the parent cell. Gram's stain, × 1000.

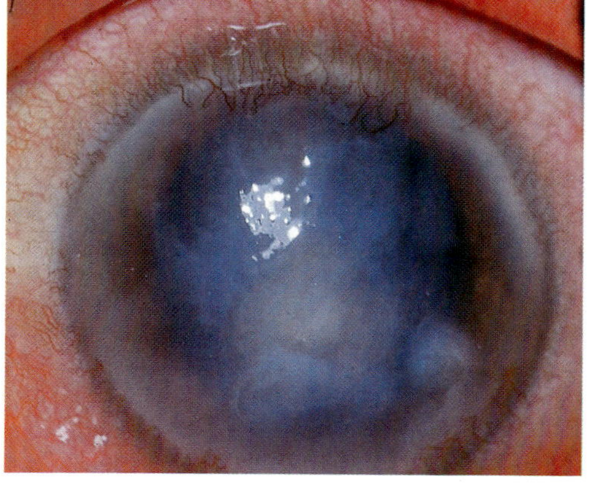

4–62A Fungal corneal ulcer due to *Aspergillus* spp. This patient developed a central corneal ulcer from *Aspergillus* spp. following trauma to the cornea and treatment of the resultant inflammation with glucocorticoids. The fuzzy (hyphate) edges of the central ulcer and the satellite infiltrates are very suggestive of a fungal corneal ulcer. Keratic precipitates can be seen under the central lesion. The lines represent folds in Descemet's membrane. Superficial corneal neovascularization is also evident.

4–62B Scraping of *Aspergillus* corneal ulcer. Large, branching, septate hyphae are seen in this scraping. The *Aspergillus* organisms demonstrate dichotomous branching, which helps to identify this group of fungi. Giemsa stain, ×1000.

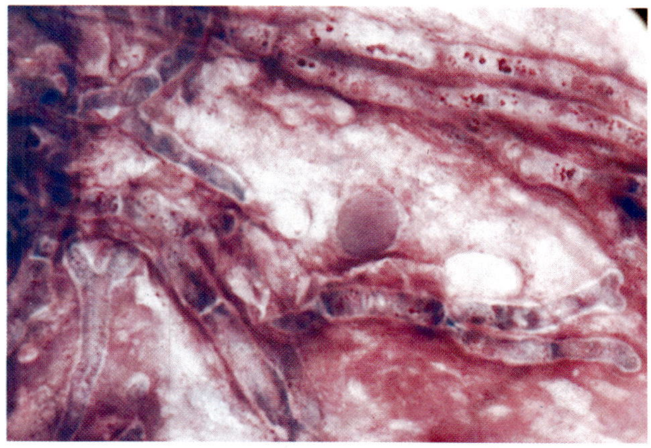

4–63A *Fusarium* corneal ulcer. This patient developed a *Fusarium* corneal ulcer following prolonged treatment of a herpes simplex keratitis with antivirals and glucocorticoids. A beginning immune ring is evident in the photograph.

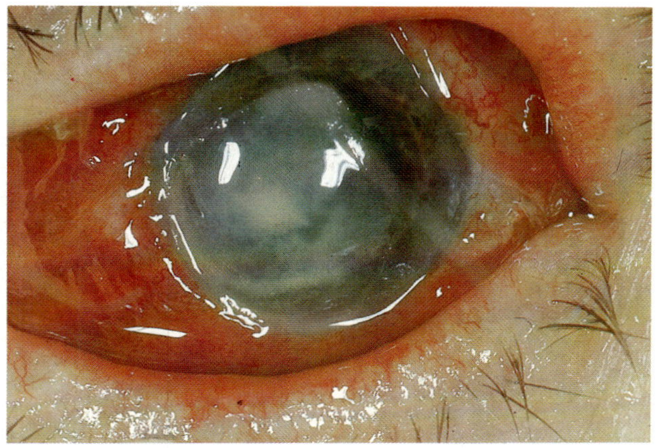

4–63B Scraping of *Fusarium* corneal ulcer. The large septate hyphae shown here establish the diagnosis of a fungal infection, but it is not sufficient to identify the fungus as *Fusarium* spp. Giemsa stain, ×1000.

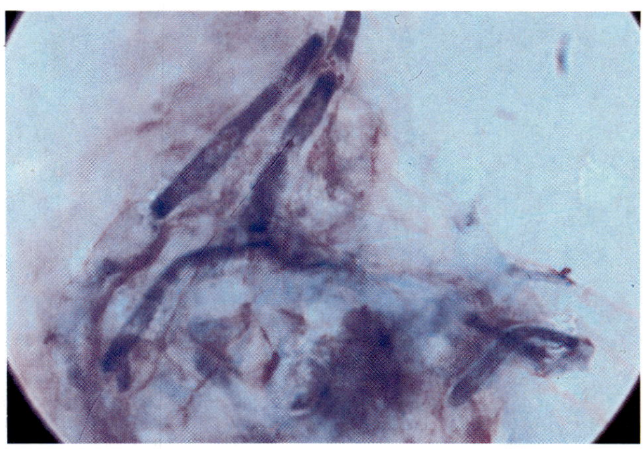

4–64A *Helminthosporium* corneal ulcer. This 61-year-old ophthalmologist developed a corneal abrasion while cutting his lawn. He was treated with antibiotics and glucocorticoids then three weeks later noted an infiltrate in the cornea. Scrapings and cultures revealed *Helminthosporium* spp. The failure of the ulcer to progress centrally, the corneal neovascularization, and the elevated base of the ulcer are all suggestive of a fungal infection.

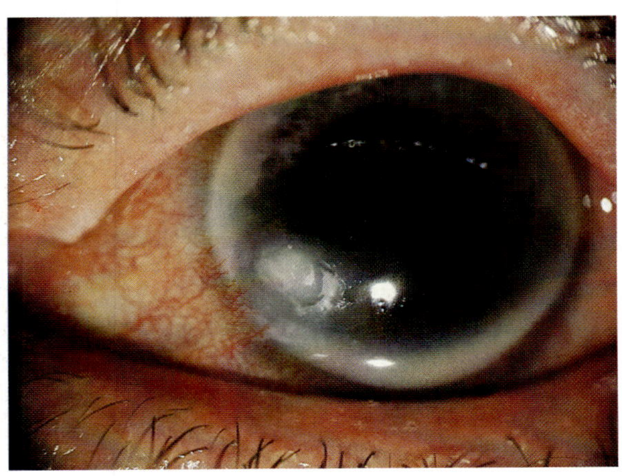

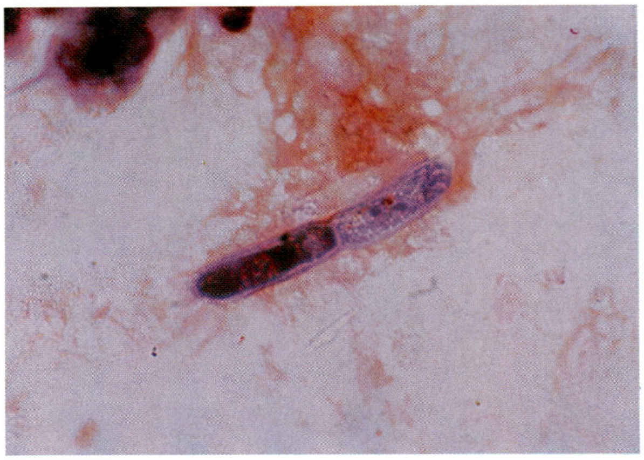

4–64B Scraping from *Helminthosporium* corneal ulcer. A fragment of a hypha is shown here. This fragment was sufficient to allow a diagnosis of fungal keratitis, and cultures later confirmed the diagnosis of *Helminthosporium* spp. Gram's stain, × 1000.

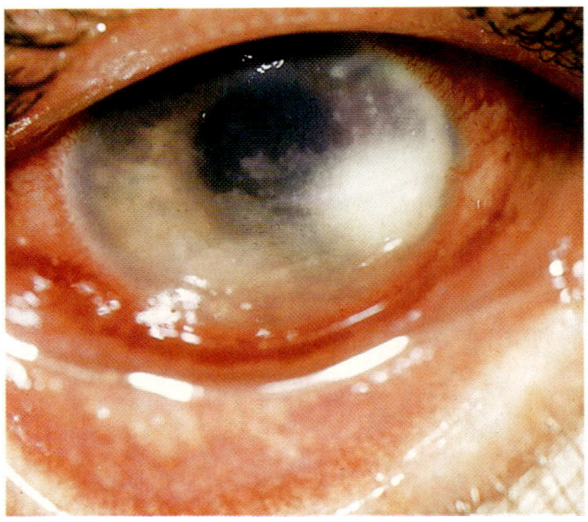

4–65 *Aspergillus* corneal ulcer. This 24-year-old male was air-evacuated to the San Francisco Bay area from Vietnam after developing a corneal ulcer. He had scratched the eye while crossing through a barbed wire fence and was treated with a combination antibiotic-glucocorticoid preparation. Four weeks later he was seen by the authors for his corneal ulcer. Many of the characteristics of a fungal infection are evident, including satellite lesions, fuzzy edges to the lesions, endothelial plaque, and marked inflammation.

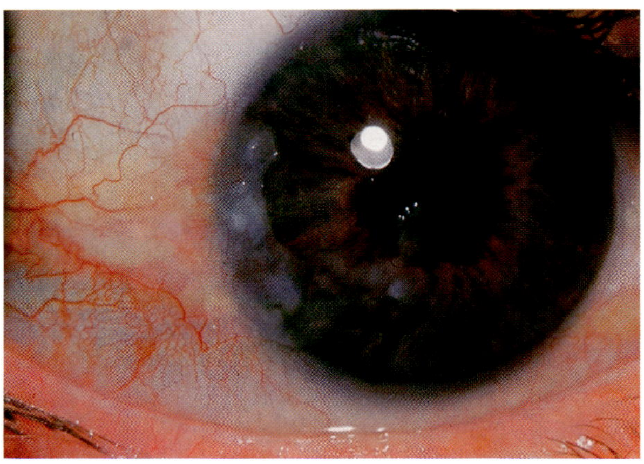

4–66 Leukoplakia of the cornea. Leukoplakia is a major cause of an elevated lesion of the cornea. The lesion appears thickened, white, or gelatinous and typically contains fronds of blood vessels growing perpendicular to the surface of the cornea. The lesion usually begins within the interpalpebral area of the cornea. In this patient, the fronds of vessels are apparent in the conjunctiva, while the corneal lesion appears semiopaque and homogeneous. (Photograph courtesy of Dr. Phillips Thygeson.)

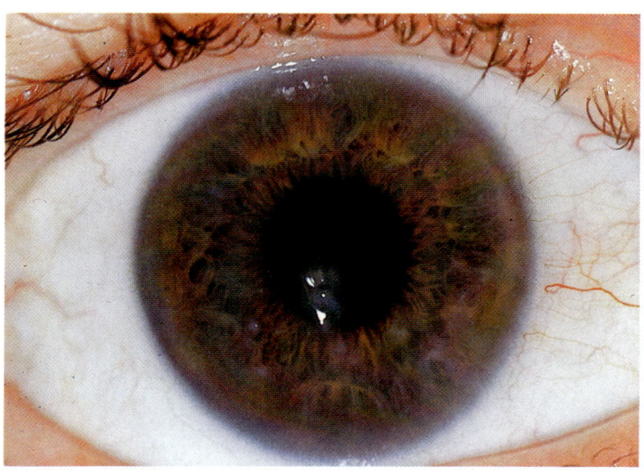

4–67 Salzmann's nodular degeneration. The nodules of Salzmann's nodular degeneration are elevated and appear bluish-gray in color. They represent newly formed collagen and are usually found near areas of corneal scarring. This patient has several nodules near the visual axis and another nodule near the 8:00 position.

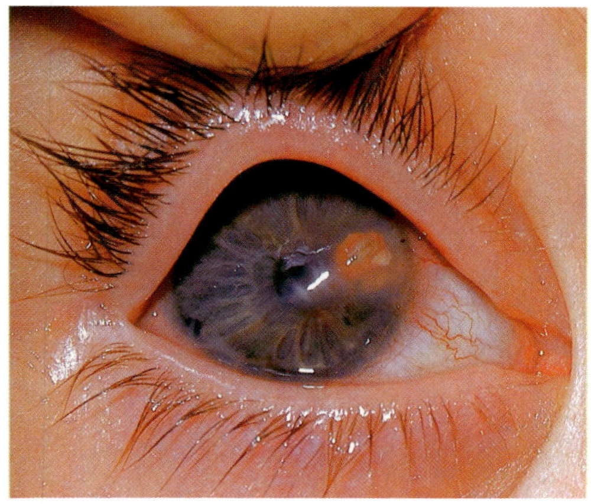

4–68 Granuloma of the cornea. This patient developed a granuloma of the cornea following a perforating injury. The granuloma is elevated, vascularized, and has a fleshy appearance.

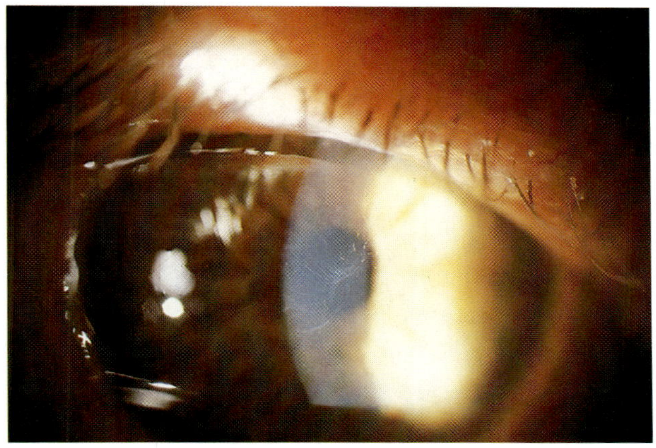

4–69 Fingerprint lines in anterior membrane dystrophy. Anterior membrane dystrophy is characteristically composed of fingerprint lines, maps, and/or dot-like opacities at the level of the basement membrane of the corneal epithelium. The fingerprint lines and some dots are visible over the visual axis in this patient. (Photograph courtesy of Dr. David M. Meisler.)

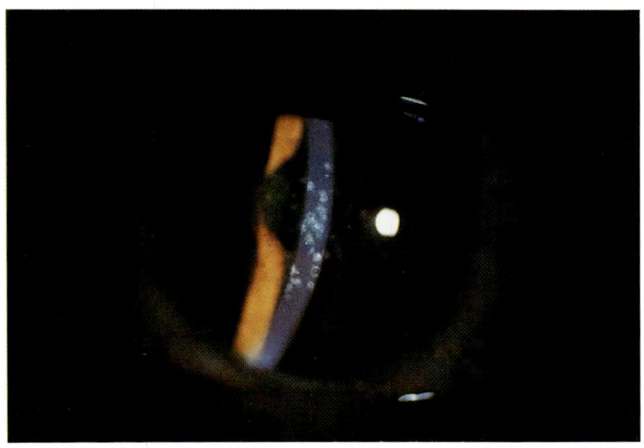

4–70 Granular dystrophy of the cornea. The lesions comprising granular corneal dystrophies occur at the level of the anterior stroma and involve the central cornea. Characteristically, they have sharp, irregular margins, making them resemble bread crumbs. The stromal areas between the lesions are clear; the peripheral cornea is not involved. The lesions in this patient enlarged progressively during the eight years that she was followed by the authors.

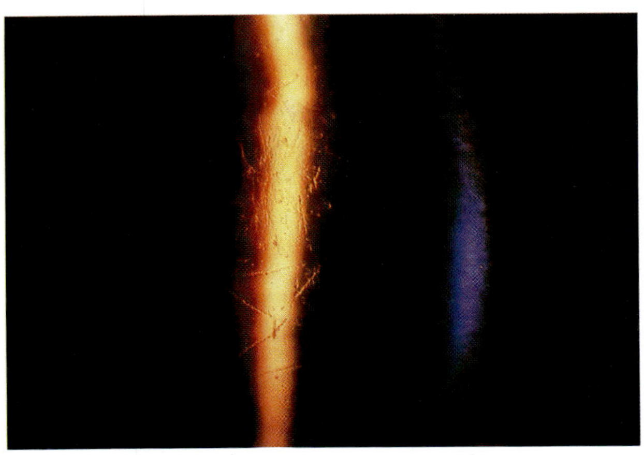

4–71 Lattice corneal dystrophy. Lattice dystrophy is characteristically composed of central refractile lines, white dots, and a central haze. The opacities become dense and the lines more radially oriented as the dystrophy increases in intensity. This slit lamp photograph distinctly outlines the linear appearance of the opacities.

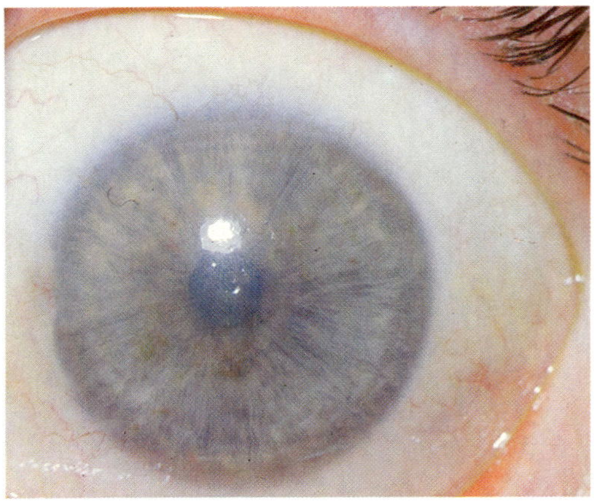

4–72 Fuchs' epithelial-endothelial dystrophy. Fuchs' epithelial-endothelial dystrophy begins in the endothelium. As the condition progresses, the stroma and eventually the epithelium become edematous because of endothelial failure. The epithelium then appears bedewed, as seen in this patient, and eventually large bullae may be formed.

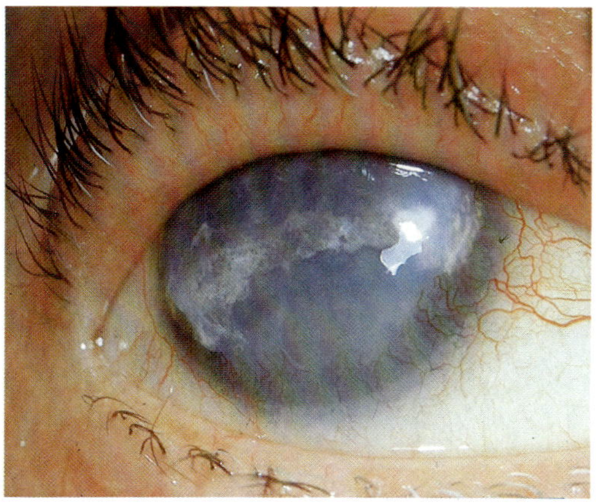

4–73 Band keratopathy. Band keratopathy has the appearance of a superficial grayish opacity interrupted by clear round zones of varying diameters. The opacity occurs in the interpalpebral area of the cornea, first in the peripheral cornea but eventually involving the central cornea. In this patient, a band keratopathy has developed in a badly scarred cornea. The gray opacity can be seen extending across the center of the cornea.

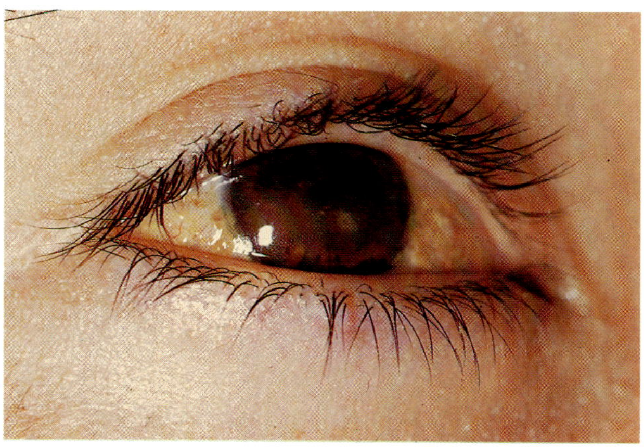

4–74 Climatic droplet (spheroidal) degeneration. Climatic droplet degeneration occurs in the interpalpebral areas of the cornea. The lesions consist of yellow-white oil-like droplets that develop subepithelially and subsequently coalesce to form a yellowish-gray subepithelial band. This patient was a 16-year-old male who developed such degenerative changes (Ahmad et al., 1977). (Reprinted with permission from *Archives of Ophthalmology.)*

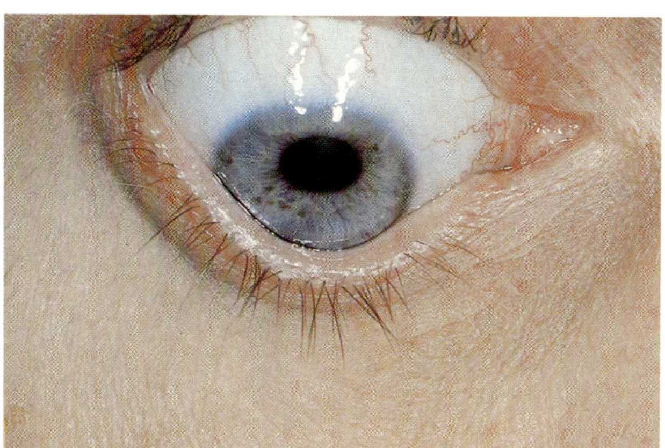

4–75 Keratoconus. The cone of keratoconus can often be seen by asking the patient to look down and then observing the lower eyelid to see if it is peaked centrally (Munson's sign), as is evident in this photograph of a patient with keratoconus.

Chapter 5

Infections and Inflammations of the Sclera and Episclera

Regardless of cause, an episcleritis or scleritis may be acute or chronic in nature. Episcleritis occurs more frequently than scleritis; it is often bilateral and is usually benign and self-limited, although recurrences are frequent. Scleritis, on the other hand, can be serious, leading to prolonged morbidity, loss of vision, and occasionally loss of the eye. Recurrences of scleritis are also frequent.

Episcleritis

Episcleritis is limited to the loose vascular connective tissue between the conjunctiva and the sclera. Except in herpes zoster, episcleritis does not spread to involve the sclera.

Classification

Clinically, episcleritis can be divided into a simple (diffuse) (Fig. 5–1) and a nodular form (Fig. 5–2). The simple form may be sectoral or may involve the entire anterior segment of the eye. The inflammatory reaction in the diffuse form is poorly circumscribed, and the involved area appears flat.

The nodular variety of scleritis appears elevated, and the inflammatory reaction is more intense than in the simple variety. The nodules are nontender, measure about 2 to 3 mm in diameter, and are freely movable over the underlying sclera. In some instances, the nodules become confluent, but they do not undergo necrosis. Nodular episcleritis is found most commonly in the interpalpebral area. Pingueculitis (Fig. 5–3) may be regarded as a nodular episcleritis.

Manifestations

The onset of episcleritis is usually acute and its manifestations include redness, tearing, and, in some cases, moderate pain. Occasionally the pain is severe, but even then it does not radiate. The injection is usually bright red (Fig. 5–4) without the bluish or violaceous hue that occurs with scleritis.

Episcleritis usually persists for two to three weeks, but may last for only five days or for many months. Characteristically, the nodular form lasts longer than the simple form; both may be recurrent. In both types, the inflammatory reaction usually recurs in a different area than the previous attack, and a nodular episcleritis may recur as a simple form or vice versa. Recurrences of episcleritis usually occur within three to six years, but have been reported to occur as late as 30 years after the initial attack.

Associated Diseases

Episcleritis occurs more commonly between the ages of 30 and 40 years and more frequently in women. In about 70 percent of cases, no etiology for the episcleritis is found. Some cases (about 5%) are associated with connective tissue diseases, especially rheumatoid arthritis (Fig. 5–5), while about 3 percent are associated with gout. About 10 percent of episcleritis is associated with systemic infections, especially herpes zoster (7%), while a few cases are caused by syphilis, herpes simplex, tuberculosis, the Epstein-Barr virus, Hansen's disease, staphylococcal blepharitis in association with acne rosacea, and coccidioidomycosis. Other causes of episcleritis include ophthalmia nodosum (which occurs from a foreign-body reaction to caterpillar hairs), sarcoid, Wegener's granulomatosis (Bullen et al., 1983) and Crohn's disease (Petrelli et al., 1982). Recently, recurrent episcleritis has also been found to be associated with Berger's disease (a primary glomerulonephritis) and other nephropathies with IgA and/or isolated C3 deposits (Sirbert et al., 1983).

Episcleritis occurring with herpes zoster ophthalmicus usually develops during the course of the skin eruption or at the time it is subsiding. Herpes simplex infection of the episclera is commonly associated with a linear or dendritic marginal corneal lesion and absent corneal sensation (see Chapter 4). An episcleritis caused by staphylococcal infection, tuberculosis, coccidioidomycosis, syphilis or the Epstein-Barr virus (infectious mononucleosis) (Fig. 5–6) is usually nondescript and probably the result of a delayed hypersensitivity reaction to antigens of the infecting organism.

Although the episcleritis associated with Hansen's disease gives nonspecific findings (Fig. 5–7), it is usually bilaterally symmetrical and occurs at the limbus. As the inflammation progresses, the episcleritis may spread either circumferentially or posteriorly.

Sequelae

The main sequelae of episcleritis are mild opacification and thinning of the adjacent cornea, which occurs in about 15 percent of cases. When glaucoma occurs, it is usually caused by the topical application of glucocorticoids, which are frequently used in the treatment of episcleritis.

Scleritis

Scleritis, unlike episcleritis, can be serious because of its tendency to become chronic and to cause severe sequelae, including severe pain, uveitis (Wilhelmus et al., 1981), thinning and perforation of the sclera, and loss of vision. It is an inflammatory process of the dense, rigid, scleral tissue, and usually involves both sclera and episclera.

Manifestations

The manifestations of scleritis (Watson, 1980) usually develop gradually and include redness, tearing, tenderness of the globe, and a deep or aching pain that is commonly referred to the forehead, jaw, or temple. More than half of the cases are bilateral. With the exception of scleromalacia perforans, a form of necrotizing scleritis that causes few or no signs of associated scleral inflammation and no pain, the pain of scleritis is often intense and probably arises from edema and distortion of the sensory nerve endings. In the necrotizing type of scleritis accompanied by signs of inflammation (see below) the pain may arise from actual destruction of the nerve endings.

Examination in natural light of a patient with scleritis reveals a bluish or violaceous-reddish hue of the involved sclera (Fig. 5–8), which results from engorgement of the deep (superficial and deep episcleral) vessels. With the aid of the slit lamp, the inflammatory edema within the sclera can be seen to displace the deep and superficial episcleral vessels anteriorly; in episcleritis only the superficial scleral vessels are displaced anteriorly.

Classification

Depending upon its location, scleritis is classified as anterior or posterior. Anterior scleritis is further divided into diffuse anterior, nodular anterior, and necrotizing anterior scleritis. Necrotizing anterior scleritis can be further subdivided into necrotizing scleritis with inflammation and necrotizing scleritis without inflammation (scleromalacia perforans).

Anterior Scleritis

Diffuse Anterior Scleritis

Diffuse anterior scleritis accounts for about 40 percent of the cases of scleritis. It occurs most commonly in women between the ages of 40 and 70 years, and about 25 percent of the patients have a systemic disease such as rheumatoid arthritis, ankylosing spondylitis, gout, or varicella-zoster ophthalmicus. The inflammatory lesion is widespread, nonelevated, poorly circumscribed, and often involves the entire anterior portion of the globe (Figs. 5–9, 5–10).

Nodular Anterior Scleritis

Nodular anterior scleritis comprises about 30 percent of cases of scleritis and occurs primarily in women aged 40 to 60 years. Its onset is insidious, and the known associated systemic diseases include rheumatoid arthritis, varicella-zoster, and gout. The nodule is fixed to the sclera, tender to touch, and does not progress to necrosis, although the sclera may appear clear beneath the severly congested episclera. The nodules frequently occur in the superior part of the globe.

Necrotizing Anterior Scleritis

The necrotizing form of anterior scleritis has a poor prognosis and 40 percent of patients develop significant loss of vision. Furthermore, unless appropriately treated with systemic immunosuppressives, about one-third of patients with necrotizing anterior scleritis die within five years following onset (Foster et al., 1984). Vasoobliterative changes have been demonstrated in necrotizing anterior scleritis by the use of anterior segment fluorescein angiography (Watson and Young, 1985).

About 15 percent of scleritis cases are of the necrotizing type; in the majority (about two-thirds) of these cases there is minimal or no surrounding inflammation. Histological examination, however, shows abundant numbers of plasma cells, lymphocytes, and mast cells (Young and Watson, 1984a and b); active fibroblasts and macrophages with phagocytized collagen fibrils; and swollen and unraveled scleral collagen fibrils (Young and Watson, 1984).

Necrotizing Scleritis with Surrounding Inflammation. Necrotizing scleritis with surrounding inflammation has a subacute onset. It usually occurs in young and middle-aged women, and more than half of all cases are bilateral. The pain increases progressively and eventually may become severe enough to require narcotics. Redness and chemosis are prominent early features, followed later by development of avascular patches with intense peripheral injection (Figs. 5–13, 5–14). The overlying conjunctiva may be absorbed as a result of the inflammatory process (Fig. 5–15). Necrotizing scleritis is frequently associated with rheumatoid arthritis and other connective tissue diseases.

The complications resulting from the inflammatory form of necrotizing scleritis include sloughing of the sclera, staphyloma (Fig. 5–16), scleral perforation (usually following trauma), scarring of the cornea (Fig. 5–17), and ring ulcer (which may be confused with Mooren's ulcer, except for the severe involvement of the sclera).

Necrotizing Scleritis without Inflammation. Necrotizing scleritis without inflammation (scleromalacia perforans) represents about 10 percent of cases of scleritis. It is characterized by lack of pain, and signs of yellow or white nontender necrotic nodules (Figs. 5–18, 5–19), which later regress to leave scleral thinning and staphyloma formation. This form of scleritis usually occurs in women over the age of 40 years, and more than half of these patients have crippling, long-standing rheumatoid arthritis.

Diseases Associated with Anterior Scleritis

Many diseases are associated with anterior scleritis. These include rheumatoid arthritis (Figs. 5–15, 5–18, 5–19), systemic lupus erythematosus, polyarteritis nodosa, Reiter's syndrome, Wegener's granulomatosis (Bullen et al., 1983; Vogiatzis, 1983), a limited form of Wegener's granulomatosis (Spalton et al., 1981), giant cell arteritis, erythema nodosum, relapsing polychondritis, other vasculitides and connective tissue diseases, gout (Fig. 5–20), necrobiotic xanthogranuloma with paraproteinemia (Robertson and Winkelmann, 1984), ulcerative colitis, and Crohn's disease (Fig. 5–21) (Petrelli et al., 1982). Anterior scleritis has also been reported to occur following cataract surgery (Salamon et al., 1982). In some instances the scleritis may precede the systemic findings, such as in rheumatoid arthritis (Kleiner et al., 1984).

Systemic infections that cause a scleritis include herpes zoster (Figs. 5–8, 5–22) (Womack and Liesgang, 1983), tuberculosis (Fig. 5–23), Hansen's disease (Hogweg and Leiker, 1983) (Fig. 5–24), syphilis, and onchocerciasis. Direct infection of the sclera without systemic disease occurs with infectious agents such as *Pseudomonas* spp., *Aspergillus* spp. (Stenson et al., 1982), *Lasiodiplodia* spp. (Slomovic et al., 1985), and *Acanthameba* spp. Direct infection of the sclera with *Mycobacterium tuberculosis* (Fig. 5–23) and *Pseudomonas* spp. (Fig. 5–25) (Cordère et al., 1981) causes scleral ulceration.

Herpes zoster causes a diffuse scleritis, often preceded by episcleritis. Like the episcleritis in herpes zoster, the scleritis occurs at about the time that the skin lesions begin to crust, suggesting an immune-complex mediated reaction. Scleritis associated with Hansen's disease usually occurs in the upper temporal quadrant and is nodular in type. It occurs in association with the lepromatous form of the diesease. The scleritis associated with episodes of syphilis, onchocerciasis, or *Acanthameba* spp. infection is diffuse in type.

Sequelae of Anterior Scleritis

Corneal changes occur in about 30 percent of cases of scleritis and consist of opacification, vascularization (Figs. 5–26A and B), and thinning. The cornea is involved in the mid or deep stroma in areas adjacent to the scleritis. The corneal thinning begins as a peripheral furrow and progresses to loss of the corneal epithelium (Fig. 5–27), marked stromal thinning, and eventual perforation. The corneal melting is usually painless.

Recurrent attacks of scleritis may occur anywhere on the globe, and the recurrent attacks may persist for more than five years. An associated iritis with findings of 1+ to 2+ cells and flare is common. In rare instances, a scleritis may present as a sclerouveitis in which the uveitis is more severe than the scleritis (Wilhelmus et al., 1981).

Thinning of the sclera may occur with diffuse and nodular forms of anterior scleritis (Womack and Liesgang, 1983) and necrotizing scleritis. The involved sclera becomes gray or blue and in some instances a rearrangement of the sclera may occur instead of true thinning. In some instances a staphyloma occurs, especially if glaucoma supervenes (Fig. 5–28). Glaucoma occurs in about 12 percent of cases of scleritis and arises from blockade of scleral outflow channels, ciliary body swelling and angle closure, or choroidal effusion, or it may be induced by the use of glucocorticoids (Wilhelmus et al., 1981).

Posterior Scleritis

Posterior scleritis is recognized in about 2 percent of cases of scleritis. In many instances it is probably missed, especially when it occurs in association with an anterior scleritis (Fig. 5–29), in which cases it represents a posterior extension of the anterior scleritis.

Manifestations

The manifestions of posterior scleritis include pain

and proptosis, limitation of ocular movement, retraction of the lower eyelid, reduced visual acuity, and shallowing of the anterior chamber. Fundus changes may include exudative retinal detachment (Fig. 5–30) (Berger and Reeser, 1981), annular choroidal detachment, a subretinal mass, chorioretinal changes, and edema of the optic nerve head and macula. Other findings include thickening of the posterior sclera (Fig. 5–31) (Rochels and Reis, 1980), and a double shadow on B-scan (Marushak, 1982).

Differential Diagnosis

The differential diagnosis of posterior scleritis includes orbital pseudotumor, intraocular tumors (Yeo et al., 1983), and uveal effusion syndrome. In some instances, a posterior scleritis is associated with a uveal effusion syndrome.

References

Berger, B, and Reeser, F: Retinal pigment epithelial detachments in posterior scleritis. *Am. J. Ophthalmol.* 90: 604–606, 1981.

Bullen, CL, Liesgang, TJ, McDonald, TJ, and Deremee, RA: Ocular complications of Wegener's granulomatosis. *Ophthalmology* 90: 279–290, 1983.

Cordère, F, Brownstein, S, and Jackson, WB: *Pseudomonas aeruginosa* scleritis. *Am. J. Ophthalmol.* 91: 706–710, 1981.

Foster, CS, Forstot, SL, and Wilson, LA: Mortality rate in rheumatoid arthritis patients developing necrotizing scleritis or peripheral ulcerative keratitis. Effects of systemic immunosuppression. *Ophthalmology* 91: 1253–1263, 1984.

Hogweg, M, and Leiker, DL: A survey on eye involvement among leprosy patients in the Netherlands. *Doc. Ophthalmol.* 56: 69–76, 1983.

Kleiner, RC, Raber, IM, and Passero, FC: Scleritis, pericarditis and aortic insufficiency in a patient with rheumatoid arthritis. *Ophthalmology* 91: 941–946, 1984.

Marushak, D: Uveal effusion attending posterior scleritis. A case report with A-scan and B-scan echograms. *Acta Ophthalmol.* 60: 773–778, 1982.

Petrelli, EA, McKinley, M, and Troncale, FL: Ocular manifestations of inflammatory bowel disease. *Ann. Ophthalmol.* 14: 356–360, 1982.

Robertson, DM, and Winkelmann, RK: Ophthalmic features of necrobiotic xanthogranuloma with paraproteinemia. *Am. J. Ophthalmol.* 97: 173–183, 1984.

Rochels, R, and Reis, G: Echographie bei skleritis posterior. *Klin. Monatsbl. Augenheilkd.* 177: 611–613, 1980.

Salamon, SM, Mondino, BJ, and Zaidman, GW: Peripheral corneal ulcers, conjunctival ulcers, and scleritis after cataract surgery. *Am. J. Ophthalmol.* 93: 334–337, 1982.

Sirbert, D, Saudax, E, Hurault de Ligny, B, Bene, MC, and Raspiller, A: A new etiology of episcleritis: Nephropathies with IgA and/or isolated C3 deposits. *J. Fr. Ophtalmol.* 6: 921–925, 1983.

Slomovic, AR, Forster, RK, and Gelender, H: *Lasiodiplodia theobromae* panophthalmitis. *Can. J. Ophthalmol.* 20: 225–228, 1985.

Spalton, DJ, Graham, EM, Page, NGR, and Sanders, MD: Ocular changes in limited forms of Wegener's granulomatosis. *Br. J. Ophthalmol.* 65: 553–563, 1981.

Stenson, S, Brookner, A, and Rosenthal, S: Bilateral endogenous necrotizing scleritis due to *Aspergillus oryzae*. *Ann. Ophthalmol.* 14: 67–72, 1982.

Vogiatzis, KV: Bilateral blindness due to necrotizing scleritis in a case of Wegener's granulomatosis. *Ann. Ophthalmol.* 15: 185–188, 1983.

Watson, PG, and Young, RD: Changes at the periphery of a lesion in necrotising scleritis: Anterior segment fluorescein angiography correlated with electron microscopy. *Br. J. Ophthalmol.* 69: 656–663, 1985.

Watson, PG: The diagnosis and management of scleritis. *Ophthalmology* 87: 716–720, 1980.

Wilhelmus, KR, Watson, PG, Vasavada, AR: Uveitis associated with scleritis. *Trans. Ophthalmol. Soc. UK* 101: 351–356, 1981.

Womack, LW, Liesgang, TJ: Complications of Herpes Zoster Ophthalmicus. *Arch. Ophthalmol.* 101: 42–45, 1983.

Yeo, JH, Jakobiec, FA, Iwamoto, T, Brown, R, and Harrison, W: Metastatic carcinoma masquerading as a scleritis. *Ophthalmology* 90: 184–194, 1983.

Young, RD, and Watson, PG: Microscopic studies of necrotizing scleritis. I. Cellular aspects. *Br. J. Ophthalmol.* 68: 770–780, 1984a.

Young, RD, and Watson, PG: Microscopic studies of necrotizing scleritis. II. Collagen degradation in the scleral stroma. *Br. J. Ophthalmol.* 68: 781–789, 1984b.

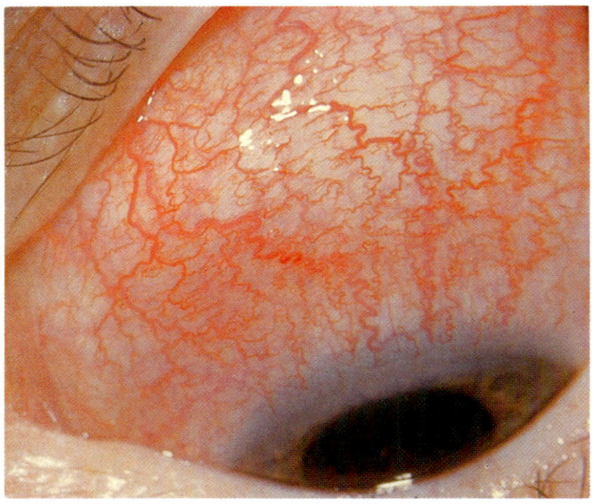

5–1 Simple episcleritis. Simple diffuse episcleritis is present in this 43-year-old female with rheumatoid arthritis. The surface overlying the episcleritis is not elevated and the margins of the inflammatory lesion are indistinct. Both the conjunctival vessels and the superficial episcleral vessels are engorged. The conjunctival appear tortuous and can be seen superficial to the superficial episcleral vessels.

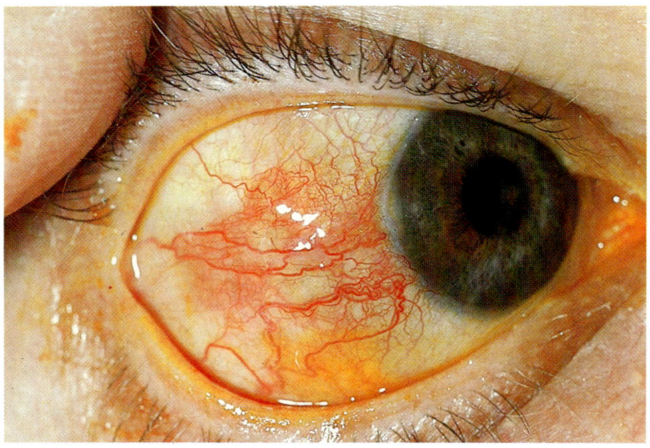

5–2 Nodular episcleritis. A nodular episcleritis has an elevated surface. The nodules are small, may be single or multiple, and may coalesce, as has occurred in this 37-year-old male. Dilated superficial vessels can be seen coursing over the nodule and superficial episcleral vessels can be seen within the nodule.

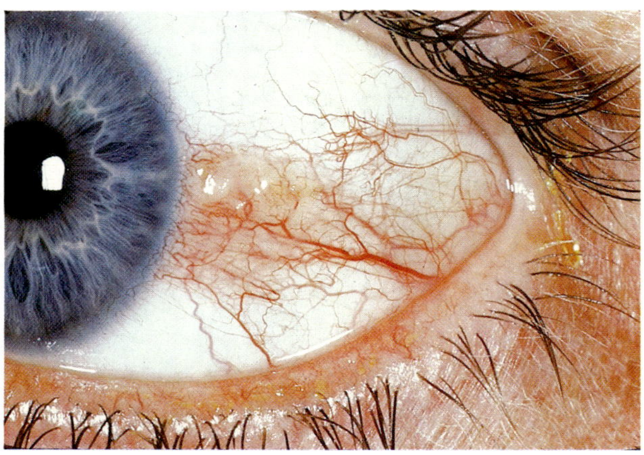

5–3 Pingueculitis. Pingueculitis represents an inflammation of the episclera underlying a pinguecula. It is probably one form of nodular episcleritis and is similar to other forms except that a pinguecula is present in the area of inflammation. In this patient, the episcleritis is readily evident, together with a large conjunctival vessel leading to the pinguecula. The underlying superficial episcleral vessels are readily seen. Some yellow crusting, which is unrelated to the pingueculitis, is visible at the lateral canthus.

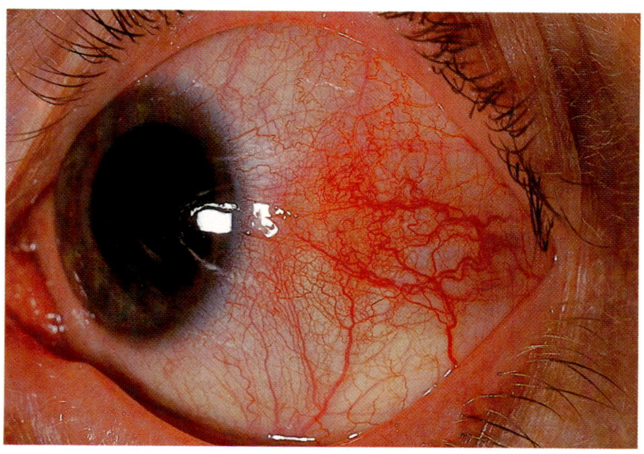

5–4 Simple episcleritis. Episcleritis is bright red or brick red in color. In this 33-year-old male with a sectoral form of simple episcleritis due to Reiter's syndrome, redness is caused by engorgement of the conjunctival vessels and the superficial episcleral vessels. Both the conjunctival and superficial episcleral vessels are visible.

5–5 Episcleritis associated with rheumatoid arthritis. Although no cause can be found for an episcleritis in about 70 percent of cases, several systemic conditions are known to cause episcleral inflammation. Rheumatoid arthritis is associated with an episcleritis in about 5 percent of cases. In this 64-year-old female, a diffuse episcleritis developed in association with severe rheumatoid arthritis. The red conjunctival vessels and the deeper more bluish-appearing superficial episcleral vessels can be readily identified. There is mild injection of the palpebral conjunctiva.

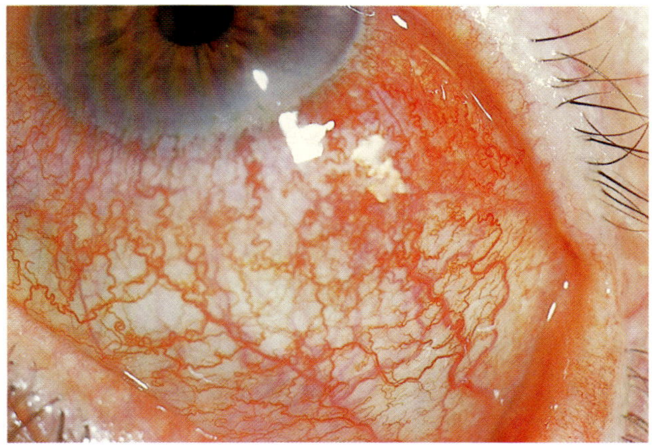

5–6 Episcleritis associated with infectious mononucleosis. The episcleritis associated with Epstein-Barr viral infections is nondescript. In this 47-year-old female, episcleritis occured in the course of infectious mononucleosis and persisted for 3½ weeks. The dilated conjunctival and superficial episcleral vessels are visible in this photograph.

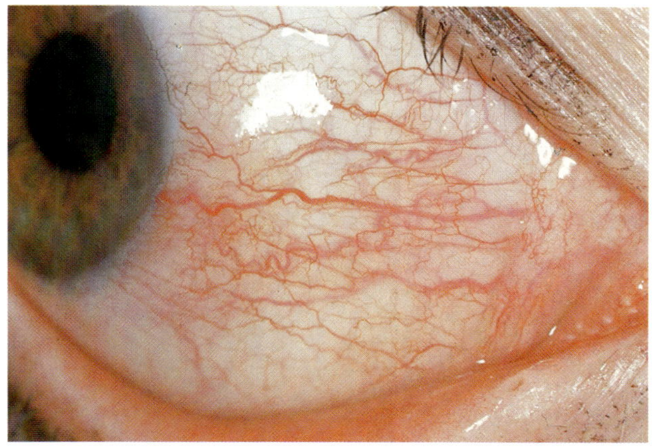

5–7 Episcleritis associated with Hansen's disease. The episcleritis associated with Hansen's disease is often bilateral and often occurs near the limbus. The simple episcleritis in this patient with Hansen's disease is intense and diffuse. Note how the inflammation abuts directly onto the limbus and extends as far posteriorly as one can see. The xanthelasma noted in the upper nasal eyelid of each eye is not related to Hansen's disease or to the episcleritis.

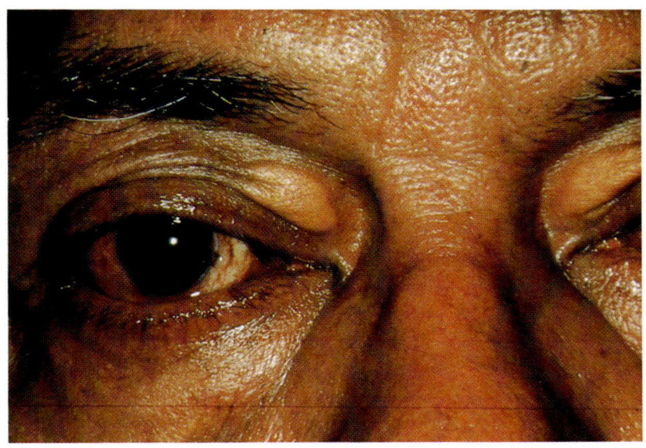

5–8 Violaceous or bluish hue associated with anterior scleritis (see Fig. 5–13). The injection associated with a scleritis has a violaceous or bluish hue when the eye is examined in daylight, which is due to the engorgement of the deep (superficial and deep) episcleral vessels. In this patient with anterior scleritis due to herpes zoster, intense injection and chemosis is noted nasally, and the violaceous hue is more readily apparent inferiorly. Early superficial vascularization of the cornea is occurring nasally and there is some irregularity of the corneal surface, which can be appreciated by the distortion of the light reflex.

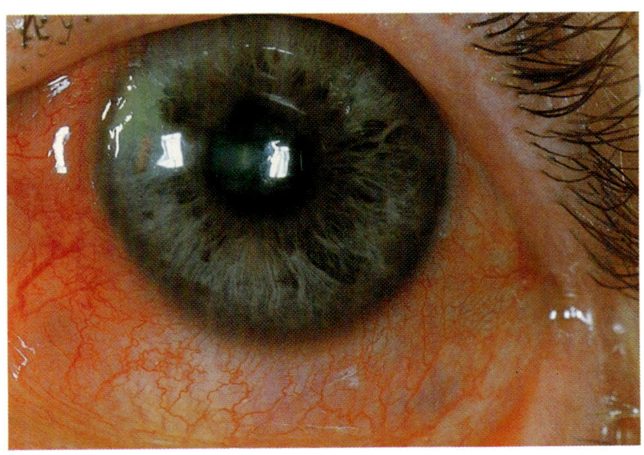

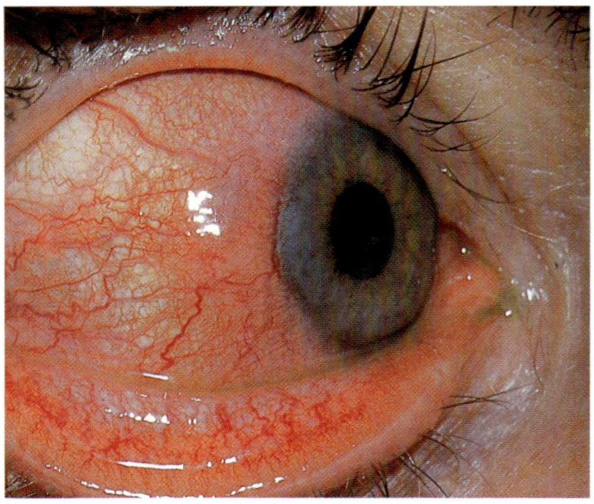

5–9 Diffuse anterior scleritis. A diffuse anterior scleritis is flat, poorly demarcated, and may involve the entire anterior segment of the globe. Diffuse violaceous injection and dilation of the superficial and deep episcleral vessels is readily apparent in this 47-year-old female.

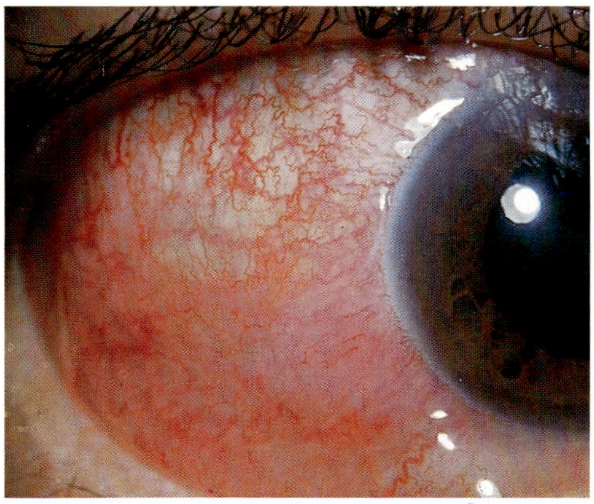

5–10 Violaceous hue in diffuse anterior scleritis. The diffuse scleral inflammation involving the entire anterior portion of the globe is apparent in this 43-year-old female. There is a violaceous hue and the overlying episcleral and conjunctival edema are readily evident.

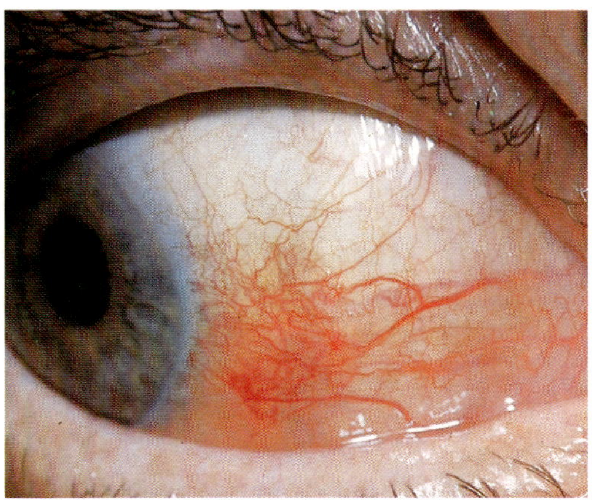

5–11 Nodular anterior scleritis. The nodules making up a nodular anterior scleritis are elevated and fixed to the underlying sclera. The inflammation is usually more intense than that occurring in diffuse anterior scleritis. The nodule in this 42-year-old male is adjacent to the limbus. Dilated conjunctival vessels and dilated deep vessels can be seen coursing toward the nodule.

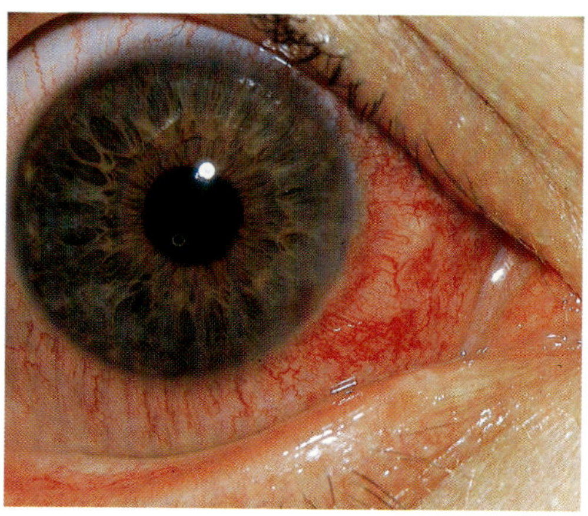

5–12 Nodular anterior scleritis due to ulcerative colitis. The nodules of anterior nodular scleritis may be single, as in this patient with ulcerative colitis, or multiple. In some instances several nodules may fuse to form a very large nodule. Superficial corneal neovascularization is visible adjacent to the nodule in this patient, and an area of hemorrhage is evident in the corneal stroma. Both deep and superficial dilated vessels are prominent in the nodule.

5–13 Necrotizing anterior scleritis with surrounding inflammation. This is associated with prominent redness and edema early in the course of the inflammation, as noted in this 67-year-old female. Subsequently, avascular patches and thinning of the sclera develop. There is intense superficial and deep injection, and scleral thinning is present medially.

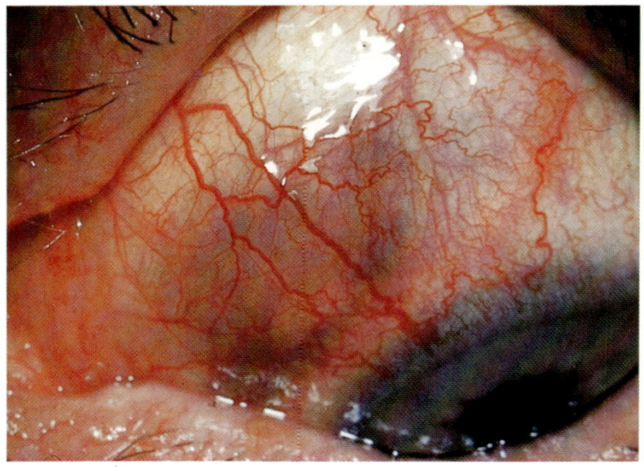

5–14 Necrotizing anterior scleritis with surrounding inflammation and staphyloma formation. Severe necrosis in necrotizing scleritis with surrounding inflammation may lead to marked thinning and eventual staphyloma formation, as has occurred in this patient. The pain is usually intense, and narcotics may be required for its relief. Evidence of scleral thinning resulting from previous inflammation can be seen superiorly.

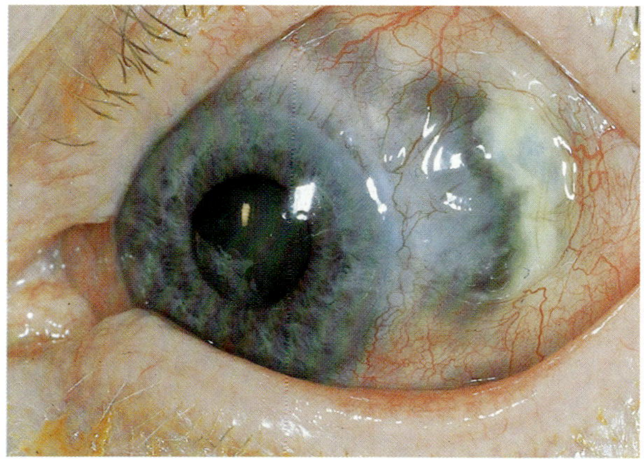

5–15 Necrotizing anterior scleritis with absorption of the overlying conjunctiva. The inflammatory process in necrotizing scleritis may be sufficiently intense to cause necrosis of the overlying conjunctiva, as has occurred in five separate areas in this 55-year-old female with severe rheumatoid arthritis and necrotizing scleritis with inflammation.

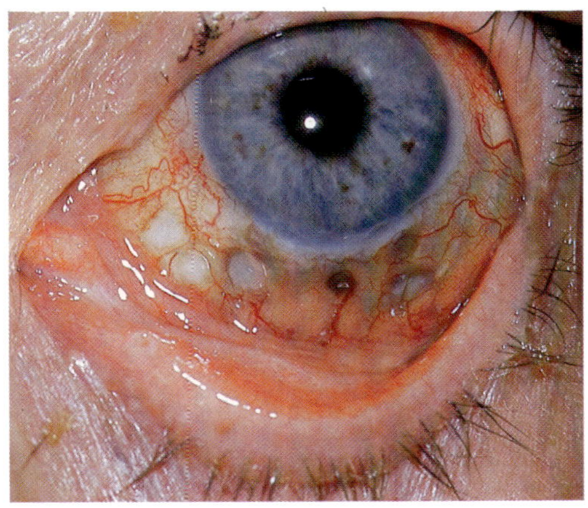

5–16 Staphyloma. (See also Figs. 5–14, 5–28.) One of the major complications of necrotizing scleritis is the formation of a staphyloma, such as is evident in this 68-year-old female with rheumatoid arthritis. The staphyloma may be located circumferentially, as in this patient. Superficial corneal neovascularization is also evident.

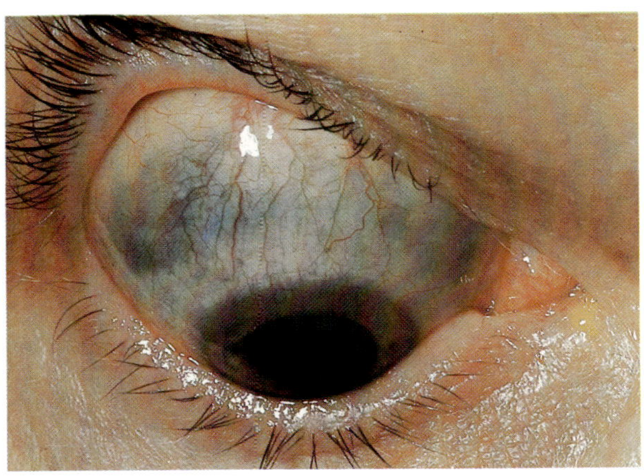

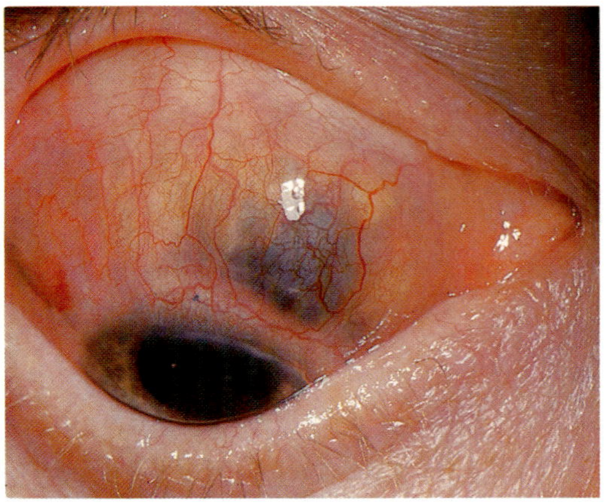

5–17 Marginal keratitis in necrotizing scleritis with inflammation. Marginal keratitis progressing to scarring of the cornea is a major complication of necrotizing scleritis. This patient with rheumatoid arthritis developed corneal involvement and a staphyloma from necrotizing scleritis. Areas of continuing necrosis are evident posterior to the staphyloma.

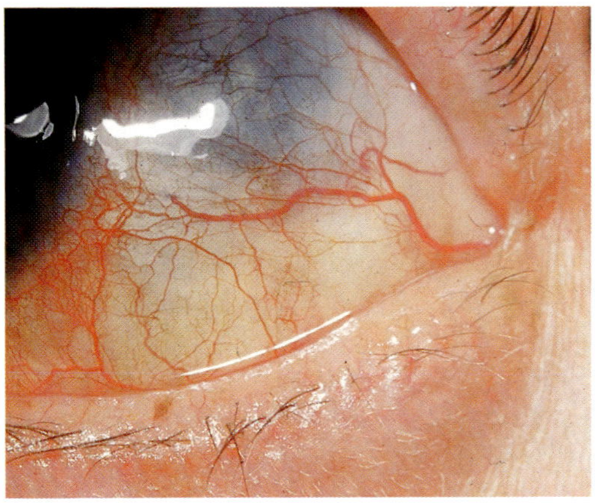

5–18 Necrotizing anterior scleritis without surrounding inflammation. This is characterized by the development of yellow or white nontender avascular nodules which become necrotic and later regress to leave scleral thinning and staphyloma. In this 72-year-old male with rheumatoid arthritis, two white nodules inferior to the area of scleral thinning probably represent rheumatoid nodules. Although there is minimal surrounding inflammation, the scleral thinning later spread to involve these nodular areas.

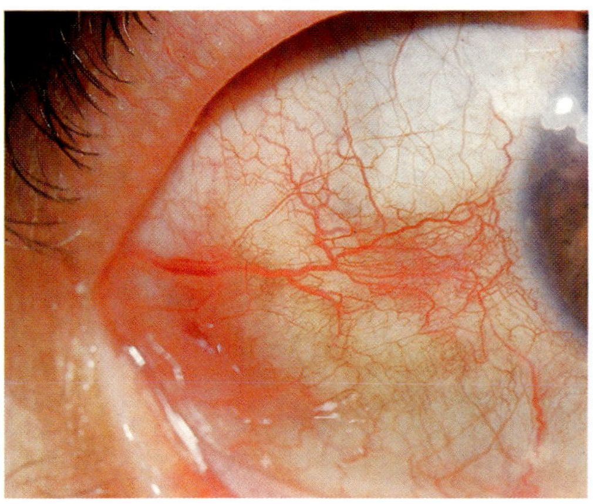

5–19 White nontender necrotic nodules of necrotizing anterior scleritis without inflammation. A large, white nontender necrotic nodule is visible just inferior to the dilated superficial and deep vessels in this 49-year-old male with rheumatoid arthritis.

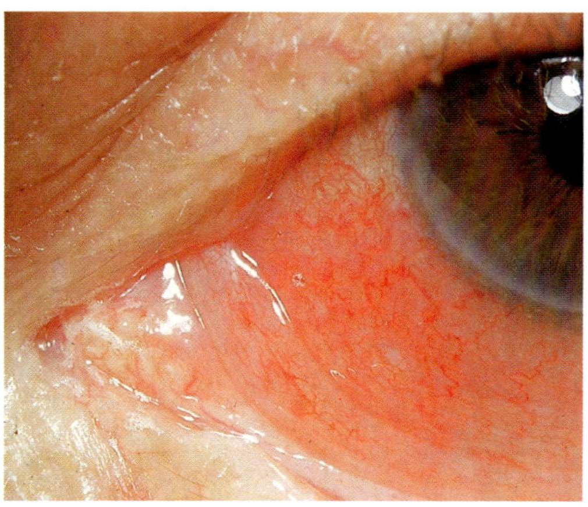

5–20 Scleritis associated with gout. This 59-year-old male developed scleritis in association with an attack of gout. There is superficial and deep vascular engorgement. Although the scleritis recurred independently of other manifestations of gout, strict control of the patient's uric acid level eventually controlled both the scleritis and the gouty arthritis.

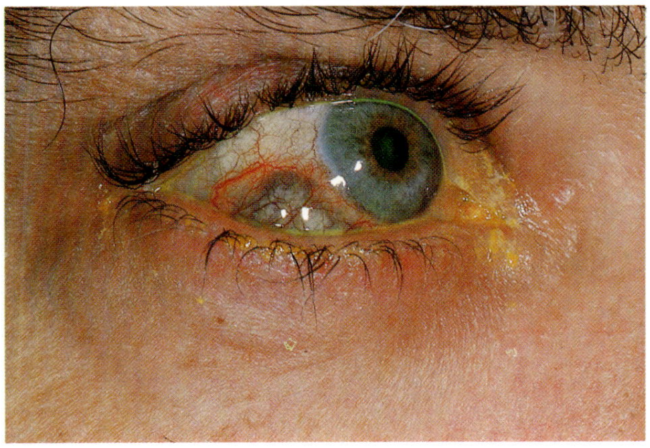

5–21 Scleritis associated with Crohn's disease. This 29-year-old male with Crohn's disease had had several attacks of necrotizing scleritis; the attacks were often unrelated to manifestations of Crohn's disease. After a particularly severe attack of scleritis, this staphyloma developed. The patient showed a mild contact hypersensitivity to the combination antibiotic-glucocorticoid drop he was using, as evidenced by the wrinkling and thickening of the skin of the lid near the medial canthus.

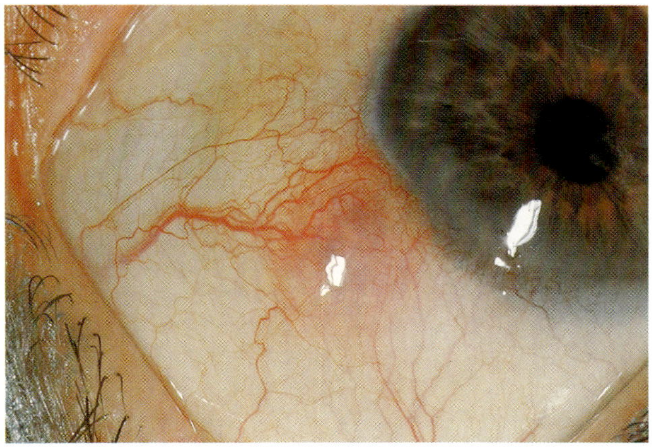

5–22 Anterior nodular scleritis associated with herpes zoster. An anterior scleritis developed in this 37-year-old female with herpes zoster at the time when all her skin lesions had either crusted or completely disappeared. Slight thinning of the sclera which became more marked as the scleritis progressed, is evident in this photograph. Both deep and superficial injection are seen.

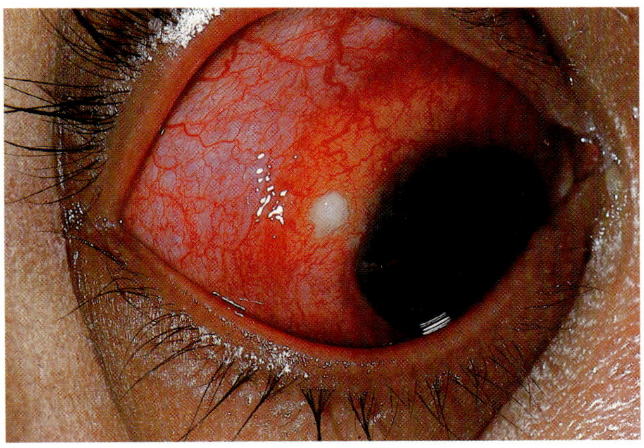

5–23 Ulcerative scleritis due to tuberculosis. This 34-year-old Filipino woman complained of redness, pain, photophobia, and blurred vision. She had a single scleral ulcer in each eye; her chest X-ray revealed cavitationary lung lesions. The scleral ulcers gradually healed after antituberculous therapy. (A photograph of her other eye is present in Chapter 3, Fig. 3–38.)

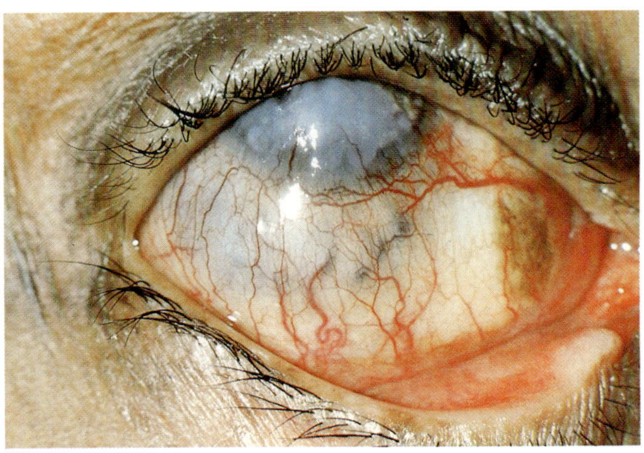

5–24 Staphyloma in Hansen's disease. The staphylomas that develop in Hansen's disease may be very large and in some instances may cause disorganization of the entire globe. In this Egyptian woman, a staphyloma is evident along with an exposure keratitis. The brown pigment occurring nasally is a racial pigmentation and is unrelated to the scleritis or the Hansen's disease.

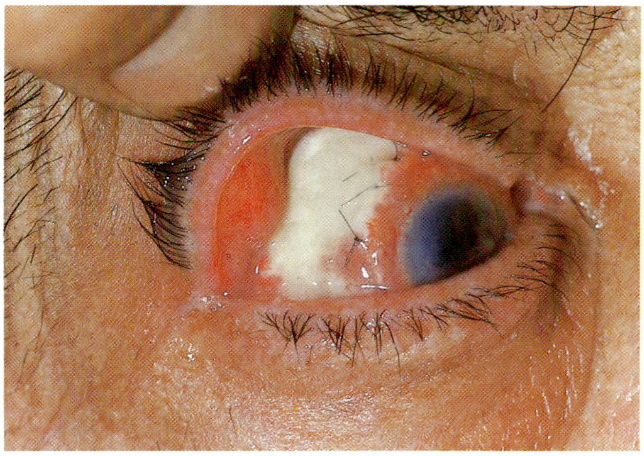

5–25 Ulcerative scleritis due to *Pseudomonas aeruginosa*. This 76-year-old male developed a scleral abscess due to an infection with *P. aeruginosa,* following the insertion of a Lincoff intrascleral sponge for a retinal detachment. The infection persisted after removal of the sponge and the administration of topical and systemic antibiotic therapy. Treatment by continuous irrigation with gentamicin led to healing. Scleral necrosis is evident together with a peripheral keratitis. The sutures were placed at the time of removal of the Lincoff sponge.

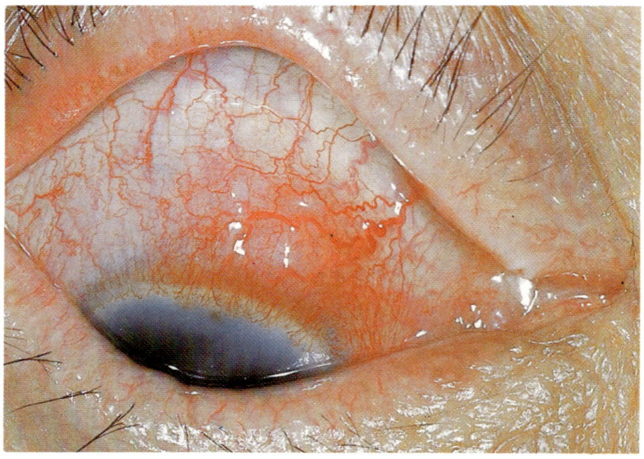

5–26A Neovascularization of the cornea in nodular scleritis. Neovascularization and opacification of the cornea may develop adjacent to an area of anterior scleritis, as in this 67-year-old patient with nodular scleritis that developed following an attack of herpes zoster ophthalmicus. The superficial corneal vessels are prominent in this photograph and mask the vessels in the mid-stroma. Early opacification is evident in the midcorneal stroma. Superficial vessels course over the nodule, while the deep vessels cannot be seen because of edema of the scleral and episcleral tissue.

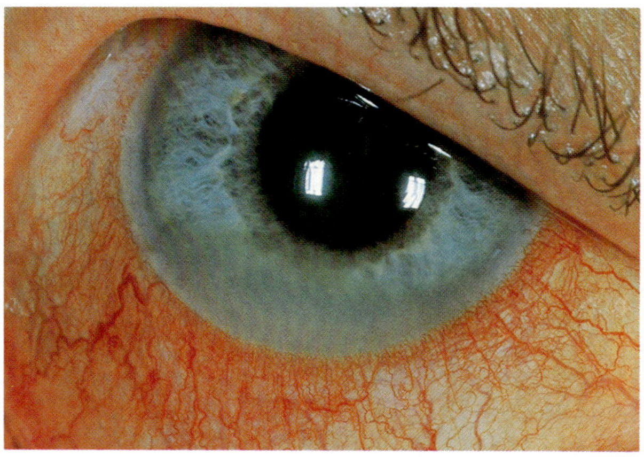

5–26B Infiltration of the anterior and midcorneal stroma in diffuse scleritis. Inflammatory infiltration of the anterior and midcorneal stroma, which later became vascularized, is evident in this 48-year-old female with a diffuse anterior scleritis.

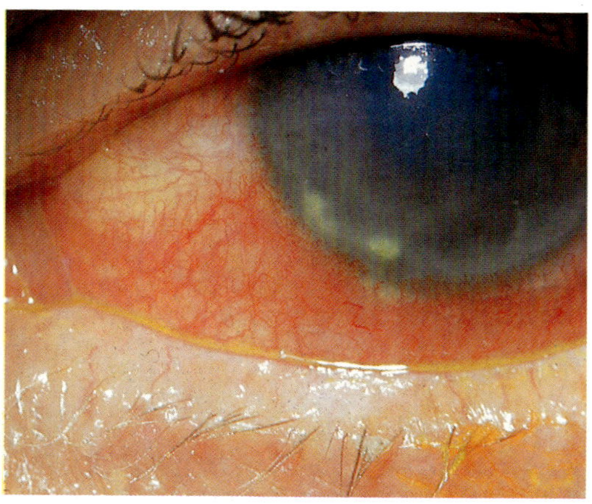

5–27 Marginal corneal furrow with loss of overlying corneal epithelium in diffuse anterior scleritis. This 57-year-old male with severe rheumatoid arthritis developed a marginal corneal furrow and ulceration (stained with fluorescein) during an acute attack of diffuse anterior scleritis. The cornea subsequently became vascularized in that area. Note the marked haziness and early superficial neovascularization of the inferior cornea.

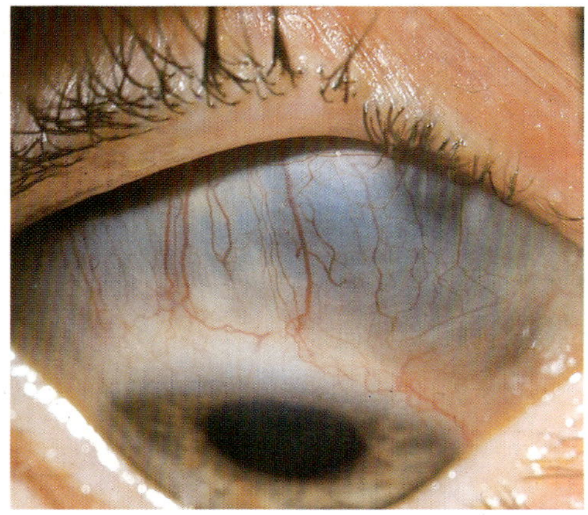

5–28 Extensive staphyloma in a patient with rheumatoid arthritis. Staphylomas may be small and localized or extensive, as in this patient who had severe rheumatoid arthritis and a necrotizing anterior scleritis. The conjunctiva is intact and conjunctival vessels course over the staphyloma.

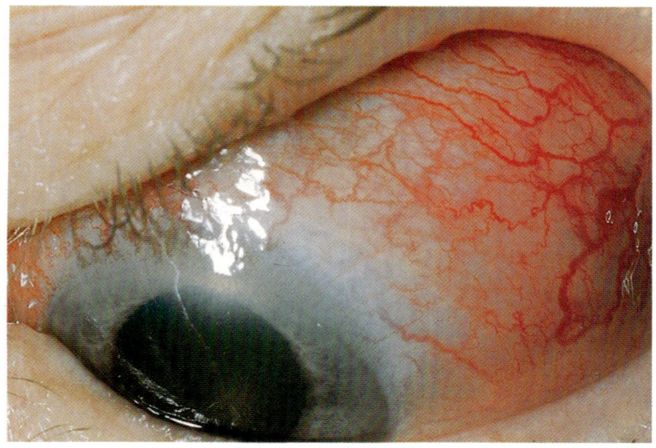

5–29 Posterior scleritis in association with an anterior scleritis. This 62-year-old physician developed pain, proptosis, limitation of extraocular movement, and decreased vision during hospitalization for treatment of an ulcerative colitis. A diffuse anterior scleritis, which is more marked towards the equator of the globe, can be seen. The posterior scleritis is, of course, not visible.

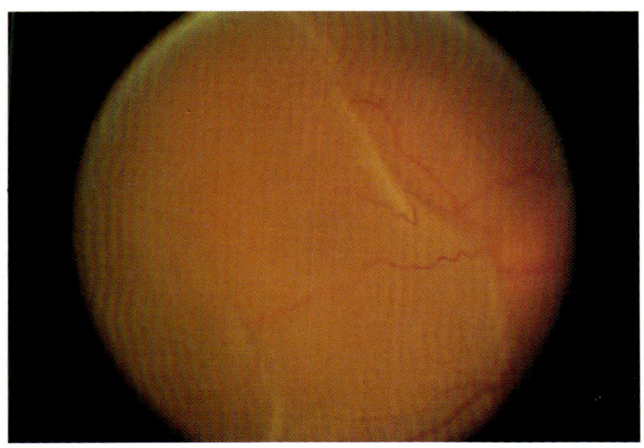

5–30 Exudative retinal detachment associated with posterior scleritis. The patient shown in Figs. 5–29 and 5–31 was noted to have an exudative retinal detachment, which accounted for his reduced vision. The retinal detachment subsided with systemic glucocorticoid treatment.

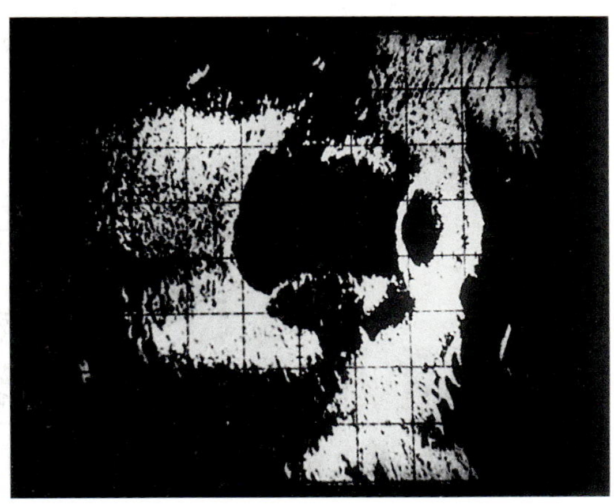

5–31 B-scan (ultrasound) examination of patient with posterior scleritis. A B-scan of the patient shown in Figs. 5–29 and 5–30 revealed marked thickening of the posterior sclera.

Chapter 6

Infections and Inflammations of the Lacrimal Apparatus

The surface of the eye is partially protected by the tears, which dilute and flush material entering the conjunctival sac and carry the material into the lacrimal sac and eventually into the nose. A valuable protective adjunct to tears is the mucus produced by the conjunctival goblet cells (Fig. 6–1), which helps protect the surface of the eye by its scavenging action. Diseases of the lacrimal apparatus may therefore threaten the integrity of the eye and cause loss of vision or even blindness. Such diseases include decreased or absent tear formation, which is common in middle-aged and older women; the uncommon infections and inflammations of the secretory portion of the lacrimal apparatus (the orbital and palpebral lobes of the lacrimal gland and the goblet cells of the conjunctiva); and the common infections and dysfunctions of the excretory system of the lacrimal apparatus.

Dacryoadenitis (Inflammation of the Lacrimal Gland)

Pain, swelling, and a sensation of fullness of the upper eyelid, together with conjunctival swelling and redness, are the major manifestations of a dacryoadenitis; when the orbital lobe of the lacrimal gland is involved, mild proptosis and restriction of ocular movements also occur. The pain, swelling, and redness (Fig. 6–2) occur in the region of the lacrimal gland. Occasionally, reduced tear formation also occurs. The swelling of the upper eyelid that occurs in dacryoadenitis causes an S-shaped curve to the lid margin (Fig. 6–3), as well as a pseudoptosis that often masks the conjunctival redness.

An acute bilateral dacryoadenitis is usually associated with systemic diseases such as mumps, infectious mononucleosis, and influenza in adults and children, and endogenous gonorrhea in adults. An acute unilateral dacryoadenitis most frequently results from introduction of a bacterial pathogen into the lacrimal gland through a penetrating injury or by a retrograde infection arising from a bacterial conjunctivitis. A bacterial dacryoadenitis may quickly evolve into a lacrimal gland abscess (Fig. 6–4). An acute unilateral dacryoadenitis may be simulated by a cellulitis of the upper eyelid, especially if it involves the lateral aspect of the eyelid (Fig. 6–5).

Chronic dacryoadenitis (whether bilateral or unilateral) is unusual, but most commonly results from sarcoid (Figs. 6–6A and B), and in some instances lacrimal gland enlargement is the initial sign of sarcoidosis (Nowinski et al., 1983). The gumma of tertiary syphilis and the tuberculoma of tuberculosis may also cause a chronic dacryoadenitis (Sen, 1980). A simple dacryops of the lacrimal gland may be produced by the larva *Cysticercus cellulosae* (Sen, 1982). A chronic bilateral swelling in the region of the lacrimal gland may result from prolapse of fat, prolapse of the palpebral lobe of the lacrimal gland (Fig. 6–7A), or a dermolipoma (Fig. 6–7B). Tumors, including lymphomas, mixed tumors of the lacrimal gland, and eosinophilic granulomas of the lateral wall of the orbit, may enlarge progressively and at the same time produce mild inflammatory signs simulating a chronic dacryoadenitis (Ameniya et al., 1983; Feldman et al., 1985).

Canaliculitis

The canaliculus is the small duct that leads from the lacrimal punctum to the lacrimal sac. Inflammation of either the upper or lower canaliculus (canaliculitis) is uncommon, but is a major cause of chronic unilateral conjunctivitis (see Chapter 3). Moreover, canaliculitis is frequently overlooked as a possible cause of a chronic conjunctivitis, and patients are often seen by several ophthalmologists before the diagnosis is made (Smith and Henderson, 1980).

The lower canaliculus (Fig. 6–8) is infected at least twice as often as the upper canaliculus (Fig. 6–9), and women are afflicted more commonly than men. The causative organism has a tendency to grow within a diverticulum of the canaliculus (Fig. 6–10) without invading tissue. The diverticulum provides a site for the organism to lodge and propagate without being flushed into the lacrimal sac and into the nose.

Patients with a canaliculitis have symptoms and signs of a chronic conjunctivitis, including a mucoid or mucopurulent discharge, tearing, and conjunctival redness that is most intense in the medial aspect of the bulbar conjunctiva (Fig. 6–8). Other signs include dilation and pouting of the affected punctum, and regurgitation of a milky or white-appearing mucoid discharge from the punctum when pressure is applied over the lacrimal sac or the involved canaliculus (Fig. 6–11) (Demant and Hurwitz, 1980). If the punctum is dilated and pressure is applied in such a way as to "milk the canaliculus" toward the punctum, concretions containing the offending organism can frequently be expressed (Figs. 6–12A and B).

The major bacterial cause of a canaliculitis is *Actinomyces israelii,* an anaerobic filamentous bacterium (Fig. 6–13). Other bacterial causes include *Enterobacter cloacae* (Chumbly, 1984) and fusobacterium (Weinberg et al., 1977). Fungal causes include *Aspergillus niger* (Fig. 6–12B) and *Candida* spp. Viral infections of the canaliculi, including herpes simplex (deKoning and van Bijsterveld, 1983) are unusual, but may cause scarring of the punctum and the distal canaliculus. Such scarring may also result from the prolonged administration of medications, including antivirals such as idoxuridine.

Dacryocystitis

An acute or chronic inflammation of the lacrimal sac (dacryocystitis) occurs in both infants and adults, but especially in women. It is usually caused by bacteria, especially by *Haemophilus influenzae* (Fig. 6–14) in infants and young children and by *Staphylococcus aureus, Streptococcus pyogenes* (Fig. 6–15), or *Streptococcus pneumoniae* in adults. The organisms are able to propagate within the lacrimal sac as a result of stagnation of tears; mucus and organisms are normally pumped through the nasolacrimal duct into the nose, but remain in the sac when the nasolacrimal duct is blocked from congenital fibrotic obstruction, trauma, or infection (Hurwitz and Rodgers, 1983).

The symptoms of dacryocystitis include tearing, discharge, pain, and redness. The signs include swelling, tenderness over the region of the involved lacrimal sac, and regurgitation of mucus or mucopurulent material if pressure is applied over the area (Fig. 6–16).

The swelling, pain, and tenderness from a dacryocystitis can be differentiated from those produced by an ethmoiditis; in ethmoiditis the major portion of the swelling and tenderness is located superior to the medial canthal ligament (Fig. 6–17), whereas in dacryocystitis the signs are located primarily inferior to the medial canthal ligament. The swelling caused by a congenital dacryocystocele (Harris and DiClementi, 1982) a mucocele of the ethmoid sinus (Fig. 6–17), or a tumor of the lacrimal sac (Fig. 6–18) may simulate a dacryocystitis.

Complications that may arise from infections of the lacrimal sac include a peridacryocystitis, abscess of the lacrimal sac (Fig. 6–19), fistula formation into the overlying skin (Fig. 6–19), an orbital cellulitis or orbital abscess, conjunctivitis of Morax (Fig. 6–20), and cellulitis of the lower eyelid. Such infection may also occasionally serve as the source of a bacteremia. The conjunctivitis of Morax is a hyperacute conjunctivitis caused by a relatively silent chronic dacryocystitis due to *Streptococcus pyogenes* (see Chapter 4).

Keratoconjunctivitis Sicca

Keratoconjunctivitis sicca (dry eye) must be considered at least briefly in any text of infections and inflammations of the external eye, since the tear film plays a major role in the defense mechanisms of the external eye. A dry eye can have any of a number of causes, including conjunctival scarring (e.g., from chemical injury), hypovitaminosis A (Fig. 6–21), and infections such as trachoma or any severe membranous or pseudomembranous conjunctivitis. It may be associated with skin eruptions such as erythema multiforme major (Fig. 6–22), or mucous membrane diseases such as cicatricial pemphigoid (Fig. 6–23). It may also occur from Sjögren's syndrome with or without connective tissue disease (primary Sjögren's syndrome) (Alarcon-Segovia, 1984; Fox et al., 1984) (Fig. 6–24), trauma to the lacrimal gland, and the Riley-Day syndrome (Fig. 6–25).

In addition to producing symptoms of pain, foreign-body sensation, burning, and blurred vision, severe keratoconjunctivitis sicca is commonly associated with loss of vision and is a major contributor to corneal scarring through dryness and infection (Fig. 6–26).

Wolff in 1954 suggested that the precorneal tear film consisted of three layers: the outer layer (a thin oily layer), the middle layer (a thicker watery layer), and the innermost layer (a thin mucoid layer). This concept is overly simplified, but allows the clinician to consider various factors and modes of therapy for keratoconjunctivitis sicca.

The outer layer of the precorneal tear film (a phospholipid) is produced by the meibomian glands and serves to retard evaporation of the watery layer of the tears. It also reduces the surface tension of the tears, allowing better spreading of the tear film. Loss of the oily layer is unusual and is seen primarily in cases in which scarring of the meibomian glands has occurred, such as in erythema multiforme major. Deficiency of the outer layer of tears is recognized by the slit lamp finding of scarring of the orifices of the meibomian gland (Fig. 6–27) and loss of the oily tear layer. A deficiency of the layer may also be detected in the electrophoretic pattern of the tears.

The middle layer (the aqueous layer) is secreted by the lacrimal gland and the accessory glands of Krause and Wolfring. The proteins within the middle layer (albumin, a "middle fraction," and lysozyme) help reduce the surface tension of tears to maintain a continuous tear film. Loss of the middle layer of the precorneal tear film occurs in Sjögren's syndrome, graft versus host disease, and conditions that cause scarring of the mucous membranes. The aqueous layer of tears may also be reduced following surgery on the lacrimal gland. Deficiency of the aqueous layer is determined by the Schirmer tear test, by rose bengal staining of epithelial defects produced by the absence of the tear film (Fig. 6–28), and by demonstration of the absence of lysozyme in the tears.

The innermost layer of the tear film is a thin mucoid layer that covers the corneal epithelium and is derived from the conjunctival goblet cells. This layer is composed primarily of glycoproteins and hexosamines and is essential for spontaneous spreading of the aqueous layer of tears over the corneal epithelium. In the early stages of Sjögren's syndrome, the mucous layer is abnormal, and abnormal strands of mucus (Fig. 6–29) and mucous filaments may be seen on the cornea (Fig. 6–30). The abnormal mucus and mucous filaments cause symptoms of foreign-body sensation and discomfort. Absence of the mucoid layer occurs primarily in the cicatrizing diseases of the conjunctiva and in the late stages of Sjögren's syndrome. The presence of the mucous layer is detected by measuring the breakup time of the tears as the patient is examined at the slit lamp.

References

Alarcon-Segovia, D: Symptomatic Sjögren's syndrome in mixed connective tissue disease. *J. Rheumatol.* 11: 582–583, 1984.

Amemiya, T, Mori, H, and Koizumi, K: Clinical and histocytopathological study of chronic dacryoadenitis. *Graefes Arch. Clin. Exp. Ophthalmol.* 220: 229–232, 1983.

Chumbly, LC: Canaliculitis caused by *Enterobacter cloacae:* Report of a case. *Br. J. Ophthalmol.* 68: 364–366, 1984.

Demant, E, and Hurwitz, JJ: Canaliculitis: Review of 12 cases. *Can. J. Ophthalmol.* 15: 73–75, 1980.

deKoning, EW, van Bijsterveld, OP: Herpes simplex virus canaliculitis. *Ophthalmologica* 186: 173–176, 1983.

Feldman, RB, Moore, DM, Hood, CI, Hiles, DA, and Romano, PE: Solitary eosinophilic granuloma of the lateral orbital wall. *Am. J. Ophthalmol.* 100: 318–323, 1985.

Fox, RI, Howell, FV, Bone, RC, and Michelson, P: Primary Sjögren's syndrome: Clinical and immunopathologic features. *Semin. Arthritis Rheum.* 14: 77–105, 1984.

Harris, GJ, and DiClementi, D: Congenital dacryocystocele. *Arch. Ophthalmol.* 100: 1763–1765, 1982.

Hurwitz, JJ, and Rodgers, KJ: Management of acquired dacryocystitis. *Can. J. Ophthalmol.* 19: 213–216, 1983.

Kim, H-B, and Ostler, HB: Marginal corneal ulcer due to β streptococcus. *Arch. Ophthalmol.* 95: 454–455, 1977.

Nowinski, T, Flanagan, J, and Ruchman, M: Lacrimal gland enlargement in familial sarcoidosis. *Ophthalmology* 90: 909–913, 1983.

Ryan, S, and Font, RL: Primary epithelial neoplasms of the lacrimal sac. *Am. J. Ophthalmol.* 76: 73–88, 1974.

Sen, DK: Tuberculosis of the orbit and lacrimal gland: A clinical study of 14 cases. *J. Pediatr. Ophthalmol. Strabismus* 17: 232–238, 1980.

Sen, DK: Acute suppurative dacryoadenitis caused by a *Cysticercus cellulosae. J. Pediatr. Ophthalmol. Strabismus* 19: 100–102, 1982.

Smith, RL, and Henderson, PN: Actinomycotic canaliculitis. *Aust. J. Ophthalmol.* 8: 75–79, 1980.

Weinberg, RJ, Sartoris, MJ, Buerger, GF, and Novak, JF: Fusobacterium in presumed actinomyces canaliculitis. *Am. J. Ophthalmol.* 84: 371–374, 1977.

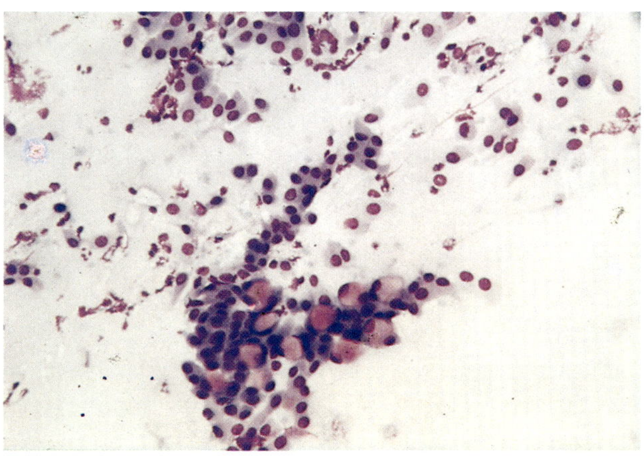

6–1 Goblet cells. The goblet cells of the conjunctiva are derived from the conjunctival epithelium; their name is derived from their goblet shape. Morphologically, the cells are distinctive — their nuclei are crowded to one side of their cells and the cytoplasm is distended with mucin. × 100.

6–2 Conjunctival hyperemia and swelling in the superior temporal quadrant near the lacrimal gland orifices. Conjunctival hyperemia and chemosis near the orifices of the lacrimal gland are commonly found in acute dacryoadenitis. This 6-year-old female had noted swelling of the outer aspect of the upper eyelid and redness of the lateral aspect of the conjunctiva for four days. Note the chemosis and hyperemia of the conjunctiva in the region of the lacrimal gland orifices.

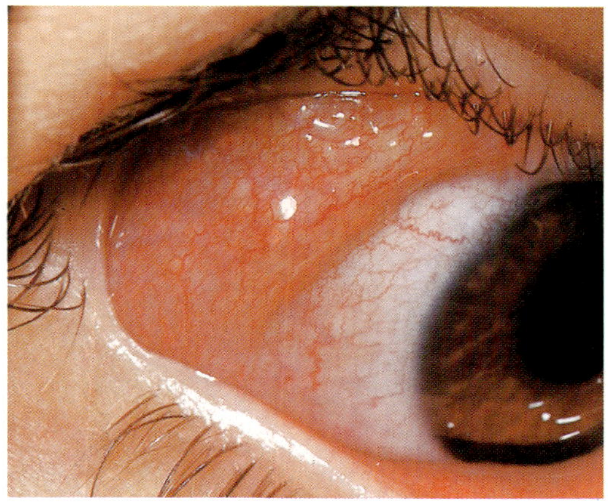

6–3 S-shaped curve of the margin of the upper eyelid in dacryoadenitis. This 17-year-old female developed an acute bilateral dacryoadenitis associated with influenza. She complained of a feeling of fullness and swelling of the upper eyelid and tenderness on rotation of the eyes. An elongated S-shaped curve of the lid margin can be outlined, beginning at the medial canthal region and following the curve of the upper eyelid to the lateral canthus. Her tear lysozyme and Schirmer tear test were normal both at this time and two weeks later when the dacryoadenitis had subsided.

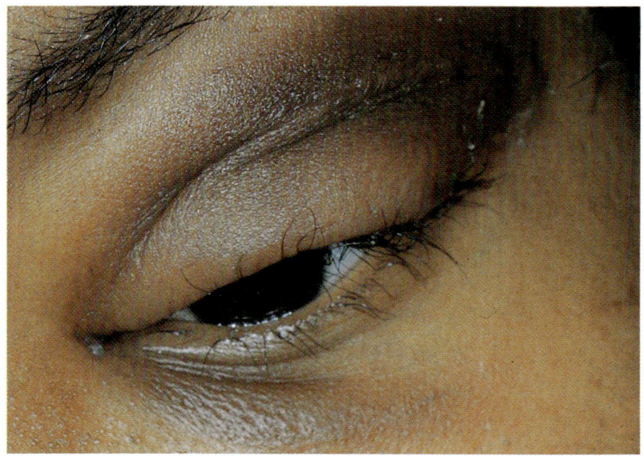

6–4 Lacrimal gland abscess associated with an acute *Haemophilus influenzae* conjunctivitis. Bacterial infections of the lacrimal gland, especially when they develop by retrograde spread of the organism from a conjunctival infection or by introduction of the organism with a penetrating injury, may be complicated by abscess formation. This child developed a retrograde infection of the lacrimal gland from a conjunctivitis due to *H. influenzae.* Marked conjunctival injection together with swelling, discharge, and early suppuration can be seen in this photograph.

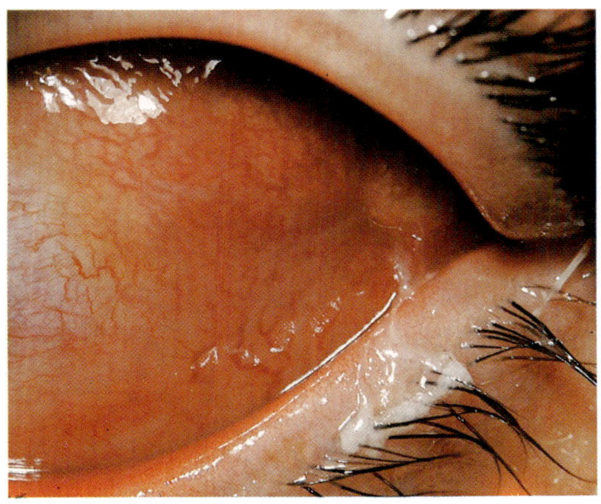

6–5 Cellulitis (preseptal cellulitis) of the upper eyelid. A cellulitis of the upper eyelid (preseptal cellulitis), especially when it involves the temporal part of the eyelid, may simulate an acute dacryoadenitis, as seen in this 27-year-old Filipino male who developed a beta-hemolytic streptococcal cellulitis. An S-shaped curve similar to that in Fig. 6–3 is present, together with edema and erythema of the outer aspect of the upper eyelid; the conjunctiva was not involved (compare this with Fig. 6–2).

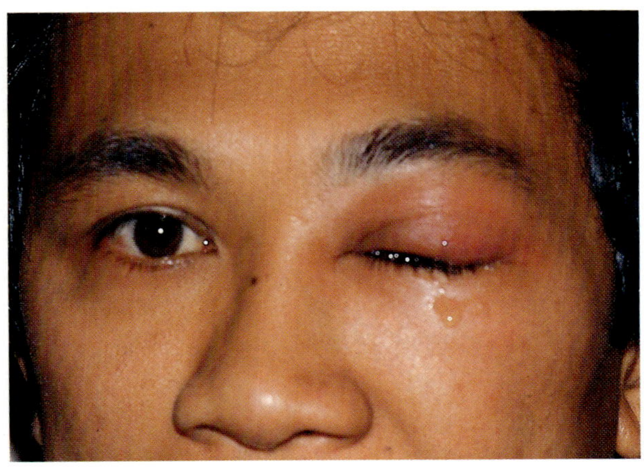

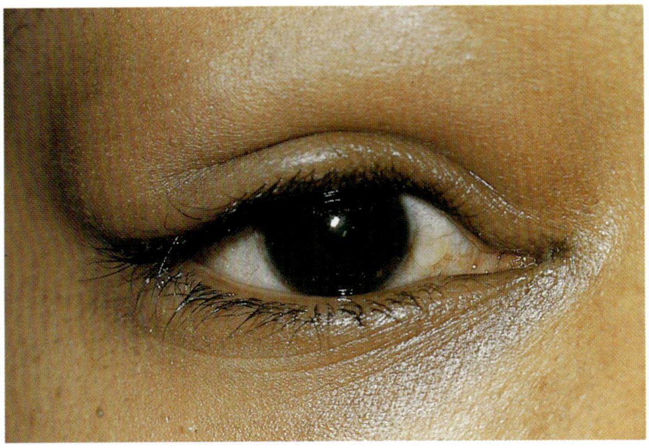

6–6A Chronic recurrent dacryoadenitis due to sarcoid. Chronic recurrent dacryoadenitis is usually bilateral and most commonly results from sarcoid involvement of the lacrimal gland. This 17-year-old female with proven sarcoid had three episodes of recurrent enlargement of the lacrimal glands. Swelling, most marked in the upper outer quadrant of the eyelid and orbit, is evident.

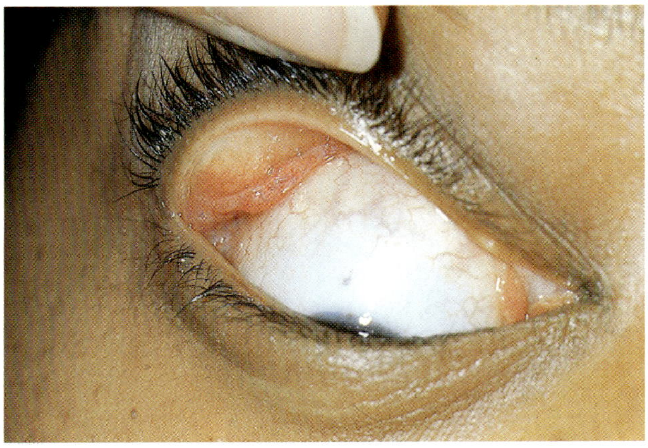

6–6B Chronic recurrent dacryoadenitis due to sarcoid, demonstrating hyperemia and nodularity of the conjunctiva. In this photograph of the same patient shown in Fig. 6–6A, the hyperemia and nodularity of the conjunctiva are readily visible.

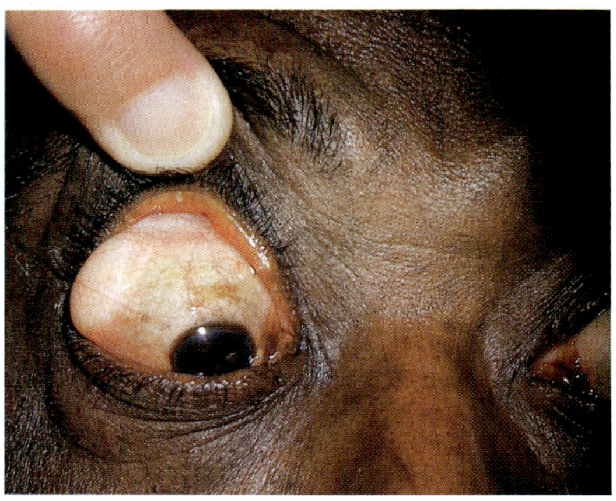

6–7A Prolapse or ptosis of the palpebral lobe of the lacrimal gland. A prolapse of fat that surrounds the lacrimal gland or a prolapse of the palpebral lobe of the lacrimal gland may simulate a chronic dacryoadenitis, as is evident in this 27-year-old male who had noted an increased fullness of the area overlying the lacrimal gland for several years. Note the globular swelling in the outer aspect of the orbit.

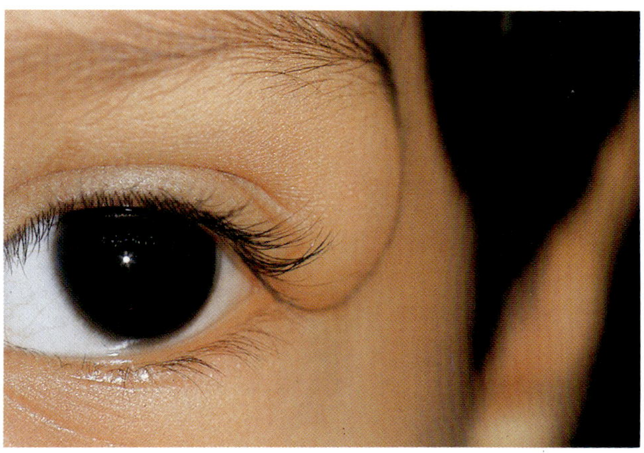

6–7B Dermolipoma in the region of the lacrimal gland. This 2½-year-old child was seen by the authors for a painless noninflammatory swelling of the outer aspect of both orbits since birth. The masses had increased in size over the past two years and at surgery were found to be dermolipomas.

6–8 Infection of the lower canaliculus. A canaliculitis occurs most commonly in the lower canaliculus. Discharge and blood can be seen at the lower punctum in this 57-year-old female — a concretion was partially expressed before the photograph was taken. The punctum is edematous, and the palpebral conjunctiva inflamed and infiltrated. Mucus is noted in the conjunctival sac. The skin of the lid is discolored and thickened as a result of the prolonged conjunctivitis.

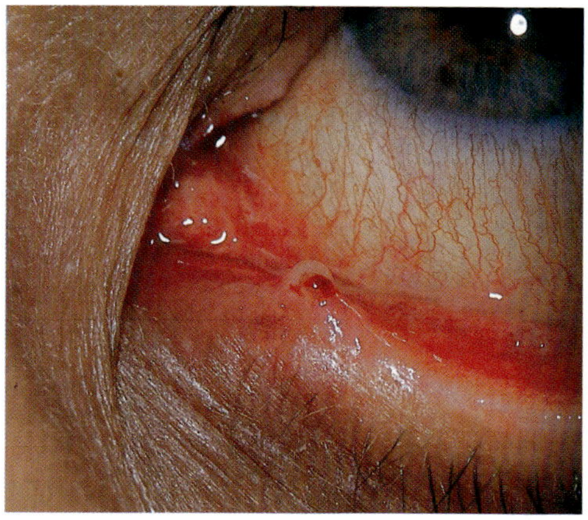

6–9 Infection of the upper canaliculus. A canaliculitis of the upper canaliculus is frequently overlooked. This 68-year-old male had had a chronic conjunctivitis for more than eight months. Pouting and inflammation of the upper punctum and a mucopurulent discharge are evident. Following expression of the actinomycotic concretions, complete relief of symptoms occurred within 36 hours.

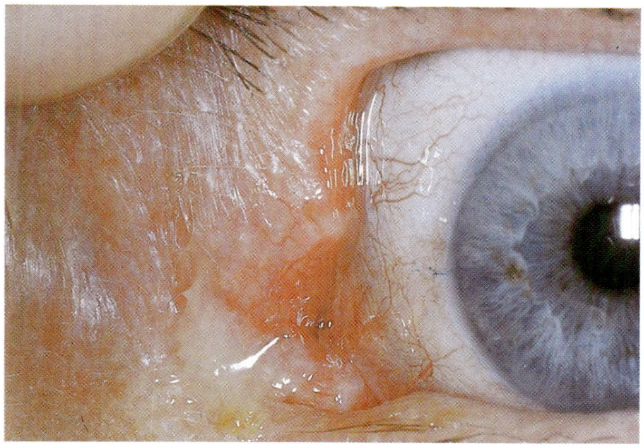

6–10 Diverticulum of the lower canaliculus. Diverticula of the canaliculi are common; bacteria or fungi can lodge and propagate within them causing a chronic conjunctivitis from shedding of the organism and its products into the conjunctival sac. This large diverticulum was demonstrated by injection of radio-opaque material into the canaliculus to visualize the excretory system. (The radio-opaque line running beyond the lateral wall of the orbit is the tube used to inject the dye into the excretory system.) (Reprinted with permission from the *American Journal of Ophthalmology.)*

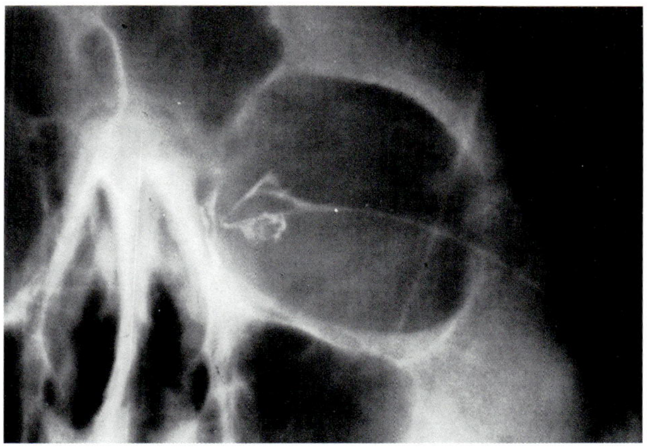

6–11 Pouting of the lower punctum, hyperemia, and infiltration of the medial conjunctiva, along with mucoid material expressed from the lower canaliculus. Redness and infiltration of the conjunctiva in chronic conjunctivitis from a canaliculitis are most intense in the medial aspect of the conjunctiva. Pouting of the lower punctum, hyperemia and infiltration of the conjunctiva, and mucoid discharge that was expressed from the lower punctum are readily visible in this 57-year-old Japanese female with an inferior canaliculitis.

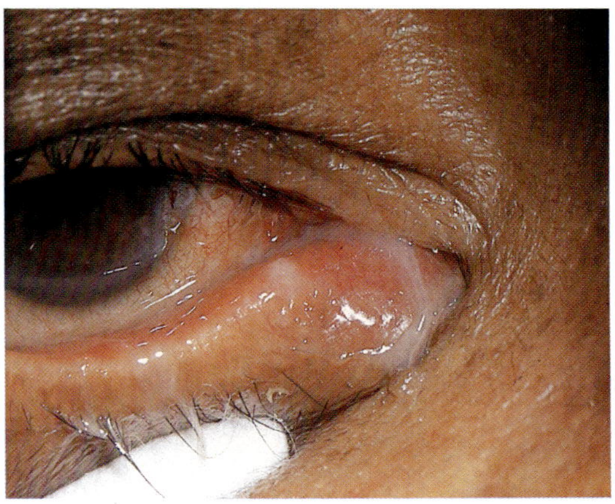

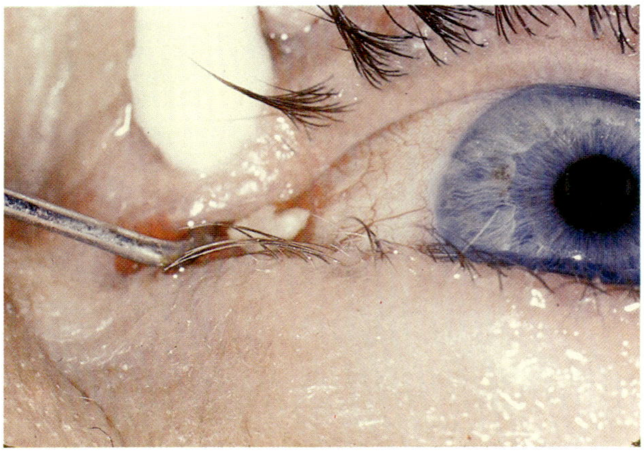

6–12A Concretions due to actinomycosis infection of the canaliculus. *Actinomyces israelii* concretions are hard and of the consistency of large grains of sand. The concretions fill the diverticulum and occasionally line the canaliculus distal to the diverticulum. One is often surprised by the size and number of the concretions. This concretion was expressed from the patient shown in Fig. 6–9 by "milking the canaliculus" toward the punctum using pressure applied on the conjunctival side with the crook of a muscle hook, and counterpressure applied on the skin side with a cotton-tipped applicator.

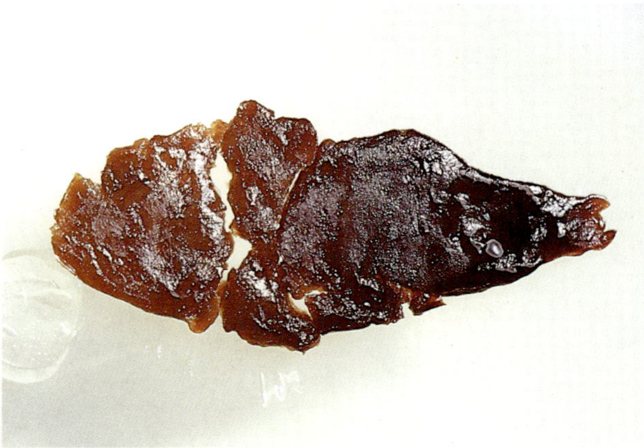

6–12B *Aspergillus niger* cast of the diverticulum. *A. niger* and *Candida* spp. may form soft rubbery casts of the diverticulum and/or the lacrimal sac that they infect. This cast was expressed from the canaliculus of a 27-year-old female who had a chronic conjunctivitis due to *A. niger* canaliculitis. The cast was recovered by carefully "milking the canaliculus" as described in Fig. 6–12A.

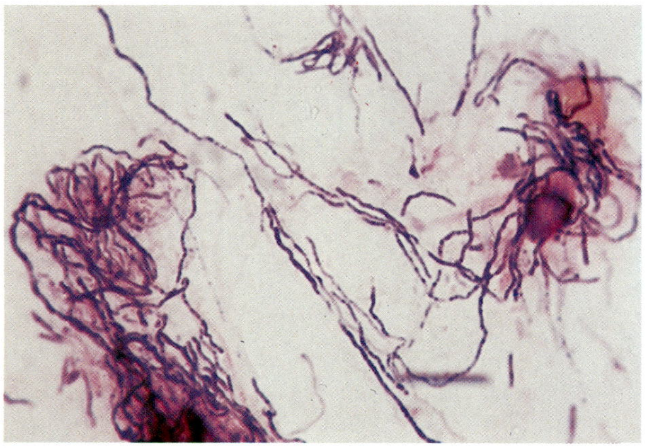

6–13 Smear from a concretion showing the filamentous *Actinomyces israelii* bacteria. This filamentous organism can be readily seen under the microscope, if the concretions are pulverized, smeared, and stained. This is a smear of the pulverized concretion from the patient in Fig. 6–9. Gram's stain × 100.

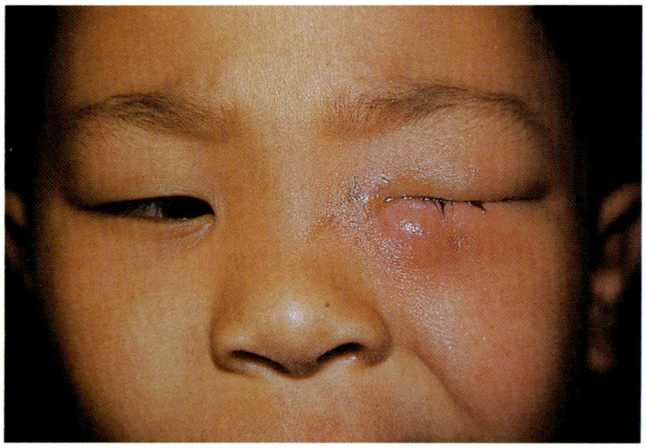

6–14 Acute *Haemophilus influenzae* dacryocystitis in a young child. A dacryocystitis in an infant or young child is most commonly caused by *H. influenzae,* as seen in this 3-year-old patient. Because they lack protective antibodies, young children are more susceptible to *H. influenzae* infections. Erythema and swelling of the skin overlying the lacrimal sac and the lower eyelid are evident; tearing is also prominent.

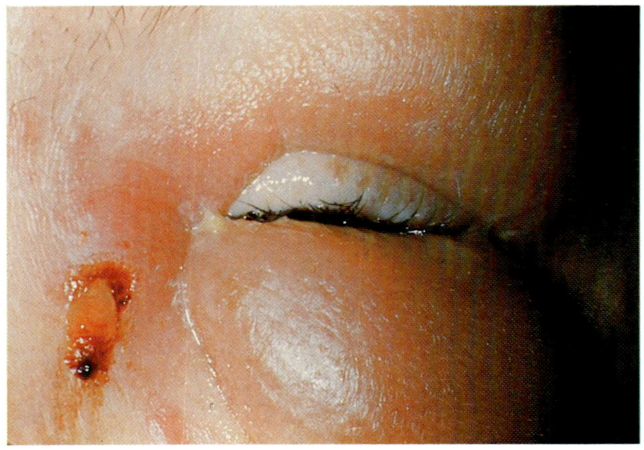

6–15 Acute dacryocystitis due to *Streptococcus pyogenes*. The most frequent causes of a dacryocystitis in the child over three years of age and in the adult are *S. pyogenes* and *S. pneumoniae.* This 21-year-old patient with Down's syndrome developed an acute dacryocystitis due to *S. pyogenes,* which progressed to form a peridacryocystitis before spontaneously draining through the skin. The fistula can be readily seen over the lacrimal sac region.

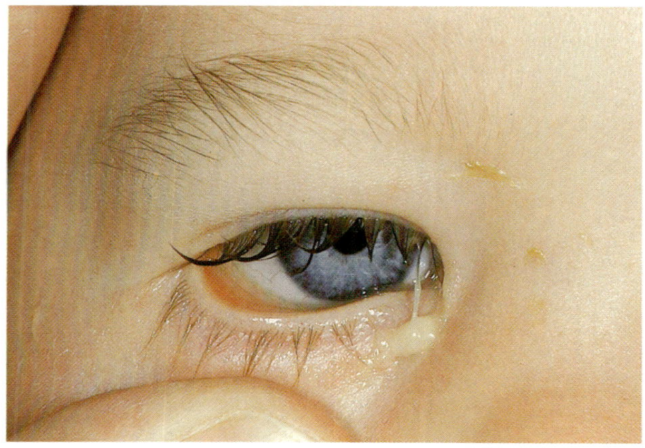

6–16 Regurgitation of mucopurulent material through the lower punctum following application of pressure over the lacrimal sac. Mucopurulent material can often be expressed easily from the lacrimal sac when there is an occlusion of the nasolacrimal duct or an acute dacryocystitis. This 1½-year-old child had had tearing since birth. Moderate mucopurulent material was easily expressed when pressure was applied over the lacrimal sac region.

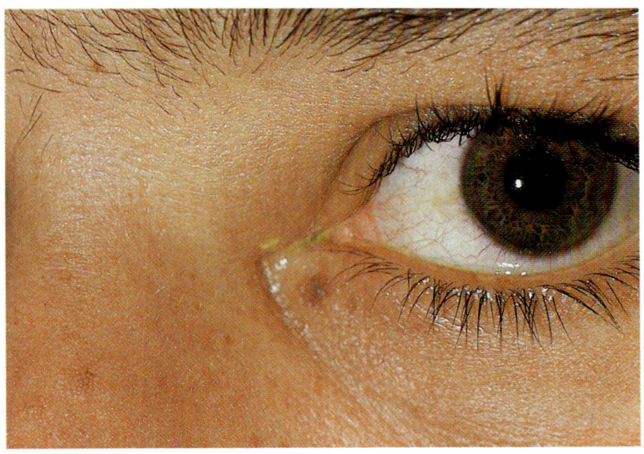

6–17 Mucocele of the ethmoid sinus. A mucocele may be mistaken for a chronic dacryocystitis. However, the major part of the swelling in a mucocele is located superior to the medial canthal ligament, whereas in a dacryocystitis the major signs are located inferior to the medial canthal ligament. In this 26-year-old male with a mucocele of the ethmoid sinus, the major part of the swelling occurred superior to the medial canthal ligament. Compare the location of the swelling in this photograph to the location of the swelling in Fig. 6–14.

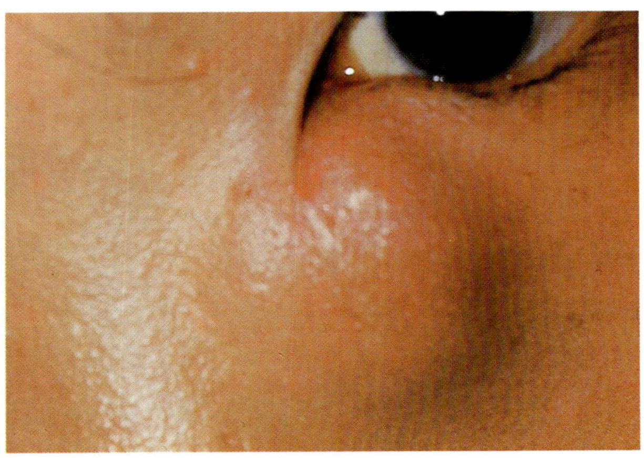

6–18 Swelling from a tumor of the lacrimal sac. A tumor of the lacrimal sac is uncommon. It causes progressive swelling of the region of the lacrimal sac and occasional tearing. When the tumor is malignant, pain may occur (Ryan and Font, 1974). This 69-year-old Chinese man had noted a mass in the region of the lacrimal sac. There was no tearing or inflammation. (The epicanthal fold is due to his race and is not related to the lacrimal sac tumor.)

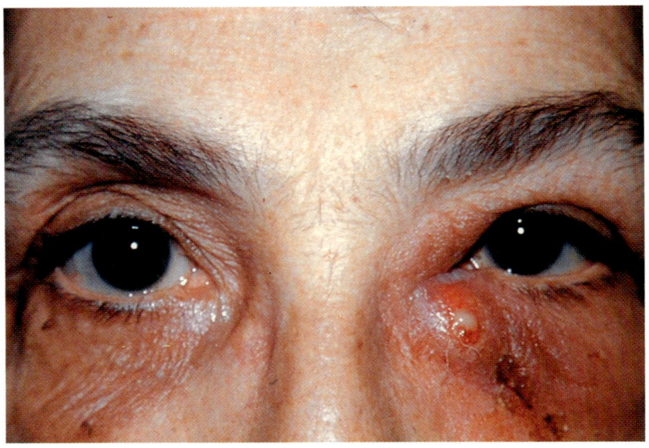

6–19 Lacrimal sac abscess due to *Streptococcus pyogenes*, showing spontaneous drainage. If untreated, a dacryocystitis may produce an abscess that spontaneously drains, as occurred in this 69-year-old female who had a chronic dacryocystitis. The patient had had chronic tearing, swelling, and discharge until one week before being seen, when she noted pain, tenderness, and redness over the lacrimal sac region. The day before this photograph was taken, spontaneous drainage of the lacrimal sac abscess occurred leaving a small draining fistula that can be seen over the region of the abscess. The patient also had a chronic dacryocystitis of the other eye as can be seen by the tearing, thickening and redundancy of the upper and lower eyelids, and swelling over the lacrimal sac.

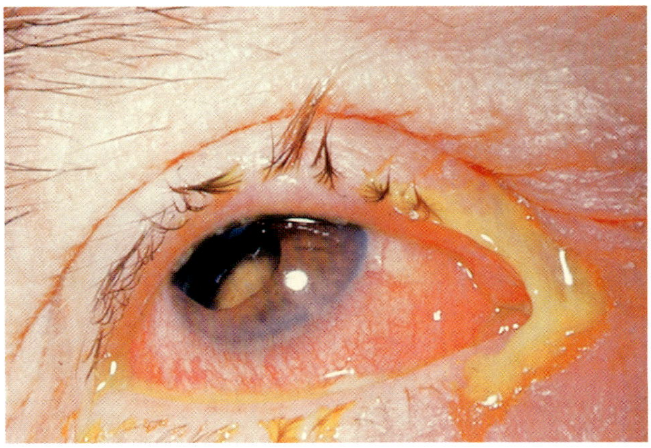

6–20 Hyperacute conjunctivitis of Morax. An acute or hyperacute conjunctivitis arising from a beta streptococcus infection was described in 1931 by Morax and has been called a conjunctivitis of Morax. The source of the infection is usually a relatively silent dacryocystitis (Kim and Ostler, 1977), and the conjunctivitis responds poorly to conventional therapy unless the dacryocystitis is also treated. This 72-year-old female had developed a hyperacute conjunctivitis three days previously. The conjunctivitis responded only after the dacryocystitis was treated by repeated irrigation of the lacrimal system and eventual dacryocystorhinostomy. Hyperemia and edema of the eyelids and a discharge are readily seen. The dislocated lens and surgical coloboma of the iris are unrelated to the conjunctivitis. The eye has been blind for more than 10 years.

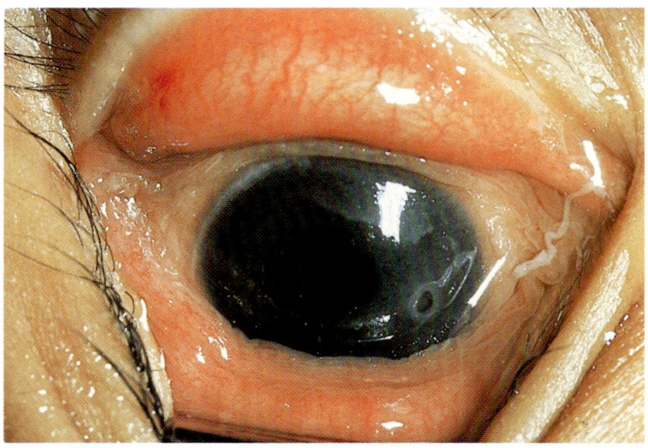

6–21 Keratomalacia in hypovitaminosis A. Loss of conjunctival goblet cells, deficient secretion of the aqueous portion of the tears, and keratinizing metaplasia are common findings in vitamin A deficiency. Dryness and early keratinization of the conjunctiva together with loss of corneal luster and breakdown of the corneal epithelium are evident in this patient. (Photograph courtesy of Dr. A. Summers.)

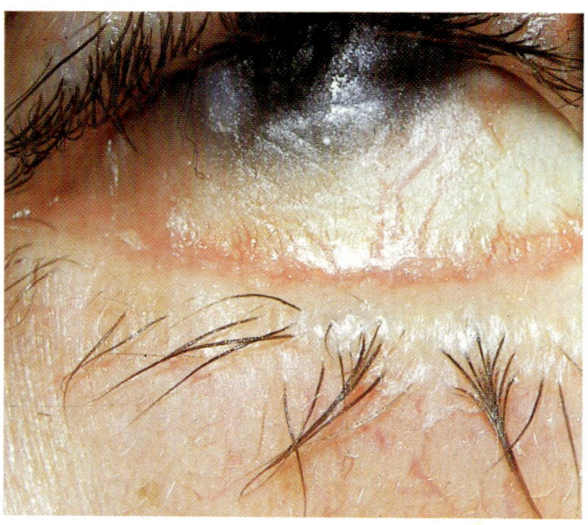

6–22 Dry eye, total symblepharon, and cicatrization of the conjunctiva from erythema multiforme major (Stevens-Johnson syndrome). Erythema multiforme major frequently causes scarring of the conjunctiva and in some instances, such as in this 54-year-old female who developed Stevens-Johnson syndrome following exposure to long-acting sulfonamides 24 years earlier, may cause complete obliteration of the fornices and a totally dry eye. Note the marked dryness of the conjunctiva and cornea and the total symblepharon of the lower eyelid and outer aspect of the upper eyelid. As a rule of thumb, erythema multiforme major occurs before the age of 45 years.

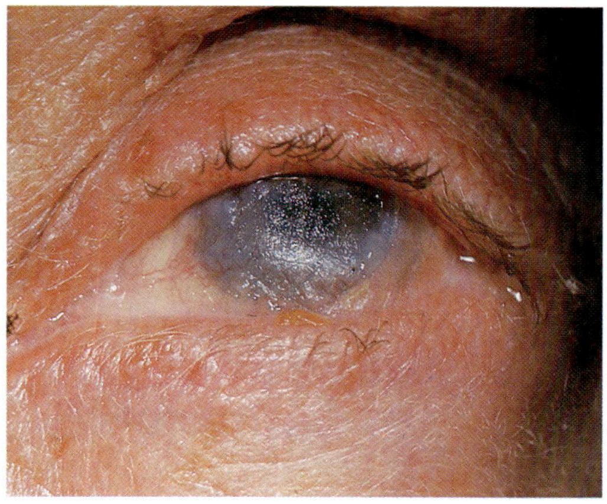

6–23 Dry eye and total symblepharon in cicatricial pemphigoid. Cicatricial pemphigoid frequently causes obliteration of the lower and in some instances the upper fornix. This 64-year-old female developed cicatricial pemphigoid two years previously and has total symblepharon formation of the lower eyelid of each eye. The upper fornix is still present, and even though some tearing occurs, proper wetting of the cornea and conjunctiva is absent because of loss of the goblet cells as a result of conjunctival scarring. As a rule of thumb, cicatricial pemphigoid begins after the age of 45 years.

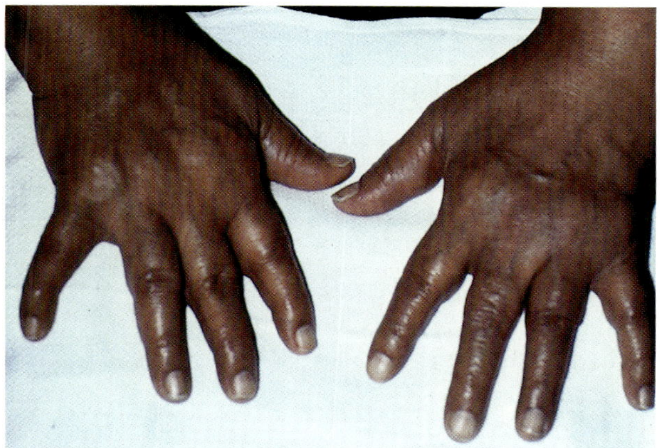

6–24 Early rheumatoid arthritis of the hands in Sjögren's syndrome. Sjögren's syndrome is commonly associated with connective tissue disease, as is evident in this 47-year-old female with early rheumatoid arthritis. The tapered fingers and the fusiform swelling of the proximal interphalangeal joints are characteristic of early rheumatoid arthritis.

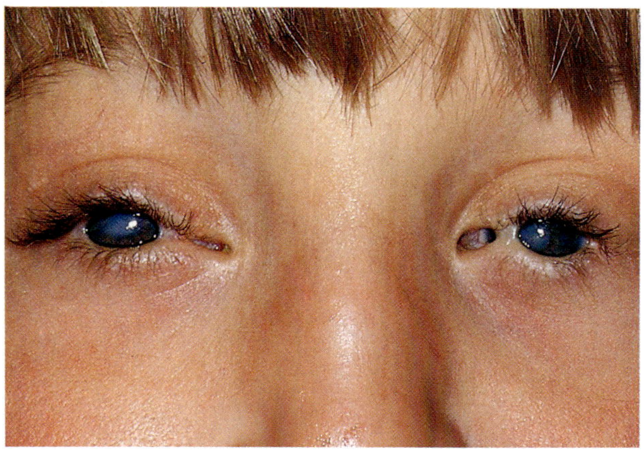

6–25 Riley-Day syndrome. Congenital alacrima occurs in the Riley-Day syndrome. This 6-year-old child had congenital alacrima and absent corneal sensation. He was noted to scratch the corneas frequently during infancy. Lid adhesions were placed in an effort to preserve the corneas from dryness and from trauma due to scratching. The lid adhesions and corneal scarring are readily evident.

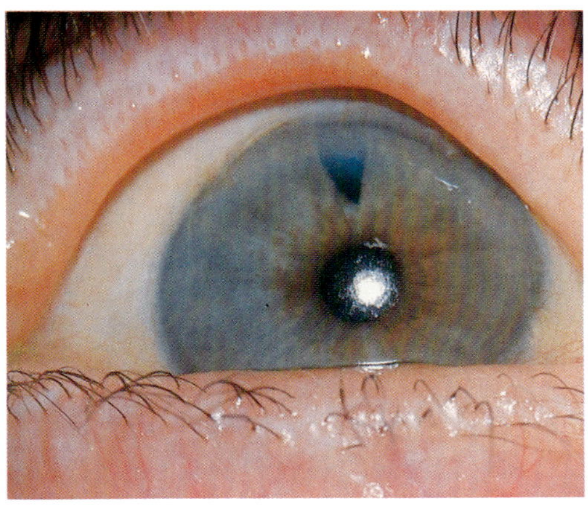

6–26 Dryness of the cornea in Sjögren's syndrome. Loss of luster of the cornea, as evidenced by distortion of the light reflex and a haziness of the pupil and iris, is apparent in this 67-year-old female who developed Sjögren's syndrome three years previously. The patient had had an uneventful cataract extraction and a peripheral iridectomy five years previously.

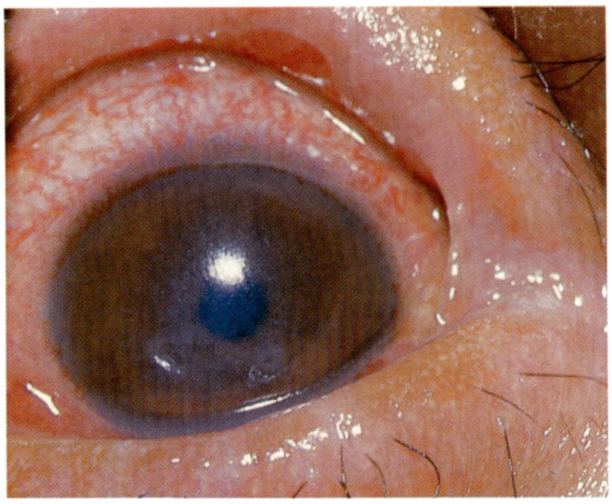

6–27 Early scarring of the orifices of the meibomian glands in erythema multiforme major. Although this patient still shows signs of inflammation and activity from erythema multiforme major, scarring of the orifices of the meibomian glands, early symblepharon formation, and dryness of the cornea with formation of two trophic corneal ulcers are evident. The patient developed erythema multiforme major three weeks previously in response to a trigger of sulfonamides.

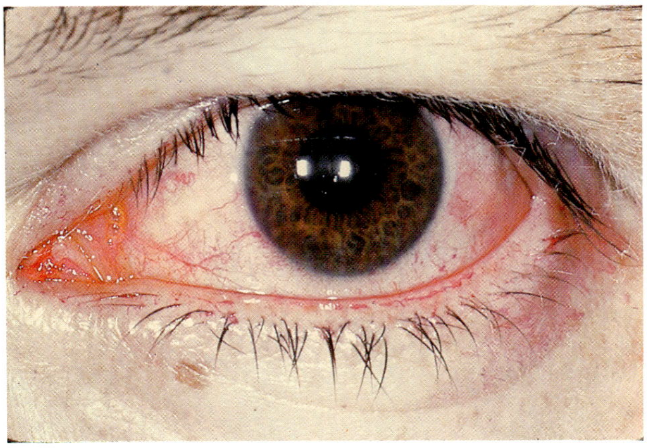

6–28 Staining of epithelial defects in the exposure area of the conjunctiva with rose bengal. Staining of epithelial defects in the exposure area of the conjunctiva and the lower cornea following the instillation of rose bengal, as seen in this 43-year-old female, is highly suggestive of an aqueous deficiency of the precorneal tear film such as occurs in Sjögren's syndrome. Two small filaments can be seen centrally, as well as some mucus near the caruncle.

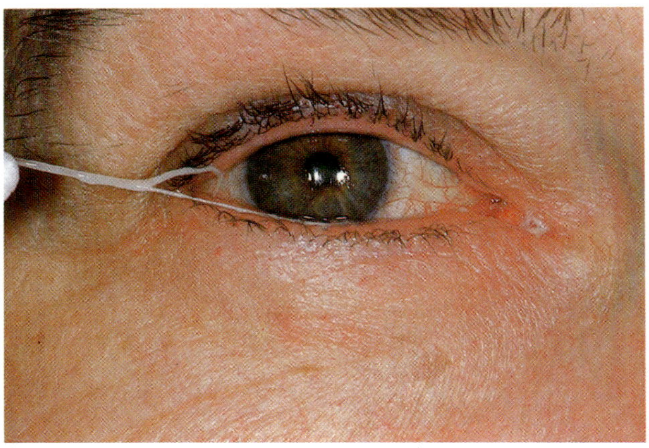

6–29 Abnormal mucous strands. Symptoms of foreign-body sensation and discomfort commonly occur from abnormal mucous strands in Sjögren's syndrome. Abnormal mucous strands were almost constant findings in this 38-year-old female with Sjögren's syndrome. The tenacity of the mucous filaments is evident in this photograph, and an abnormal tear film is readily seen — there is no tear meniscus at the margin of the lower eyelid and there is an irregular light reflex on the cornea.

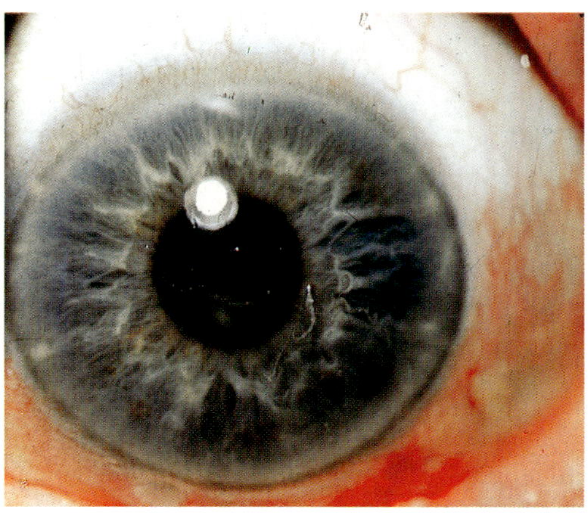

6–30 Corneal mucous filaments. Corneal mucous filaments are common in Sjögren's syndrome. The filaments may be long and multiple and usually occur in the lower half of the cornea. In this patient with Sjögren's syndrome, several long mucous filaments are evident centrally and paracentrally.

Chapter 7

Infections and Inflammations of the Orbit

Orbital Cellulitis

An orbital cellulitis is defined as an inflammation of the periorbital structures located anterior to the orbital septa (periorbital cellulitis), of the periosteal areas of the orbit, and/or of the orbital tissue itself. Approximately 80 percent of orbital cellulitis occurs in individuals under the age of 18 years, and most cases of orbital inflammation arise from inflammations or infections in areas contiguous to the orbit (especially the paranasal sinuses), and occasionally in the eye or lacrimal apparatus. Orbital cellulitis is uncommon; when it occurs it must be promptly and properly treated to avoid serious sequelae.

Manifestations of Orbital Cellulitis

The cardinal manifestations of orbital cellulitis include severe pain around the eye, pain on rotation of the eye, tenderness of the eye, marked edema and injection of the eyelids (Figs. 7–1, 7–2), proptosis (Fig. 7–2), chemosis (Fig. 7–2), limitation of ocular movements, and systemic symptoms of chills, fever, and malaise. Other signs that are valuable but less constant include decreased visual acuity, an afferent pupillary defect, increased intraocular pressure, edema of the optic nerve, and congestion of the retinal veins. A leukocytosis may also be evident.

The primary focus of an orbital inflammation can often be determined without the need for an invasive procedure by using computed tomography (CT) and echography (ultrasound) with the standardized A-scan, especially if the A-scan is supplemented by the contact B-scan. However, echography gives poor resolution of the structures behind the globe, and both CT and echography are limited in their ability to detect retained foreign bodies made of wood.

Pathways of Orbital Infection

There are four pathways by which orbital cellulitis may arise:

1. A contiguous reaction from a paranasal sinusitis (periorbital cellulitis) (Figs. 7–3 A and B), from an infection of the skin or subcutaneous tissue (preseptal cellulitis) (Fig. 7–4), or from an endophthalmitis that spreads to the orbit to cause a tenonitis (inflammation of the episcleral space);
2. An orbital cellulitis resulting from disruption of the overlying skin and orbital septum;
3. A tenonitis resulting from various fevers, such as measles;
4. An orbital cellulitis associated with bacteremia and without other apparent foci of infection.

Spread of inflammation from the paranasal sinuses is common because more than two-thirds of the orbital cavity is contiguous with the paranasal sinuses. Morover, the orbital and the paranasal cavities are often separated by a very thin or incomplete bone, which allows contiguous spread of inflammation from the paranasal sinuses to the orbit (Mills and Kartush, 1985). Inflammation may also spread to the orbit from the paranasal sinuses or the oral cavity (Bullock and Fleishman, 1985) by way of the lymphatics, bone marrow spaces, and the venous plexuses of these structures.

Suppurative infections of the orbit are rare. They are most commonly associated with penetrating wounds (Figs. 7–5 A and B) (Crawford, 1948; Krohel et al., 1982), extension from an advanced purulent paranasal sinusitis (Harris, 1983; Shapiro et al., 1982; Wenig et al., 1983), or spread from an infection of the skin of the face. Suppurative orbital infections are usually caused by *Staphylococcus aureus* and *Streptococcus pyogenes.*

Tenonitis (inflammation of the episcleral space) may be suppurative but is usually serous in nature and presents with mild proptosis and voluntary limitation of ocular movement because rotation of the globe causes pain. Serous tenonitis occurs with gonorrheal arthritis (Fig. 7–6) or acute fevers such as those associated with influenza, measles, or mumps, and also occurs during the early stages of invasion of the extraocular muscles by *Trichinella spiralis.* It is characterized by a pale lemon-colored chemosis that is most marked over the areas of insertion of the lateral and medial rectus muscles.

The manifestations of a purulent tenonitis are similar to those of a serous tenonitis, but are more severe in nature. A purulent tenonitis may arise from a skin infection, a dacryocystitis, a bacteremia, or an endophthalmitis (Fig. 7–7).

In children and adults, orbital infections resulting from a bacteremia usually develop during upper respiratory infection from *Streptococcus pneumoniae,* whereas in young children they result from *Haemophilus influenzae* type B infections.

Chronic Orbital Inflammation

A chronic inflammation frequently results from a reaction to an infectious agent that has been only partially controlled (e.g., *Mycobacterium tuberculosis);* in some instances it represents a reaction to the toxic products of tissue destruction, including infection (e.g., the gumma of syphilis). Chronic granulomatous orbital reactions are often caused by organisms that typically produce granulomas, such as *M. tuberculosis, Treponema pallidum,* and many types of fungi and parasites.

Infectious Etiologies of Orbital Cellulitis

The Gram-positive cocci *(Staphylococcus aureus* and *Streptococcus pyogenes)* (Fig. 7–8) are the most common causative agents of orbital cellulitis, except in children under the age of three years, in whom the Gram-negative bacterium *Haemophilus influenzae* type B is the most common causative agent. Other bacteria giving rise to orbital callulitis include *Streptococcus pneumoniae, Staphylococcus epidermidis, Actinomyces* spp., the coliform bacilli, *Proteus* spp., *Pseudomonas* spp., and anaerobic bacteria such as the Gram-positive anaerobic cocci and *Clostridia* spp. (Crock et al., 1985). At one time, infection by *Mycobacterium tuberculosis,* and fusiform bacilli and the tertiary stage of syphilis were major causes of orbital cellulitis. These factors are rarely implicated today in the development of orbital infections.

The most frequent fungal cause of orbital cellulitis is the zygomycosis organism, which causes mucormycosis and may lead to death (Fig. 7–9) (Castelli and Pallin, 1978). Other causative agents are *Aspergillus fumigatus* (Dortzbach and Segrest, 1983; Maniglia et al., 1984), *Blastomyces dermatitidis, Histoplasma duboisii, Pseudallescheria boydii,* and *Sporothrix schenckii.*

The parasitic infections of the orbit, which are uncommon, include several types of metazoa: *Diphyllobothrium* spp., *Echinococcus granulosus, Schistosoma* spp., the larval form of *Taenia solium, Trichinella spiralis, Wuchereria bancrofti,* the African eye worm *(Loa loa)* (Fig. 7–10); and *Trypanosoma cruzi.* Orbital myiasis may also result from invasion of the orbit by larvae of various diptera species including *Oestrus ovis, Dermatobia noxialis, Hypoderma bovis, Wohlfahrtia magnifica,* and *Calliphora vomitoria* (Wood and Slight, 1970) (Fig. 7–11).

Other Causes of Orbital Inflammation

Exophthalmic Grave's disease frequently causes orbital inflammation. In the majority of cases, the inflammation is bilateral, but in some instances the inflammation begins unilaterally. The manifestations of exophthalmic Grave's disease include exophthalmos (Fig. 7–12), edema of the eyelids, chemosis, and restriction of extraocular movements.

Sudden proptosis and signs of inflammation may be caused by hemorrhage into an orbital lymphatic varix (Fig. 7–13), spontaneous hemorrhage into the orbit in association with a blood dyscrasia, or hemorrhage resulting from trauma to the orbit; these may in many respects simulate an orbital cellulitis. A mucocele of the paranasal sinus may cause signs of lid edema, redness of the eyelid, and even proptosis (Figs. 7–14, 7–15).

A pseudotumor of the orbit frequently presents with manifestations of orbital inflammation (Fig. 7–16) (Weisberger et al., 1985; Wilner et al., 1980). Although the etiology of a pseudotumor is usually unknown, it frequently represents an orbital cellulitis that has been only partially controlled. And orbital myositis of nonspecific etiology is also a pseudotumor; it causes orbital pain, inflammation, and proptosis (Bullen and Young, 1982; Kennerdell and Dresner, 1984). The condition is usually bilateral and the proptosis usually minimal.

Inflammations of the orbital lobe of the lacrimal gland, and especially involvement of the orbital lobe by sarcoid (Figs. 7–17), may cause proptosis and other signs of orbital inflammation.

Wegener's granulomatosis frequently causes exophthalmos, inflammation of the orbit, and sinusitis (Fig. 7–18), as well as pulmonary and renal involvement (Boukes and de Vries-Knoppert, 1985; Parelhoff et al., 1985). The inflammation is usually subacute in onset, and the reaction is of a granulomatous nature.

A neoplasm of the orbit is usually insidious in onset, rarely causing orbital inflammation. However, in rare instances, because of obstruction of the drainage channels from the paranasal sinuses or the production of secondary changes in or about the orbit (such as from necrosis of the tumor or orbital fat), inflammatory symptoms and signs may be prominent and simulate an orbital cellulitis.

Cavernous sinus thrombosis must always be considered as a possible complication of orbital cellulitis. Orbital inflammation usually accompanies a cavernous sinus thrombosis, but cavernous sinus thrombosis may occur without orbital cellulitis. Cavernous sinus thrombosis is usually bilateral, causing axial proptosis, ligneous hardness of the lids and orbital tissues, and distended veins in the lids and conjunctiva (Fig. 7–19). The veins appear bluish because of stasis of circulation. Cranial nerve palsies of the third, fourth, and sixth nerves develop rapidly. Pain is a prominent feature of the disease, and blindness or death may supervene (Geggel and Isenberg, 1982).

Complications

The complications of orbital inflammation and especially orbital cellulitis can be threatening to the vision and even to life (Newell and Leveille, 1984). Suppuration within the orbital apex commonly carries a poor prognosis for vision. Other complications include periorbital abscess formation; gangrene of the eyelids; corneal exposure, ulceration, and perforation; optic nerve atrophy; choroidal and retinal vessel infarction; meningitis; cavernous sinus thrombosis; brain abscess; and death.

References

Boukes, RJ, and de Vries-Knoppert, WA: Lacrimal gland enlargement as one of the ocular manifestations of Wegener's granulomatosis. *Doc. Ophthalmol.* 59: 21–26, 1985.

Bullen, CL, and Younge, BR: Chronic orbital myositis. *Arch. Ophthalmol.* 100: 296–298, 1982.

Bullock, JD, and Fleishman, JA: The spread of odontogenic infections to the orbit: Diagnosis and management. *J. Oral Maxillofac. Surg.* 43: 749–755, 1985.

Castelli, JB, and Pallin, JL: Lethal rhinocerebral phycomycosis in a healthy adult: A case report and review of the literature. *Otolaryngology* 86: 696–703, 1978.

Crawford, WJ: Friedlander's bacillus infection following perforating wound of orbit. Report of a case treated with streptomycin. *Am. J. Ophthalmol.* 31: 1293–1296, 1948.

Crock, GW, Heriot, WJ, Janakiraman, P, and Weiner, JM: Gas gangrene infection of the eyes and orbits. *Br. J. Ophthalmol.* 69: 143–148, 1985.

Dortzbach, RK, and Segrest, DR: Orbital aspergillosis. *Ophthalmic Surg.* 14: 240–244, 1983.

Geggel, HS, and Isenberg, SJ: Cavernous sinus thrombosis as a cause of unilateral blindness. *Ann. Ophthalmol.* 14: 569–574, 1982.

Harris, GJ: Subperiosteal abscess of the orbit. *Arch. Ophthalmol.* 101: 751–757, 1983.

Kennerdell, JS, and Dresner, SC: The nonspecific orbital inflammatory syndromes. *Surv. Ophthalmol.* 29: 93–103, 1984.

Krohel, GB, Krauss, HR, and Winnick, J: Orbital abscess. Presentation, diagnosis, therapy, and sequelae. *Ophthalmology* 89: 492–498, 1982.

Maniglia, AJ, Kronberg, FG, and Culbertson, W: Visual loss associated with orbital and sinus diseases. *Laryngoscope* 94: 1050–1059, 1984.

Mills, RP, and Kartush, JM: Orbital wall thickness and the spread of infection from the paranasal sinuses. *Clin. Otolaryngol.* 10: 209–215, 1985.

Newell, FS, and Leveille, AS: Management and complications of bacterial periorbital and orbital cellulitis. *Metab. Pediatr. Syst. Ophthalmol.* 6: 209–214, 1984.

Parelhoff, ES, Chavis, RM, and Friendly, DS: Wegener's granulomatosis presenting as orbital pseudotumor in children. *J. Pediatr. Ophthalmol. Strabismus* 22: 100–104, 1985.

Shapiro, ED, Wald, ER, and Brozanski, BA: Periorbital cellulitis and paranasal sinusitis: A reappraisal. *Pediatr. Infect. Dis.* 1: 91–94, 1982.

Weisberger, EC, Zauel, DW, Gilmor, RL, and Yune, H: Otolaryngologists' role in diagnosis and treatment of orbital pseudotumor. *Otolaryngol. Head Neck Surg.* 93: 536–549, 1985.

Wenig, BL, Goldstein, MN, and Abramson, AL: Frontal sinusitis and its intracranial complications. *Int. J. Pediatr. Otorhinolaryngol.* 5: 285–302, 1983.

Wilner, HI, Bupta, KL, and Kelly, JK: Orbital pseudotumor: Association of orbital vein deformities and myositis. *Am. J. Radiol.* 1: 305–309, 1980.

Wood, TR, and Slight, JR: Bilateral orbital myiasis. Report of a case. *Arch. Ophthalmol.* 84: 692–693, 1970.

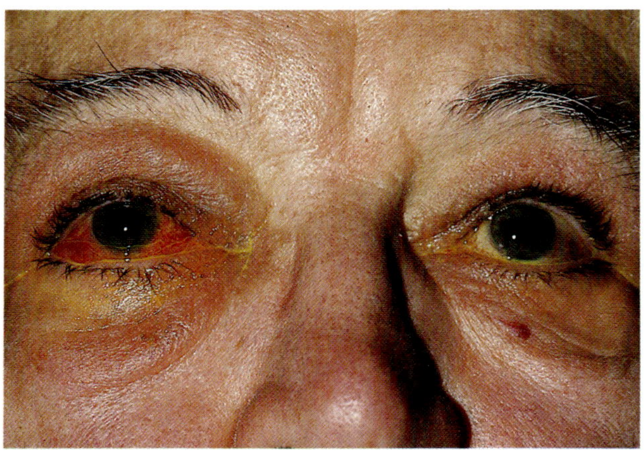

7–1 Edema and injection of the eyelid and chemosis of the conjunctiva. Edema and injection of the eyelid, chemosis of the conjunctiva, and proptosis are considered to be cardinal signs of orbital cellulitis. This 64-year-old female developed a *Streptococcus pyogenes* orbital cellulitis, which extended from the paranasal sinuses. Edema and redness of the eyelid and chemosis of the conjunctiva are evident. (Photograph courtesy of Dr. Devron Char.)

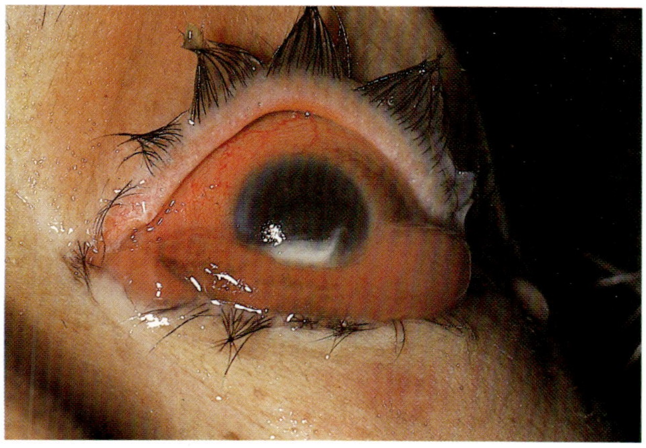

7–2 Proptosis, edema and injection of the eyelid, chemosis of the conjunctiva, and corneal ulcer. Proptosis, edema and injection of the eyelid, and chemosis of the conjunctiva are all cardinal signs of orbital cellulitis. In this 43-year-old female the chemosis and proptosis are quite severe. The pneumococcal corneal ulcer has developed as a result of corneal exposure, which allowed the pneumococcal organism to gain access to the corneal stroma.

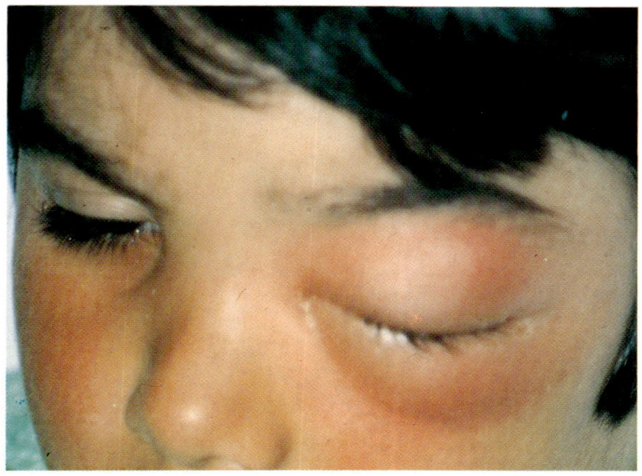

7–3A Orbital cellulitis arising from an ethmoidal sinusitis. This 3-year-old child developed an orbital cellulitis from an ethmoidal sinusitis. Marked edema of the upper and lower eyelid is evident. The child was moderately febrile. The CT scan (Fig. 7–3B) is almost diagnostic of sinus involvement. Once the sinus infection was treated and appropriate antibiotics were instituted for the *Haemophilus influenzae* infection, the orbital cellulitis quickly subsided. (Photograph courtesy of Dr. Devron Char.)

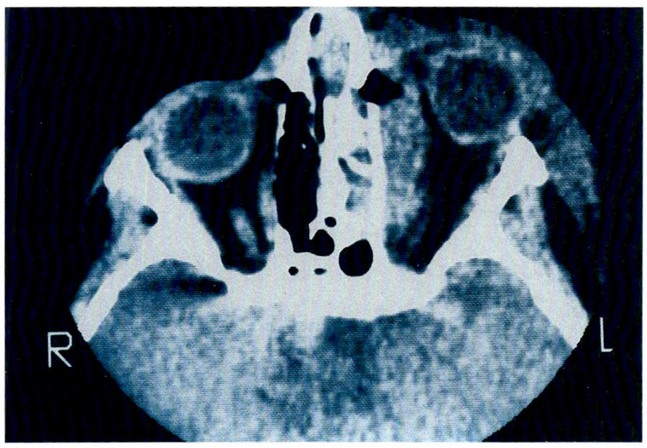

7–3B CT scan of a child (see Fig. 7–3A) with orbital cellulitis arising from ethmoidal sinusitis. The CT scan was performed the day of admission to the hospital. Proptosis and swelling of the eyelid are evident, together with inflammation of the medial aspect of the left orbit. (Photograph courtesy of Dr. Devron Char.)

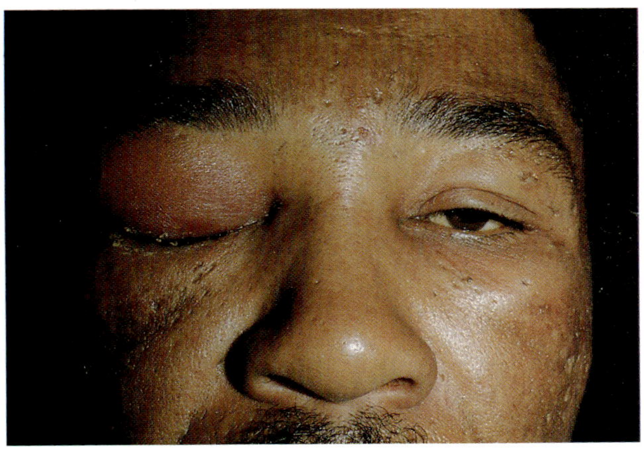

7–4 Preseptal cellulitis. A preseptal cellulitis is limited to the skin and subcutaneous tissue anterior to the orbital septum. This 42-year-old male had been struck in the region of the brow four days previously and noted increasing pain, tenderness, swelling, ptosis, and redness until he was adequately treated. Cultures of material taken from the cellulitis revealed a mixed anaerobic infection.

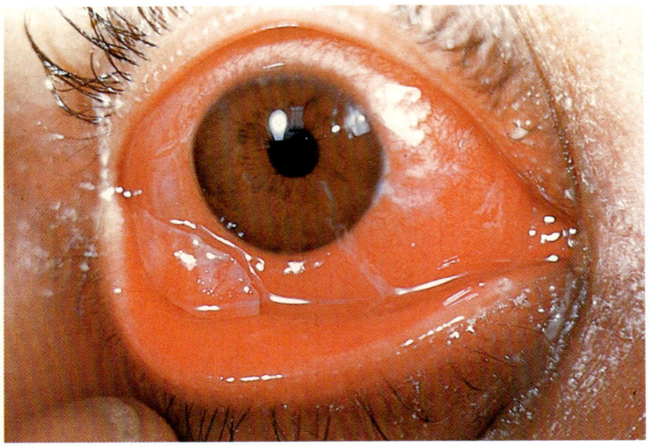

7–5A Suppurative infections of the orbit due to *Klebsiella pneumoniae*. Suppurative infections of the orbit are most commonly associated with a penetrating injury of the orbit, such as occurred in this patient who had a pencil (Fig. 7–5B) lodged in the orbit. Culture of the discharge revealed *Klebsiella pneumoniae*. (Photograph courtesy of Dr. Walter Crawford and reprinted with permission from the *American Journal of Ophthalmology*.)

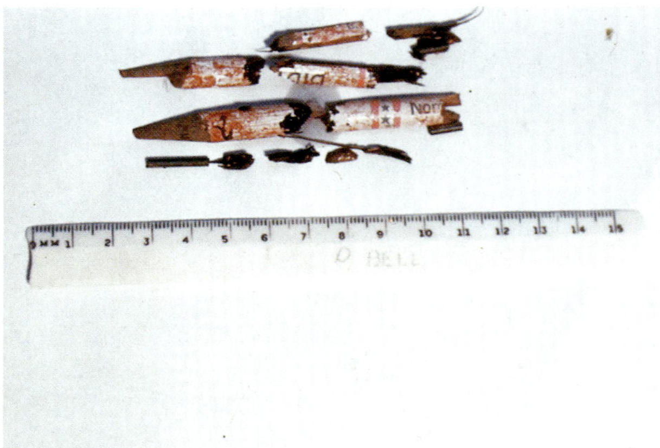

7–5B Fragments of pencil removed from orbit of patient with suppurative infection. The patient seen in Fig. 7–5A had had a persistent draining sinus of the orbit; *K. pneumoniae* could be repeatedly cultured from the discharge. He recalled having been "stabbed" in the orbit, but thought the entire pencil had been removed. (Photograph courtesy of Dr. Walter Crawford and reprinted with permission from the *American Journal of Ophthalmology*.)

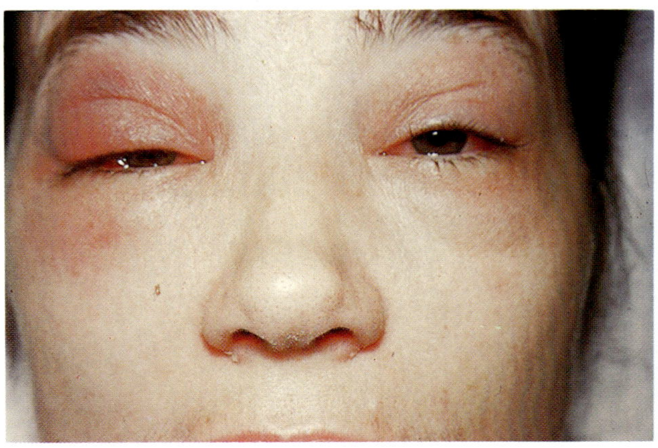

7–6 Serous tenonitis associated with gonorrheal arthritis. A serous tenonitis or inflammation of the episcleral space is uncommon. This woman who had developed a gonorrheal arthritis three days previously developed redness and edema of the eyelids, chemosis of the conjunctiva, and pain on rotation of the eyes. Systemic treatment of her gonorrhea resulted in complete resolution of her orbital findings. (Photograph courtesy of Dr. Phillips Thygeson.)

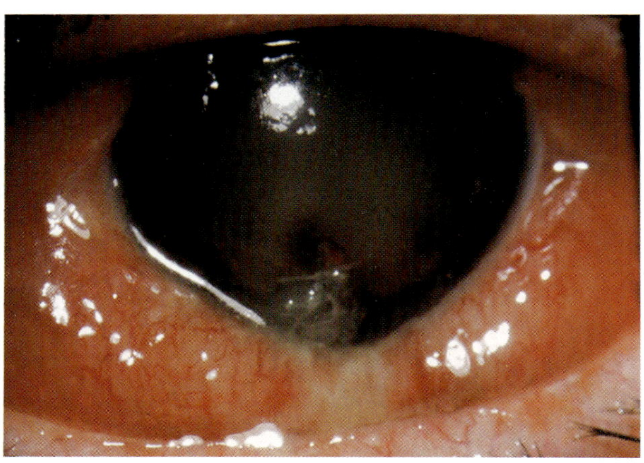

7–7 Purulent tenonitis arising from an uncontrolled endophthalmitis. A purulent tenonitis may be an early sign of beginning panophthalmitis. This patient had been struck in the eye with a piece of chicken wire three days previously. The patient had an obvious endophthalmitis from which we were able to culture *Staphylococcus aureus*. Within two days, the patient developed severe edema of the lids, chemosis, and increasing pain and exudate. Note the chemosis, exudate, obvious corneal perforation, and cataract.

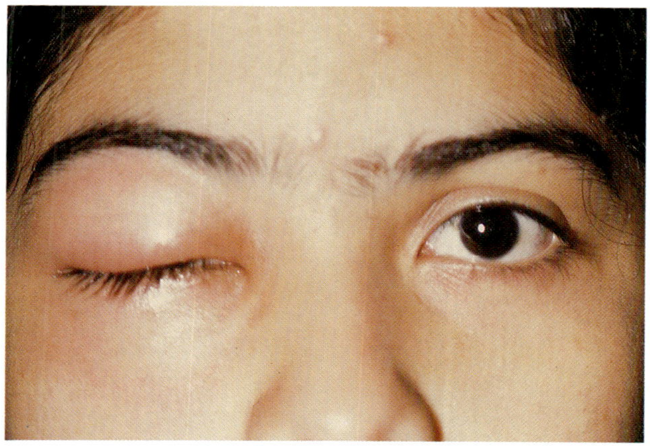

7–8 *Streptococcus pyogenes* orbital infection. This 22-year-old male developed an orbital cellulitis due to *Streptococcus pyogenes*. He gave a history of chronic frontal sinusitis, with sudden onset of pain, ptosis, edema of the lids, proptosis, and redness. Cultures taken from the ostea of the sinuses revealed *S. pyogenes*. The tenderness was most marked over the frontal sinus. The patient responded readily to treatment with systemic penicillin and drainage of the frontal sinus. (Photograph courtesy of Dr. Devron Char.)

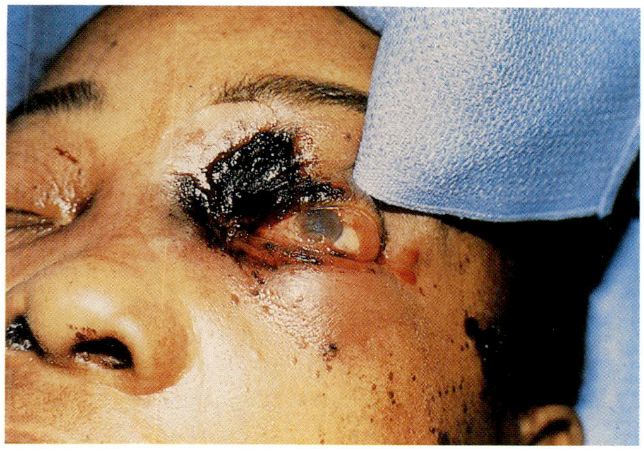

7–9 Phacomatosis of the orbit. This 54-year-old diabetic male developed mucomycosis of the left orbit, paranasal sinuses, and nose. His diabetes had been poorly controlled and he was in acidosis at the time of admission. Although the patient was treated by controlling his acidosis, by administration of systemic amphotericin B, and by extensive debridement of the affected areas, he died one day after this photograph was taken. (Photograph courtesy of Drs. William V. Good and David McCartney.)

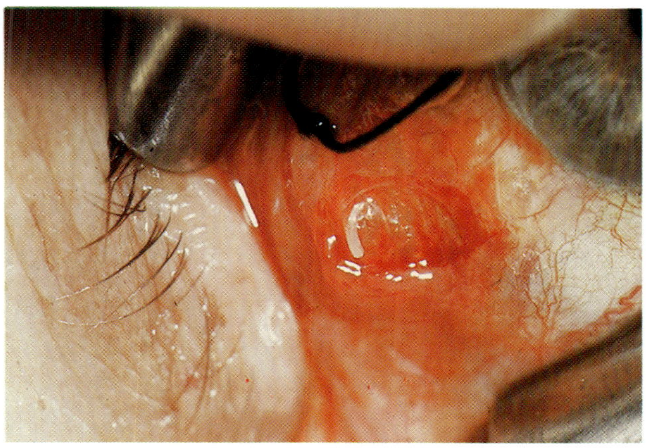

7–10 The African eye worm *(Loa loa)* at the time of removal from the subconjunctival tissue area. This 46-year-old Frenchman had spent over ten years in Africa and during that time had had an African eye worm removed from his orbit. The day that we saw him, he had noted irritation and burning of the eye and called to say that he had a "worm in his eye". The parasite was located, 4% cocaine eyedrops were instilled into the conjunctival sac in an effort to paralyze the worm, and the conjunctiva and the worm underlying the conjunctiva were then grasped with a toothed forceps. A suture was tied around the area, the conjunctiva was opened, and the *Loa loa* grasped and removed.

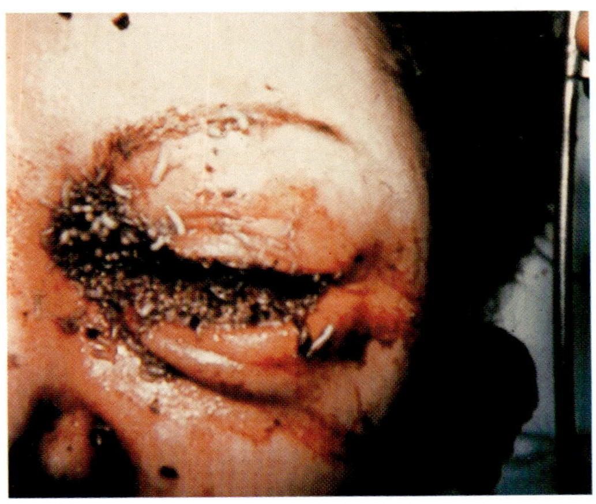

7–11 *Calliphora vomitoria* invading the orbit. This woman was found unconscious in her home and taken to the emergency room where she was found to have the maggots of *Calliphora vomitoria* invading her orbit. She died within six hours without regaining consciousness; it was thought that she had been infected during a period of drunkeness. Photograph courtesy of Dr. T. Rodman Wood and reprinted with permission from Archives of Ophthalmology.

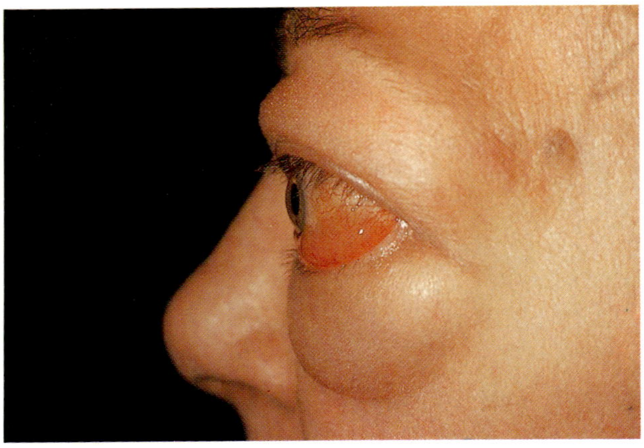

7–12 Proptosis, chemosis, and edema of the eyelids in exophthalmic Grave's disease (lateral aspect). This 61-year-old female had had exophthalmic Grave's disease for four months. The proptosis, chemosis, and lid edema are prominent signs of orbitopathy. The proptosis measured 24 mm using a Hertel exophthalmometer.

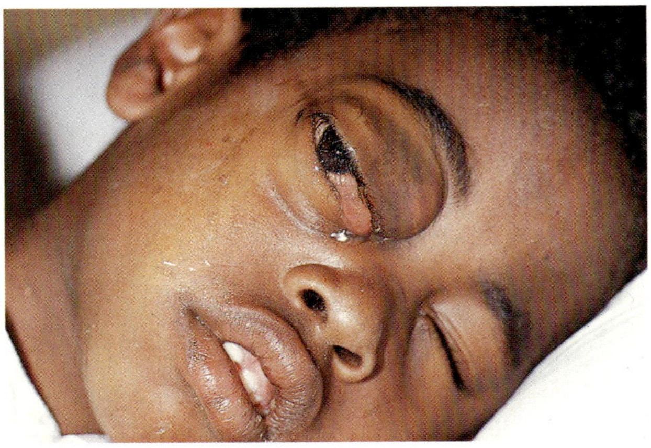

7–13 Sudden bleeding into an orbital lymphatic varix. This 8-year-old child had had surgery three years previously for bleeding into an orbital lymphatic varix, as can be seen from the lateral canthal scar. He had no further problem until three days prior to this photograph, when he developed a sudden onset of proptosis, edema of the eyelid, chemosis, and limitation of ocular movement. The morning that this photograph was taken, the patient had no light perception and the pupil was unresponsive to light. Drainage of the blood and ligation and destruction of the orbital varix was performed; the visual acuity returned to 6/15. To authors' knowledge there has been no further recurrence of his orbital problems.

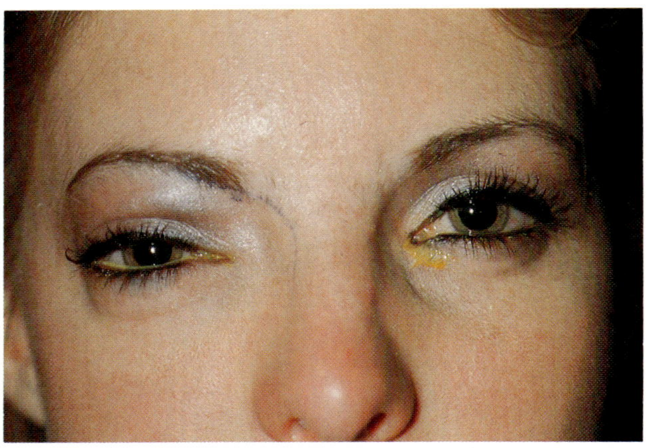

7–14 Mucocele of right ethmoid sinus. This 28-year-old female was seen with the complaint of chronic swelling of the upper eyelid and the medial aspect of the right orbit. The swelling was nontender and only slightly red. (The medial extent of the fluctuant swelling is marked with a pen.) (Photograph courtesy of Dr. Devron Char.)

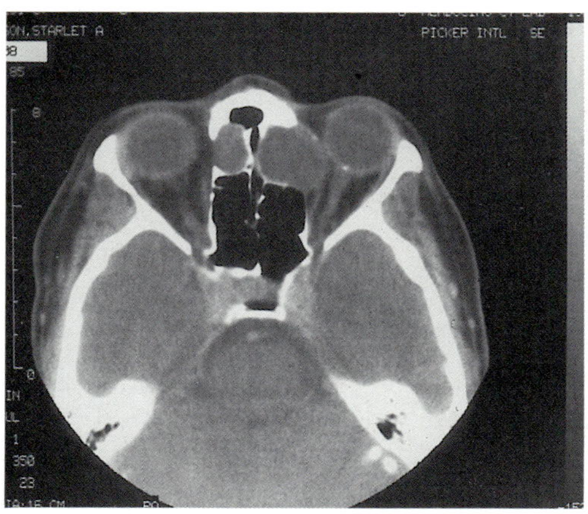

7–15 CT scan of mucocele of left ethmoid sinus. This CT scan of a patient with a mucocele of the ethmoid sinus shows marked soft tissue enlargement and erosion of the left ethmoid bone. (The CT scan is not from the patient shown in Fig. 7–14.) (Photograph courtesy of Dr. Devron Char.)

7–16 Bilateral pseudotumor of the orbit. This patient presented with a history of bilateral proptosis of three months duration. The patient first noted symptoms of redness, proptosis, and some discomfort of the left eye, which was followed in two weeks by involvement of the right eye. Proptosis of both eyes is evident, with minimal signs of edema. There was no orbital tenderness. (Photograph courtesy of Dr. Devron Char.)

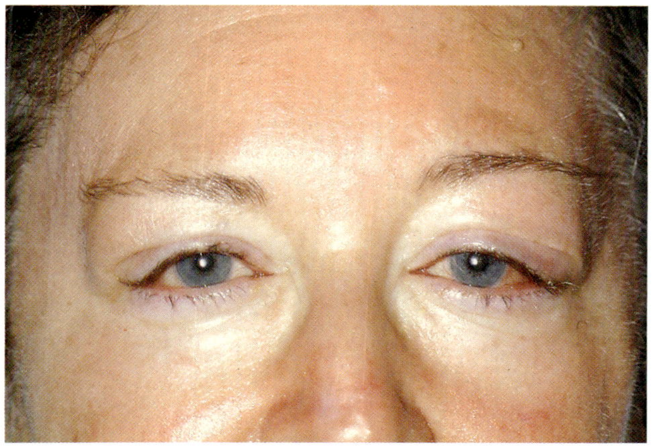

7–17 Inflammation of the orbital lobe of the lacrimal gland. This patient developed proptosis of the left eye together with edema of the left eyelid and downward displacement of the eye. He was found to have redness and edema of the orifices of the lacrimal gland. Subsequently, the patient was found to have sarcoidosis. (Photograph courtesy of Dr. Devron Char.)

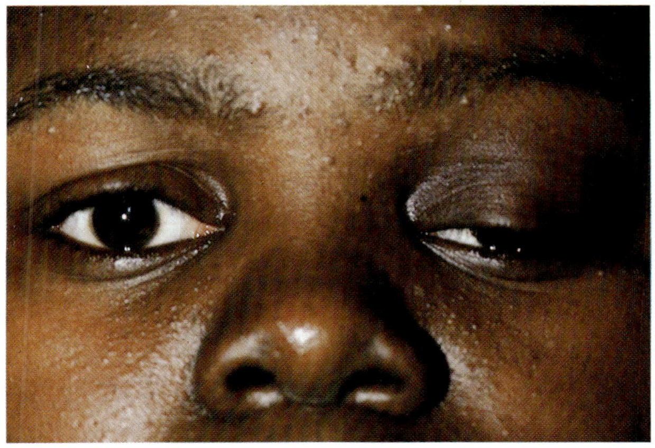

7–18 Wegener's granulomatosis with mild proptosis on the left side. Wegener's granulomatosis and midline granuloma may present with proptosis as the earliest and major complaint. This patient was found to have Wegener's granulomatosis two years previously. She had had recurrent proptosis along with some tenderness of the area of the upper eyelid whenever her immunosuppressive therapy was decreased. The skin lesion in the midline of the forehead is quite characteristic of this condition. Swelling over the area of the ethmoidal sinuses is also evident.

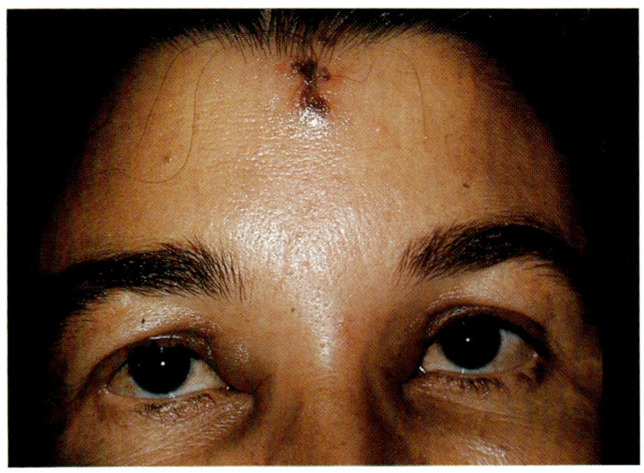

7–19 Engorged and prominent conjunctival vessels in thrombophlebitis of the orbit. Obstruction of the venous outflow of the orbit, whether due to cavernous sinus thrombosis, thrombophlebitis, pressure from an orbital tumor, or another cause, results in distention and prominence of the conjunctiva. A bluish discoloration of the vessels is often evident, as seen in this 45-year-old female with thrombophlebitis of the orbit.

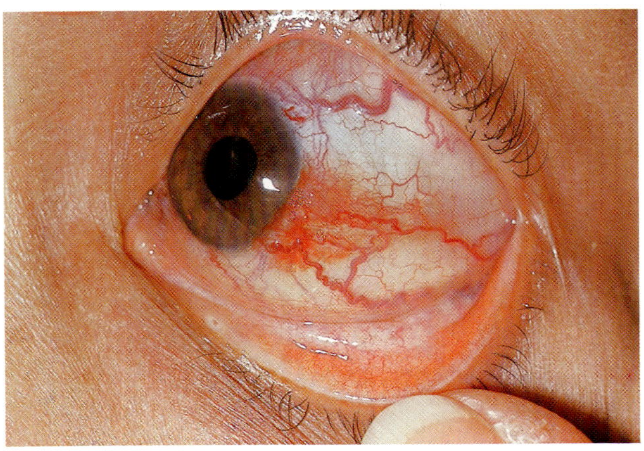

Chapter 8

Endophthalmitis

Endophthalmitis is an inflammatory process involving the internal eye. The inflammation usually involves several coats of the eye (retina, uvea, and/or sclera) and their adjacent cavities (vitreous, posterior chamber, and/or anterior chamber). Panophthalmitis, on the other hand, is an inflammatory process involving the internal eye and the soft tissue of the orbit surrounding the eye. Endophthalmitis and panophthalmitis are usually caused by infections, but may arise from reaction to a foreign body or to denatured lens material, necrosis of an intraocular tumor, or anterior segment ischema.

Sources of Endophthalmitis

Endophthalmitis most frequently arises from exogenous sources, but may also arise from endogenous sources.

Exogenous Sources of Endophthalmitis

The major source of an endophthalmitis is a penetrating injury of the eye, such as from surgery or trauma. There is a far greater risk that an endophthalmitis will develop following trauma than following surgery (Figs. 8–1A and B). However, the frequency of intraocular surgery is much greater than the frequency of trauma and it is therefore the most common cause of endophthalmitis (Ho and McMeel, 1983). Less common exogenous sources include infection of a filtering bleb (Fig. 8–2), infection by way of a vitreous wick (Maguire et al., 1985), infection following removal of a suture, and infection developing from an uncontrolled corneal ulcer or an uncontrolled orbital cellulitis.

Endogenous Sources of Endophthalmitis

Endogenous endophthalmitis is uncommon. Possible sources include hematogenous spread, as from intravenous drug abuse (Gallo et al., 1985) (Fig. 8–3) or prolonged hyperalimentation; spread from a septic embolus (Farber et al., 1985); and spread from a meningitis (metastatic endophthalmitis). Other causes of endogenous endophthalmitis are usually not infectious in origin. These include spread of inflammation from the optic nerve, inflammation arising from necrosis of an intraocular tumor, and an inflammatory reaction to lens material, such as a hypermature lens.

Etiology

More than 50 percent of all endophthalmitis is caused by the Gram-positive cocci *Staphylococcus aureus* (Fig. 8–4A) and *S. epidermidis* (Fig. 8–4B). Other Gram-positive organisms, such as *Streptococcus pneumoniae* (Figs. 8–5A, B and C), other *Streptococcus* spp. (Figs. 8–6A and B), *Bacillus* spp. and *Nocardia asteroides*, are infrequent causes of endophthalmitis.

The Gram-negative bacteria account for more than 25 percent of cases of endophthalmitis, with *Pseudomonas aeruginosa* being the most important in this group. Other Gram-negative bacteria, such as *Escherichia coli, Klebsiella pneumoniae, Proteus* spp., *Moraxella* spp. (Figs. 8–7A and B), and *Serratia marcescens*, are relatively uncommon causes.

Metastatic bacterial endophthalmitis is rare; the causative bacteria include *Neisseria meningitidis* (Hull et al., 1982), *Haemophilus influenzae* type b (Taylor et al., 1980) *Mycobacterium tuberculosis, Listeria monocytogenes, Staphylococcus aureus, Streptococcus pneumoniae* and the other *Streptococcus* spp., *Actinomyces israelii*, and *Serratia marcescens*.

Fungal endophthalmitis rarely occurs and most commonly develops following surgery. The fungal causes of exogenous and metastatic endophthalmitis include *Candida* spp. and the filamentous fungi, including the *Aspergillus* spp. (Michelson et al., 1982) and many of the opportunistic fungi.

Manifestations

The symptoms arising from a bacterial endophthalmitis may develop as soon as 24 hours or as long as several months after introduction of the organism into the eye. The intensity and time of onset of symptoms vary with the virulence of the organism, the size of inoculum, and the use of immunosuppressive agents, especially glucocorticoids. Decreased vision, photophobia, pain, and circumcorneal redness are common symptoms in exogenous bacterial endophthalmitis. In the occasional case, however, pain is not present (Deutsch and Goldberg, 1984). In endogenous (metastatic) bacterial endophthalmitis, the patient may complain only of blurred vision.

The characteristic signs of bacterial endophthalmitis include edema of the eyelids (Fig. 8–8); chemosis and injection of the conjunctiva (Fig. 8–9); loss of corneal luster (Fig. 8–10); severe anterior chamber reaction, including hypopyon formation

(Fig. 8–11); miosis; severe vitreous reaction; and loss of the red reflex. The severity of the signs, like the severity of the symptoms, varies with the virulence of the organism and the use of immunosuppressive drugs, especially glucocorticoids. With the exception of relatively avirulent bacterial infections (e.g., *Staphylococcus epidermidis),* suppuration occurs early in bacterial endophthalmitis.

If the lens-iris diaphragm is intact, bacterial infections beginning in the vitreous cavity or in the anterior chamber usually remain confined to that particular cavity (Beyer et al., 1984, 1985), except in the late stages of untreated infections. In metastatic endophthalmitis, therefore, a severe vitreous reaction and retinitis are characteristically found, while very few signs of infection are noted anteriorly (Boldrey, 1981; Farber et al., 1985).

The symptoms of a fungal endophthalmitis, which usually begin insidiously weeks or even months after onset of the infection, consist of reduced vision, pain and redness. Fungal endophthalmitis is usually nonsuppurative, and therefore the signs develop insidiously; when fully developed, the signs include those found in bacterial endophthalmitis. In fungal infections of the vitreous cavity, small round inflammatory vitreous foci develop, gradually enlarge, and as they approach the iris cause a severe anterior chamber reaction (Fig. 8–12). As the infection continues unabated, progressive narrowing of the chamber angle and occlusion of the pupil occurs, producing secondary glaucoma.

Differential Diagnosis

Severe inflammation of the eye may arise without infection. It can usually be differentiated from a true infection by its rapidity of onset (within hours) and its tendency to quickly reach a maximum intensity and to remain at that leval or begin to subside. A true infection, on the other hand, usually begins 24 hours or more following trauma and continues to worsen unless properly treated.

Inflammatory reactions arising from necrosis of an intraocular tumor are usually less severe than a true infection; the hypopyon formation and the keratic precipitates are large and often resemble "lumps of mashed potatoes." A lens-induced inflammatory reaction is most intense around the lens and lens products, and the total inflammatory reaction is less intense than an inflammation caused by a true infection.

Anterior segment ischemia is uncommon, but may occur following detachment of several recti muscles at the time of retinal detachment or of squint surgery. Anterior segment ischemia may also arise during an acute attack of angle closure glaucoma (Fig. 8–13), or during an episode of herpes zoster ophthalmicus. The major characteristics are corneal edema, moderate anterior chamber reaction, and iris atrophy. Cataractous changes tend to develop later in the course of the process.

Disorganization of the eye and marked inflammatory reaction may arise from a retained foreign body (Fig. 8–14) (Meyers et al., 1975). In most instances, the inflammation continues unabated until the foreign body is sequestered or extruded.

Complications

The complications of endophthalmitis are commonly severe. They include retinal detachment (Nelson et al. 1985), the development of an inflammatory membrane, loss of retinal function following death of retinal cells, orbital cellulitis, meningitis, metastatic spread of infection, loss of the eye, and death.

References

Beyer, TL, Vogler, G, Sharma, D, and O'Donnell, FE Jr: Protective barrier effect of the posterior lens capsule in exogenous bacterial endophthalmitis: An experimental primate study. *Invest. Ophthalmol. Vis. Sci.* 25: 108–112, 1984.

Beyer, TL, O'Donnell, FE, Goncalves, V, and Singh, R: Role of the posterior capsule in the prevention of postoperative bacterial endophthalmitis: Experimental primate studies and clinical implications. *Br. J. Ophthalmol.* 69: 841–846, 1985.

Boldrey, EE: Bilateral endogenous aspergillus endophthalmitis. *Retina* 1: 171–174, 1981.

Deutsch, TA, and Goldberg, MF: Painless endophthalmitis after cataract surgery. *Ophthalmic Surg.* 15: 837–840, 1984.

Farber, BP, Weinbaum, DL, and Drummer, JS: Metastatic bacterial endophthalmitis. *Arch. Intern. Med.* 145: 62–64, 1985.

Gallo, J, Playfair, J, Gregory-Roberts, J, Grunstein, H, Clifton-Bligh, P, and Billson, F: Fungal endophthalmitis in narcotic abusers. Medical and surgical therapy in 10 patients. *Med. J. Aust.* 142: 386–388, 1985.

Ho, PC, and McMeel, JW: Bacterial endophthalmitis after retinal surgery. *Retina* 3: 99–102, 1983.

Hull, DS, Patipa, M, and Cox, F: Metastatic endophthalmitis: A complication of meningococcal meningitis. *Ann. Ophthalmol.* 14: 29–30, 1982.

Maguire, LJ, Frantz, J, Packer, AJ, and Kaufman, H: Bacterial endophthalmitis associated with vitreous wick after penetrating keratoplasty. *Am. J. Ophthalmol.* 100: 854–855, 1985.

Meyers, R, and Ritchie, CL: Migration of wooden foreign body into the lens. Report of a case. *Canad. J. Ophthalmol.* 10: 408–411, 1975.

Michelson, JB, Freedman, SD, and Boyden, DG: Aspergillus endophthalmitis in a drug abuser. *Ann. Ophthalmol.* 14: 1051–1054, 1982.

Nelson, PT, Marcus, DA, and Bovino, JA: Retinal detachment following endophthalmitis. *Ophthalmology* 92: 1112–1117, 1985.

Taylor, JR, Cibis, GW, and Hamtil, LW: Endophthalmitis complicating *Haemophilus influenzae* type B meningitis. *Arch. Ophthalmol.* 98: 324–326, 1980.

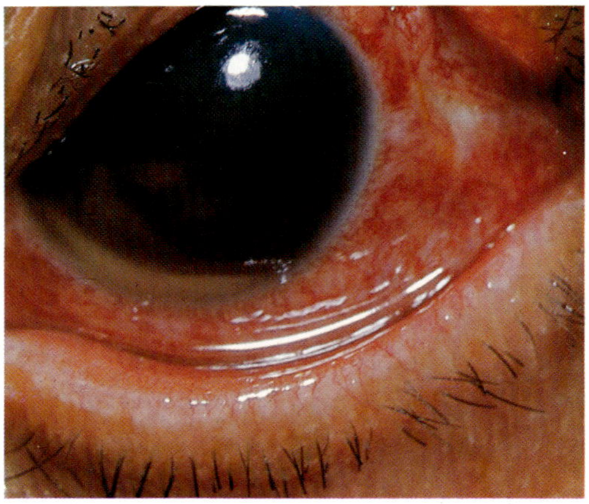

8–1A Endophthalmitis following cataract extraction. Because of the large number of intraocular surgical cases now being performed, endophthalmitis occurs most frequently following surgery. However, penetrating injuries of the eye are still common causes of (and carry a greater risk of) endophthalmitis. This patient developed a *Staphylococcus aureus* endophthalmitis three days after cataract surgery. Note the loss of luster of the cornea, and the hypopyon and haziness within the anterior chamber.

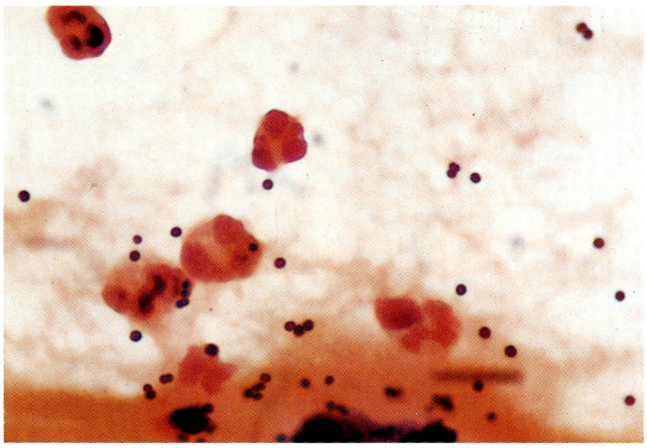

8–1B Smear of the vitreous aspirate from patient with endophthalmitis following cataract surgery. This Gram-stained smear taken from the patient shown in Fig. 8–1A shows a typical staphylococcus morphology. Most of the cocci occur singly, a few in pairs, and several in small clusters of two or more cocci. There are also a few polymorphonuclear granulocytes. Gram's stain, ×1000.

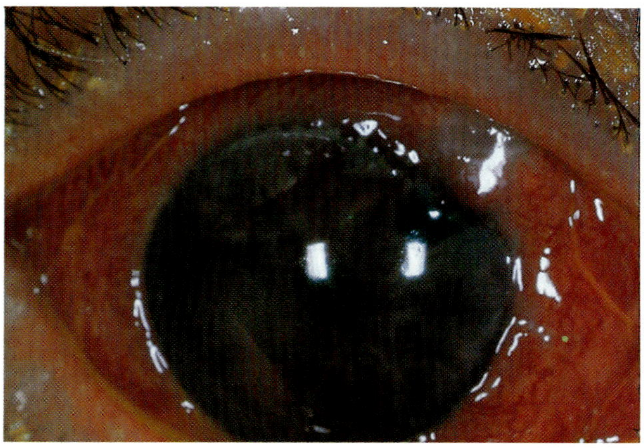

8–2 Endophthalmitis following infection of a filtering bleb. A filtering bleb may serve as a source of infection of the internal eye. This patient developed a *Haemophilus* spp. conjunctivitis followed in two days by infection of a filtering bleb and early endophthalmitis. The infected filtering bleb can be seen at the 2:00 position, along with marked injection of the globe, haziness of the cornea, and congestion of the iris. (The peripheral coloboma of the iris was made at the time of the glaucoma surgery two years previously.)

8–3 Metastatic endophthalmitis confined primarily to the vitreous cavity. Metastatic endophthalmitis may occur from intravenous drug abuse, such as occurred in this 26-year-old male who admitted to the intravenous use of mood-altering drugs. His major complaint was that of loss of vision, and as is visible in the photograph, very little reaction was present in the anterior segment of the eye. The photograph was taken after a vitreous biopsy was performed for diagnosis of the infectious agent. Note the hemorrhage on the face of the iris and vitreous and the mass in the vitreous.

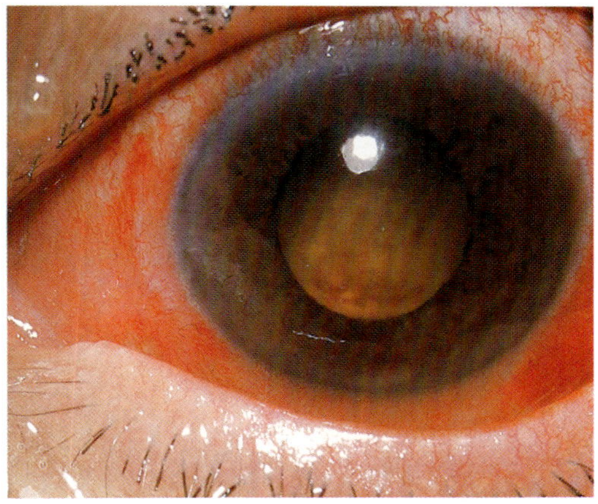

8–4A Endophthalmitis due to *Staphylococcus aureus*. This 63-year-old physician was operated upon for a retinal detachment. Forty-eight hours after surgery, he complained of pain and blurred vision and was noted to have the severe hypopyon and vitreous clouding seen in this photograph. Infiltrates are evident in the sclera and cornea, along with a very large hypopyon. *S. aureus* was recovered during vitrectomy.

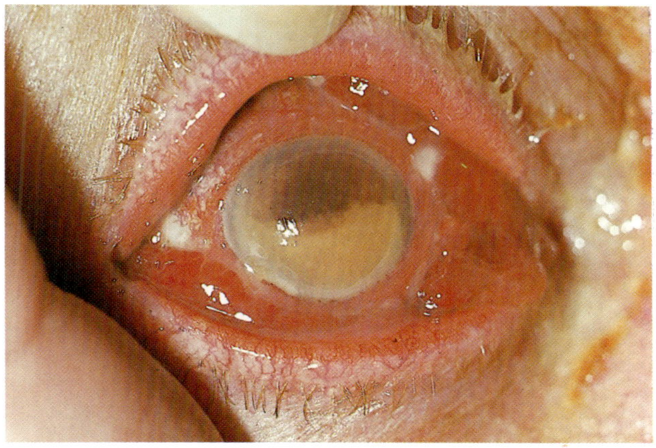

8–4B *Staphylococcus epidermidis* endophthalmitis frequently begins many days, weeks, or even months following surgery. In this 74-year-old female mild symptoms of endophthalmitis occurred, developing four weeks after surgery. Injection of the conjunctiva, hypopyon, and clouding of the anterior chamber are visible.

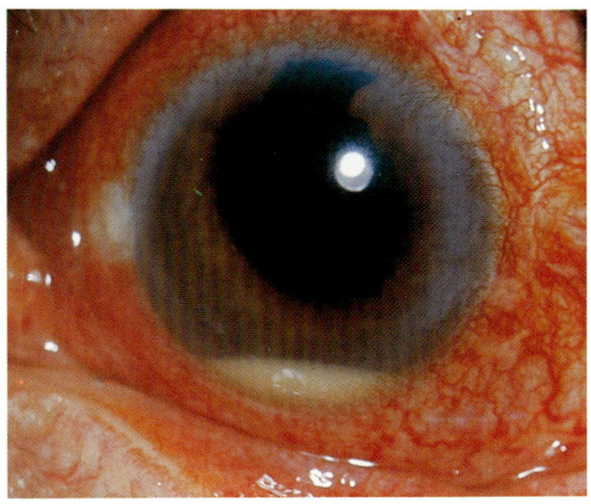

8–5A Bilateral *Streptococcus pneumoniae* endophthalmitis following glaucoma surgery (right eye). This 4-year-old child developed bilateral *S. pneumoniae* endophthalmitis following glaucoma surgery three days earlier. The patient was reprepped and redraped, and an entirely new setup of instruments and gowns was used between each procedure. The source of the organism was probably the child's nose.

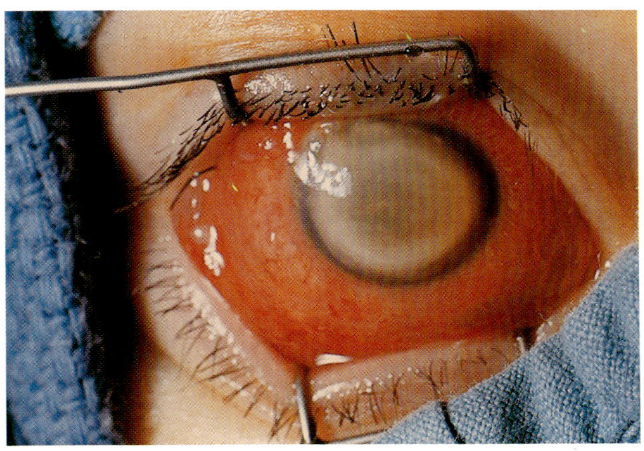

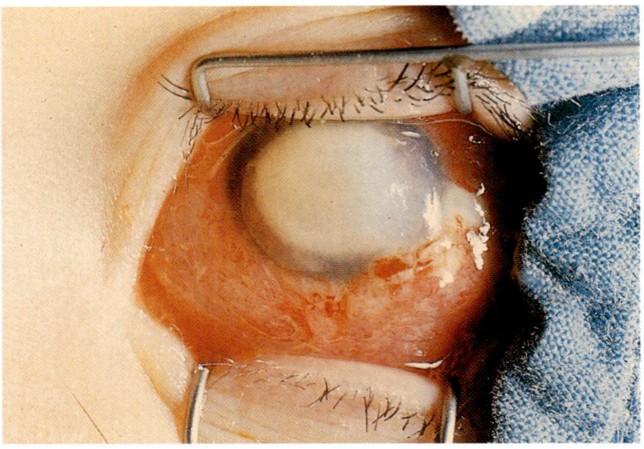

8–5B Bilateral *Streptococcus pneumoniae* endophthalmitis following glaucoma surgery (left eye). This photograph shows the same patient pictured in Fig. 8–5A.

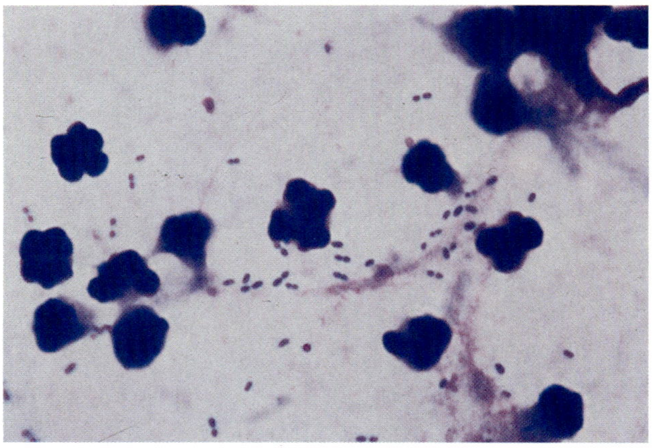

8–5C Smear of aqueous showing *S. pneumoniae.* This smear was taken from the patient shown in Figs. 8–5A and B. Organisms are generally difficult to detect in an aqueous smear, but many lancet-shaped diplococci along with a number of polymorphonuclear leukocytes can be seen in this photograph, providing an easy and rapid diagnosis. Giemsa stain, × 1000.

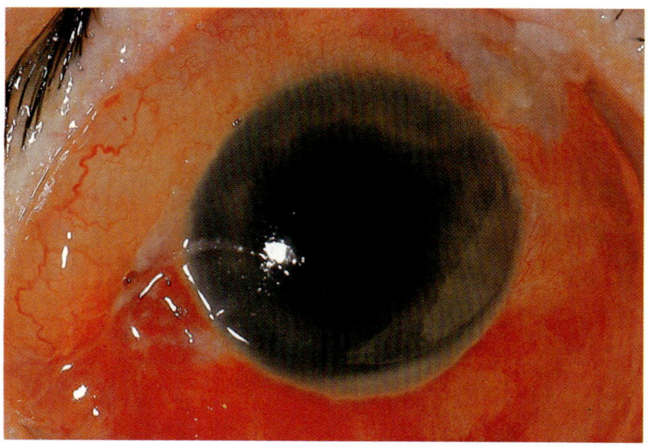

8–6A *Streptococcus faecalis* endophthalmitis. This 67-year-old female developed an endophthalmitis almost exactly one year after cataract surgery. She had developed a small filtering bleb after surgery and had been scheduled to have the filtering bleb closed surgically. She then noted pain, blurred vision, and redness of the eye and was found to have an endophthalmitis. The photograph was taken after she had been given a subconjunctival injection of methicillin. The filtering bleb is partially masked by mucopurulent material, the cornea is very hazy, and a small hypopyon is evident along with a very turbid anterior chamber.

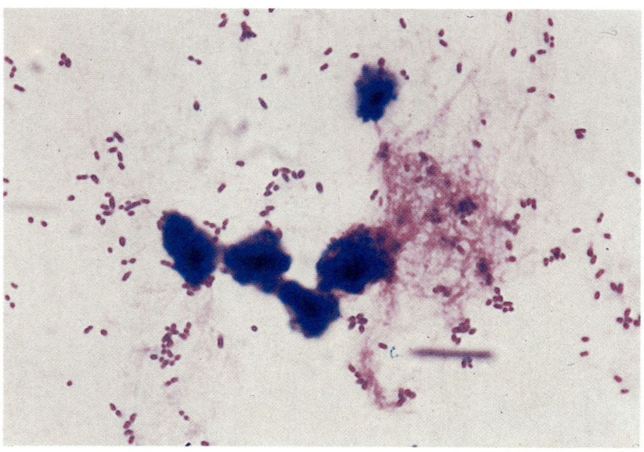

8–6B Smear of *Streptococcus faecalis* from vitreous aspirate. Streptococci in aqueous or vitreous smears usually occur in long chains. *S. faecalis* is an exception; here it can be seen as diplococci or as single cocci. Because of its morphology, this organism is sometimes confused with the pneumococcus. Giemsa stain, × 1000.

8–7A *Moraxella* spp. infection of filtering bleb. Endophthalmitis due to *Moraxella* spp. is extremely unusual. This 54-year-old male developed infection of a filtering bleb that had been made three years previously for glaucoma. Fortunately, he was seen and treated early; the infection within the bleb and the endophthalmitis were readily controlled. Purulent material can be seen in the bleb. The anterior chamber contains some fibrin, which is readily visible over the pupillary area.

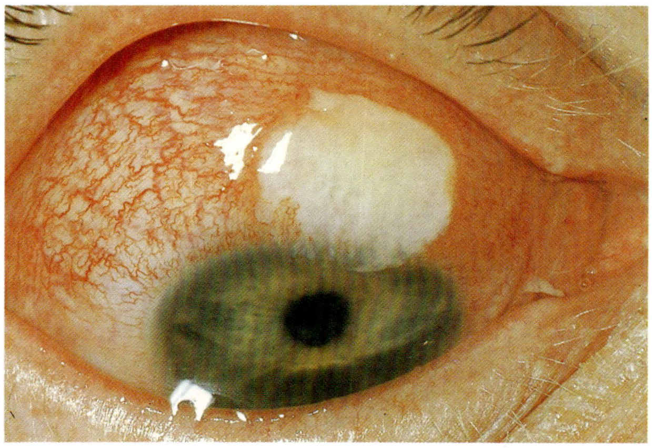

8–7B Smear of *Moraxella* spp. from filtering bleb. Large diplobacilli typical of *Moraxella* are shown in this smear. This is a Giemsa-stained slide, and the organisms therefore appear blue. Giemsa stain, × 1000.

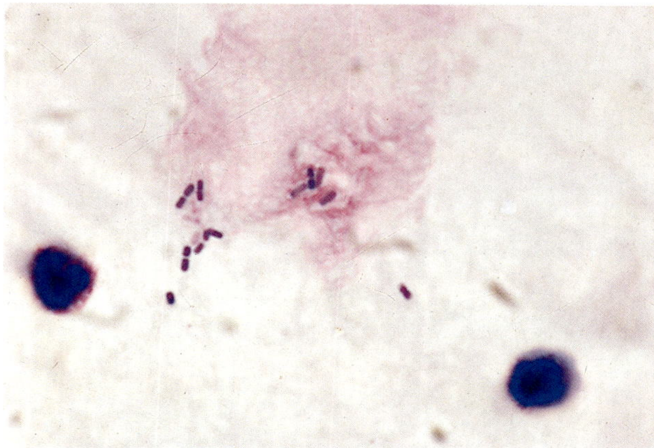

8–8 Edema and injection of the eyelids in a severe endophthalmitis. Two major signs of endophthalmitis are edema and injection of the eyelids. In this patient, who developed a beta-hemolytic streptococcal endophthalmitis three days previously, the lid edema and injection are moderately severe. The conjunctiva is injected and a hypopyon fills the anterior chamber.

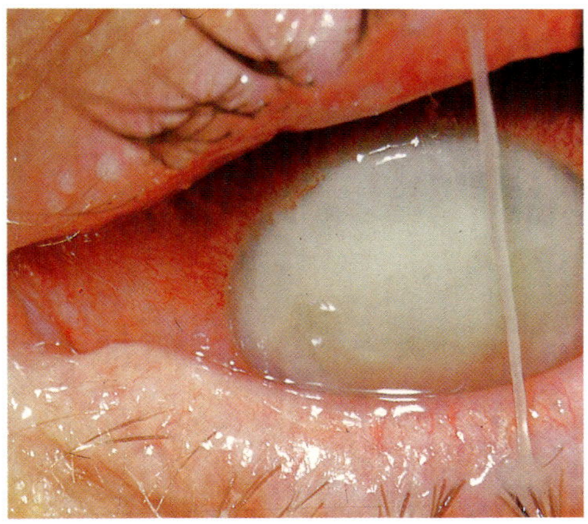

8–9 Injection of the conjunctiva in endophthalmitis. In endophthalmitis, injection of the conjunctiva occurs especially in the area surrounding the limbus. In this patient with an infected filtering bleb, one can readily see the injection of the conjunctiva, edema of the eyelids, and early loss of corneal luster.

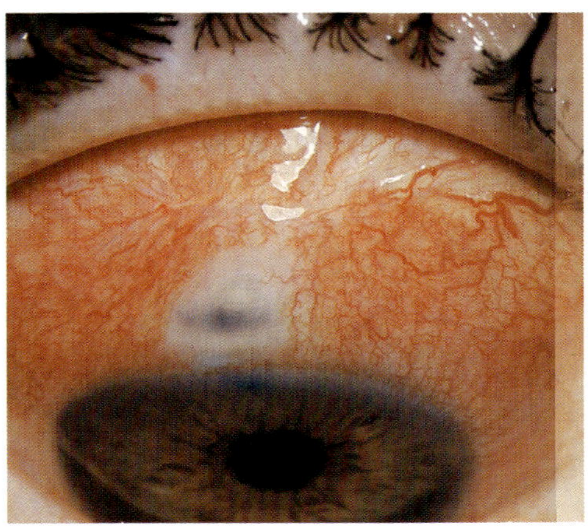

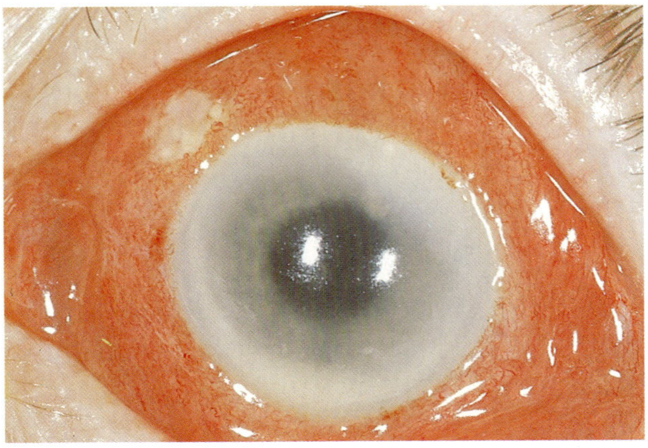

8–10 Loss of corneal luster. One major sign of endophthalmitis is the loss of corneal luster. This photograph shows one of three patients who underwent cataract extraction on the same day and who all developed a beta-hemolytic streptococcal endophthalmitis. Edema of the eyelids and conjunctival injection are also prominent.

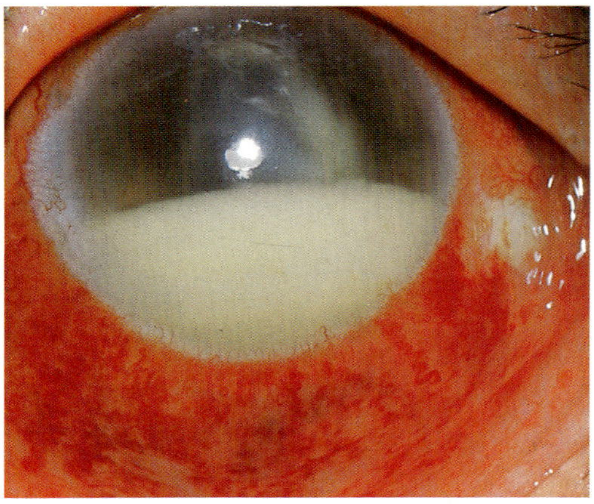

8–11 Severe anterior chamber reaction and hypopyon formation. This photograph shows the same patient pictured in Fig. 8–4B, who had developed endophthalmitis following cataract extraction. A marked anterior chamber reaction and a large hypopyon are evident, both of which are signs of endophthalmitis.

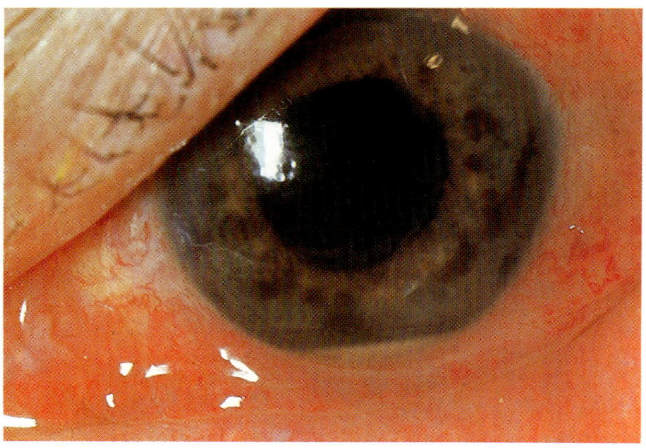

8–12 Fungal endophthalmitis due to *Aspergillus* spp. A fungal endophthalmitis may develop weeks or months following introduction of the organism into the eye. This patient developed pain, redness, and some photophobia two months after cataract surgery. He later developed vitreous clouding and some "snowballs" in the vitreous. (The tiny snowballs, together with vitreous strands, can be seen in the pupillary area.) A small hypopyon is beginning to develop.

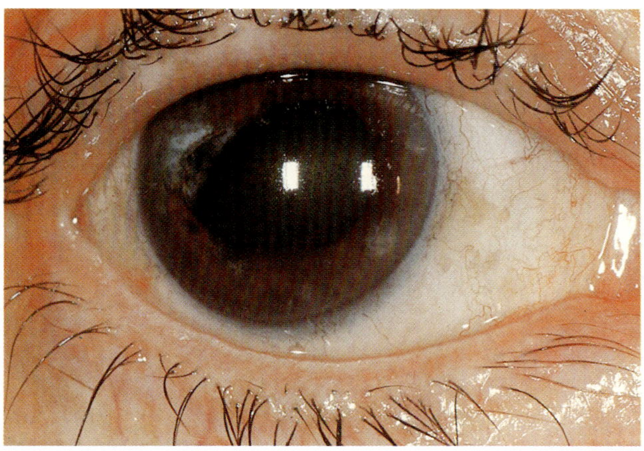

8–13 Anterior segment ischemia. Anterior segment ischemia may develop from various causes, including detachment of the rectus muscles, prolonged and marked elevation of intraocular pressure, and an attack of herpes zoster ophthalmicus. In this patient, who developed anterior segment ischemia following a severe attack of acute glaucoma, one can see iris atrophy, pigment deposition on the endothelium, subsiding corneal edema, and early cataractous changes.

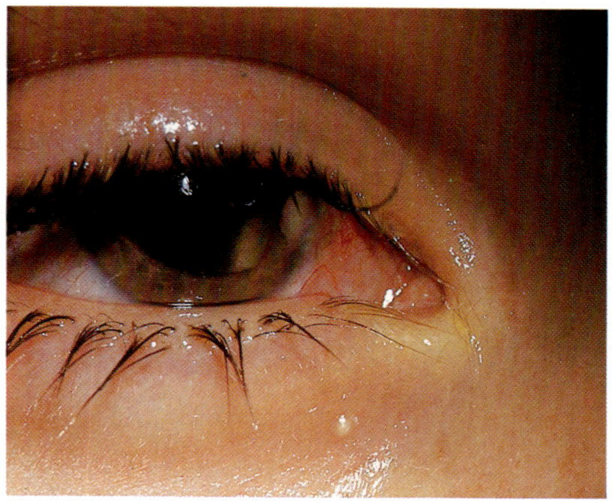

8–14 Retained intraocular foreign body. A retained intraocular foreign body usually produces persistent inflammation until it is either extruded or sequestered. This 7-year-old child had a piece of wood lodged in the vitreous. He developed a moderate inflammatory reaction that persisted until the foreign body extruded into the anterior chamber. Repeated attempts with echography to localize the foreign body or even to prove its presence were unsuccessful. The area where the wood penetrated and the intravitreal mass are both evident. (Reprinted with permission from the *Canadian Journal of Ophthalmology.*)

Chapter 9

Uveitis

The term uveitis includes any inflammation of the uveal tract, and may be subdivided into anterior uveitis (iritis, iridocyclitis, and cyclitis); posterior uveitis (choroiditis, chorioretinitis, and retinochoroiditis); and panuveitis. Anterior uveitis and panuveitis may simulate inflammations or infections of the external eye; anterior and posterior uveitis and panuveitis may simulate an endophthalmitis.

Iritis is an inflammation that affects primarily the iris; most of the inflammatory signs (cells and flare) occur in the anterior chamber. Cyclitis affects primarily the ciliary body, and the major sign of inflammation is the presence of inflammatory cells in the retrolental space and anterior vitreous. Iridocyclitis (inflammation of the iris and ciliary body) is the most common form of anterior uveitis. The inflammatory signs occur with about equal intensity in the anterior chamber and in the retrolental space and anterior vitreous.

In posterior uveitis (choroiditis, chorioretinitis, and retinochoroiditis), inflammation occurs principally in the choroid and retina. When the inflammation spreads from the choroid to involve the retina, it is usually called a chorioretinitis; when the inflammation begins in the retina and spreads to the choroid (e.g., toxoplasmosis), it is termed a retinochoroiditis.

Panuveitis is uncommon. The inflammation is of equal intensity both posteriorly and anteriorly.

Manifestations

The manifestations of an anterior uveitis include photophobia, tearing, redness, blurred vision, and miosis. There is muddy appearance or engorgement of the iris; flare and cells in the anterior chamber, retrolental space, or anterior vitreous; and keratic precipitates on the posterior surface of the cornea. The manifestations of a posterior uveitis are usually limited to blurred vision, an occasional mild redness, cells and inflammatory products in the vitreous, and edema of the choroid and retina.

The photophobia and tearing in anterior uveitis vary from mild to intense, depending on the rapidity of onset and the intensity of the inflammation. The inflammation arises from stimulation of the sensory nerve endings in the iris and/or the ciliary body: light striking the retina sets up a reflex arc that causes the muscles within the inflamed iris and/or ciliary body to contract, which in turn stimulates the sensory nerve endings. The resultant pain is a dull boring ache, which is referred to the temple, periorbital region, or other areas supplied by the trigeminal nerve.

The blurred vision of a uveitis usually results from exudation of cells and protein into the media (aqueous, retrolental space, and vitreous), which serves to change the refractive power of the media. A severe or prolonged inflammatory reaction may also cause blurring of vision by producing miosis and/or changes in the lens. In addition, a posterior uveitis may cause blurred vision by producing distortion or destruction of the visual elements of the retina.

The redness of the eye in uveitis is primarily circumcorneal (Fig. 9–1) and violaceous in hue, and develops from engorgement of the deep (superficial and deep episcleral) vessels. The pupil is miotic, and the iris is engorged (Fig. 9–1) from congestion of the iris vessels as they participate in the inflammatory reaction. The muddy appearance of the iris results from the vascular engorgement and the decrease in clarity of the iris is caused by turbidity in the overlying aqueous.

Table 9–1 Grading the Degree of Cells and Flare in the Anterior Chamber*

	Flare		Cells
Trace	Tyndall effect present (iris details not obscured)	Occasional	Rare cell visible under high power
1+	Minimal obscuration of iris	1+	Occasional cells
2+	Mild obscuration of iris	2+	10–20 cells
3+	Moderate obscuration of iris	3+	20–30 cells
4+	Severe obscuration of iris	4+	30–40+ cells

To determine the cell and flare, the high power lens of the slit lamp with a beam that is 15 × 2 units in size, and the 900 Haag-Streit slit lamp should be used.

* Modified from Hogan et al. 1959.

Table 9–2 Grading of Cells in the Retrolental Space and Anterior Vitreous

Grade	Retrolental Space	Anterior Vitreous
Mild	1 to 10 cells	1–10 cells
Moderate	10 to 25 cells	10–60 cells
Severe	More than 25 cells	More than 60+ cells

The number of cells in the retrolental space and the anterior vitreous should be determined after dilation of the pupil.

The cells and flare occurring in the anterior chamber, retrolental space, and vitreous arise from the inflammation, and the clinician, by grading the cells and flare, can therefore determine the intensity of the uveitis and follow its progress. The cells are primarily inflammatory cells, but clumps of pigment cells and red cells may also be seen circulating in the anterior chamber.

The flare represents a Tyndall phenomenon arising from the outpouring of protein into the media during the inflammation; once the iris and ciliary vessels are damaged by the inflammation, a mild flare and (rarely) a few cells may remain after the inflammation has apparently entirely subsided. The number of anterior chamber cells and the degree of flare should be determined with the aid of the slit lamp before dilation of the pupil or instillation of fluorescein into the eye.

The number of cells in the retrolental space and vitreous should be determined after the pupil is dilated, and can best be appreciated with the aid of a Hruby lens or a contact lens (Goldmann, 1968). However, it may also be useful to visualize details in the retina with a direct ophthalmoscope. The method for grading the cells and flare in the anterior chamber is shown in Table 9–1, the method for grading the number of cells in the retrolental space in Table 9–2, and the method for grading the vitreous haze in Table 9–3.

Table 9–3 Grading of Clarity of the Vitreous

Grade	Details of Retina with Direct Ophthalmoscope
Mild	Must focus
Moderate	Details hazy
Severe	Unable to visualize

In some instances, the aqueous appears to be "frozen" because of its heavy content of fibrin; this has been termed a plasmoid aqueous. A plastic iritis appearing as a clot of fibrin may also be seen if there is a large amount of fibrin in the anterior chamber. A hypopyon may also occur (Fig. 9–2).

Keratic precipitates (KP) are deposits on the posterior surface of the cornea. They usually occur in a triangular pattern, with the base of the triangle directed inferiorly. They arise from the deposition of material (cells or cell residue) onto the endothelium, and are given the descriptive terms of fibrinous, fine, medium (Fig. 9–3), large, and giant. They may be further classified according to color: white, pigmented (Figs. 9–4, 9–5), mutton-fat, or hyalinized. The size of the keratic precipitates depends on the type of cells from which they are formed; fine KPs consist of polymorphonuclear leukocytes and lymphocytes, medium KPs consist of lymphocytes and mononuclear cells, and large and giant KPs consist of epithelioid and histiocytic mononuclear cells.

Mutton-fat KPs (Fig. 9–6) are usually large and are so named because of their greasy appearance. They are usually found in granulomatous uveitis. Hyalinized KPs have the appearance of clear glass (as in a water glass) and represent KP residue. Keratic precipitates that have been present for long periods of time are usually pigmented, but the presence of pigment can not be used as an indicator of the age of the KP (Fig. 9–7). As a general rule, pigmentation of the KP reflects the degree of pigment released into the aqueous from the inflammatory process.

Koeppe and Bussacca nodules occur in granulomatous uveitis; they represent large cellular precipitates on the iris. Koeppe nodules are located at the pupillary margin. Posterior synechiae (see below) frequently occur at the sites of Koeppe nodules. Bussacca nodules, on the other hand, are located on the surface of the iris.

Synechiae, which may occur as sequelae to any inflammation in the anterior segment, are adhesions of the iris to the cornea (anterior synechiae) or of the posterior iris to the anterior lens capsule (Fig. 9–8) or to the vitreous face if the eye is aphakic (posterior synechiae). As noted previously, posterior synechiae commonly occur in areas where Koeppe nodules are present in the iris.

Iris atrophy is occasionally seen in uveitis, especially a focal iris atrophy arising from focal herpes simplex infection of the iris (Figs. 9–9 A and B) or a segmental iris atrophy in herpes zoster ophthalmicus.

Table 9–4 Classification of Uveitis

	Nongranulomatous	Granulomatous
Anterior Uveitis		
Onset	Acute (eye red and painful)	Insidious (eye white)
KP	Small to medium, white (non-mutton-fat)	Medium to large (mutton-fat)
Fibrin	May be marked in anterior chamber	Minimal or none
Nodules	None	Surface of iris; deep in iris
Posterior Uveitis		
Onset	Acute	Insidious
Choroidal or retinal involvement	Common; nodular lesions	Rare; diffuse; edema; pigmentary changes
Vitreous	Heavy exudate, veils	None or fine punctate opacities

Classification

Uveitis has traditionally been classified into nongranulomatous and granulomatous types. However, a patient may have a uveitis that is intermediate between a granulomatous and nongranulomatous type. Although this classification of uveitis does not indicate etiology, since a granulomatous and a nongranulomatous uveitis may result from the same disease, it is useful as a means of describing the uveitis.

Nongranulomatous Uveitis

A nongranulomatous uveitis usually has an acute onset causing marked symptoms; the patient is acutely aware of the time of onset. The attack usually lasts three to six weeks and the inflammation is usually intense, much greater than in granulomatous uveitis (Table 9–4). The results of a general workup in nongranulomatous uveitis are usually not rewarding.

Granulomatous Uveitis

A granulomatous uveitis is insidious in onset. The patient complains of blurring of vision and is usually unaware of when the blurring started. Characteristically, there is minimal or no redness or pain. Large KPs and nodules may be seen in the iris, choroid, retina, or vitreous (Table 9–4).

In Hansen's disease, the uveitis may be granulomatous or nongranulomatous; iris pearls (Fig. 9–10) are often seen and are pathognomonic for the disease. Iris pearls represent tiny lepromata that gradually work their way through the interstices of the iris to lie on the face of the iris.

Fuchs' Heterochromia

Fuchs' heterochromia (Fig. 9–11) is a special form of uveitis that is insidious in onset, mild in degree, and causes few sequelae except for posterior synechiae and cataracts. The condition is usually unilateral; depigmentation and blunting of the anterior iris leaf may be seen.

Etiology

Although the classification of a uveitis into nongranulomatous and granulomatous forms does not help to establish etiology, since some known organisms may cause both types of reaction (Kimura et al., 1959), it is sometimes worthwhile to know what types of reactions various organisms might cause. Table 9–5 lists the reactions usually encountered with a variety of etiologies.

Table 9–5 Reactions Usually Encountered with Various Etiologies of Uveitis*

Etiology	Anterior		Posterior	Other Manifestations
	Nongranulomatous	Granulomatous		Comments
BACTERIAL				
Tuberculosis		Iritis	Necrotizing retinochoroiditis; miliary choroiditis; overlying vitreous opacities	Subacute endophthalmitis
Syphilis				
Tertiary	Iritis	Iritis		
Secondary	Iridocyclitis		Focal (1 mm diameter) choroiditis	Skin lesions
Congenital			Focal or geographic; chorioretinitis; optic atrophy	Hutchinson's triad; retinal pigmentation
Hansen's disease	Iritis			Granulomas of iris and ciliary body; iris atrophy, pinpoint pupils; iris pearls
Brucellosis	Iritis			Severe panuveitis
Leptospirosis	Iritis			Occasional panuveitis, occurs late
VIRAL				
Herpes simplex Virus (HSV)				
Newborn	Iritis	Iritis	Chorioretinitis; retinal folds; focal pigmented scars, usually bilateral	Corneal scarring (Type 2 HSV)
Adult	Iritis; focal iritis	Iritis	Chorioretinitis	Endotheliitis; focal iris atrophy, glaucoma
Varicella zoster (VZ)	Iridocyclitis		Occlusive vasculitis; retinal hemorrhages	Skin lesions; corneal scarring; glaucoma; iris atrophy
Cytomegalovirus (CMV)				
Newborn			Diffuse chorioretinitis, bilateral	Neurosensory defects
Adult			Focal and geographic chorioretinitis; occlusive retinal vasculitis and adjacent hemorrhage	Immunosuppressed patients
Rubella, congenital			Diffuse chorioretinitis	Microphthalmos; cataract; glaucoma; deafness; heart lesions
Subacute sclerosing panencephalitis			Focal retinitis; folds in retina; retinal edema	Neurologic involvement occurs months or years after infection, leads to death
FUNGAL				
Candida	Iridocyclitis		Multifocal retinochoroiditis	Endophthalmitis; snowball opacities in vitreous; glaucoma
Sporotrichosis			Extensive retinal necrosis	Massive destruction, anterior uvea

Table 9–5 Reactions Usually Encountered with Various Etiologies of Uveitis*

Etiology	Anterior		Posterior	Other Manifestations
	Nongranulomatous	Granulomatous		Comments
Cryptococcus	Iridocyclitis		Multifocal chorioretinitis; retinal detachment	Simultaneous central nervous system involvement; secondary cataract
Aspergillosis			Multifocal choroiditis	Fulminant endophthalmitis
Coccidioidomycosis		Iritis	Multifocal choroiditis	Granuloma formation on iris; secondary cataract
Histoplasmosis				
Presumed			Small punched out spots; subretinal neovascular network	No active inflammation; organisms never found
Endoplasmic form			Active choroiditis	Endophthalmitis; organisms have been found
PARASITES				
Toxoplasmosis		Iritis	Exudative retinochoroiditis; focal necrotizing lesions, usually in macula (near pigmented scars); sheathing of vessels; juxtapapillary lesions	Many cells in overlying vitreous
Toxocariasis			Chronic cyclitis	Pseudoglioma of posterior pole; endophthalmitis; leukocoria
Onchocerciasis	Iridocyclitis		Chorioretinitis	Located near optic nerve head
Trypanosomiasis	Iridocyclitis		Hemorrhagic retinitis	
Amebiasis				
Entamoeba histolytica			Central choroiditis; cystic lesions retina	Never verified
Acanthamoeba	Iridocyclitis			Corneal ulcer; glaucoma
Wuchereria bancrofti	Iritis			Organism in anterior chamber
Brugia malayi	Iritis			Organism in anterior chamber
Taenia solium	Iritis		Retinal granuloma	Organism in anterior chamber; organism in retina
Echinococcus	Iritis			Organism in anterior chamber
Schistosoma haematobium	Iritis			Organism in anterior chamber
Loa loa			Retinal granuloma	Organism in retina
UNKNOWN ETIOLOGY				
Fuchs' heterochromic cyclitis	Iritis			Color changes in iris; blunting of iris markings; cataract; secondary glaucoma

Table 9–5 Reactions Usually Encountered with Various Etiologies of Uveitis*

Etiology	Anterior		Posterior	Other Manifestations
	Nongranulomatous	Granulomatous		Comments
Behçet's disease	Iritis		Occlusive retinal vasculitis; vitreous hemorrhage; optic atrophy; vitreous hemorrhage	Hypopyon; aphthous ulcers; skin lesions; genital ulcers; GI, CNS involvement; systemic vascular lesions; arthritis; HLA B5 associated
Sarcoidosis	Iritis	Iridocyclitis	Focal retinitis; optic atrophy; snowball opacities; vitreous strands	Skin and lymph node involvement; cerebral involvement; conjunctival nodules; prismatic cornea; cataract
Reiter's syndrome	Iritis			Arthritis of weight-bearing joints; nongonococcal urethritis; conjunctivitis; hypopyon; keratodermia blenorrhagica; HLA B27 association
Vogt-Koyanagi-Harada syndrome	Iridocyclitis	Iridocyclitis	Multifocal choroiditis; peripapillary edema; extensive infiltration; serous renital detachment; mottled scarring; macular edema; retinal phlebitis	HLA BW-54 association; poliosis; vitiligo; tinnitus; vertigo; headache; secondary glaucoma
Pars planitis Intermediate uveitis				White snowbanking in pars plana region; posterior subcapsular cataract
Birdshot choroidopathy			Multiple cream-colored or pigmented spots	
Uveal effusion			Nonrhegmatogenous retinal detachment; depigmented flecks	
Glaucomatocyclitic crisis	Mild iritis			Dilation of pupil; glaucoma; corneal edema
Sympathetic ophthalmia		Iridocyclitis	Dalen-Fuchs' nodules	Bilateral; history of trauma to exciting eye
Lens-induced uveitis	Iritis	Iritis		Centered primarily around lens or lens fragments
Rheumatoid arthritis	Iridocyclitis			Associated with scleral or corneal involvement
Anklyosing spondylitis	Iridocyclitis		Cystoid macular edema	HLA B27 association
Juvenile rheumatoid arthritis				
Pauciarticular	Chronic iridocyclitis			Seen in young girls; leukocoria due to band-shaped keratopathy
Multiarticular	Iridocyclitis			Seen in young boys

Table 9–5 Reactions Usually Encountered with Various Etiologies of Uveitis*

Etiology	Anterior		Posterior	Other Manifestations
	Nongranulomatous	Granulomatous		Comments
Ulcerative colitis	Iridocyclitis			Synchronized with colitis and episcleritis
Polyarteritis nodosa	Iridocyclitis		Massive retinal exudation and hemorrhages; optic atrophy; retinal exudates	Associated with corneal changes, peripheral corneal thinning
Psoriasis	Acute iridocyclitis			Psoriatic changes in skin; peripheral corneal thinning
Serum sickness	Acute iridocyclitis			
Acute retinal necrosis syndrome	Iridocyclitis		Massive retinal necrosis; retinal exudate; retinal holes; retinal detachment	Associated with varicella zoster organism: necrosis occurs early
Necrotic and metastatic tumors				Flare and cells; mashed potato KPs
Anterior segment ischemia				Flare and cells; iris atrophy; corneal edema
Juvenile xanthogranuloma				Cellular proliferation on iris; vitreous cells; spontaneous anterior chamber hemorrhage
Acute multifocal posterior placoid epitheliopathy (AMPPE)	Iridocyclitis		Multiple plaques; pigment disturbance in retinal pigment epithelium	Vitreous cells
Retinal detachment				Vitreous cells
Retinitis pigmentosa			Retinal pigment epithelial changes (pigment clumping)	Vitreous cells; optic atrophy; narrowing of arterioles
Sorsby's macular degeneration			Symmetrical bilateral edema; hemorrhage; exudates in macula	Vitreous cells

* Compiled from O'Connor, 1983; Schlaegel, 1985; Uchida and Fukuka, 1967; Walkowicz et al. 1969/1970; Darrell, 1967; and Schlaegel and O'Connor, 1981.

Abbreviation used: CNS, central nervous system; GI, gastrointestinal; HLA, human leukocyte antigen

References

Darrell, RW: Acute tuberculosis panophthalmitis. *Arch. Ophthalmol.* 78: 51–54, 1967.

Goldmann, H: Biomicroscopy of the eye. *Am. J. Ophthalmol.* 66: 789–804, 1968.

Hogan, MJ, Kimura, SJ, and Thygeson, P: Signs and symptoms of uveitis. I. Anterior uveitis. *Am. J. Ophthalmol.* 47: 155–170, 1959.

Kimura, SJ, Thygeson, P, and Hogan, MJ: Signs and symptoms of uveitis. II. Classification of the posterior manifestations of uveitis. *Am. J. Ophthalmol.* 47: 171–176, 1959.

O'Connor, GR: Endogenous uveitis. Part I. In Kraus-Mackiw, E, and O'Connor, GR (eds.): *Infectious Entities in Uveitis: Pathophysiology and Therapy.* Thieme-Stratton Inc., New York, 1983.

Schlaegel, TF Jr, and O'Connor, GR: Tuberculosis and syphilis: Two forgotten diseases. *Arch. Ophthalmol.* 99: 2206–2207, 1981.

Schlaegel, TF Jr.: Etiologic diagnosis of uveitis. In Duane, TD, and Jaeger, EA (eds.): *Clinical Ophthalmology,* vol 4, sec 41, pp 1–5. Harper and Row, Philadelphia, 1985.

Uchida, Y, and Fukuka, T: Etiological classification of uveitis. *Ophthalmology (Tokyo)* 9: 940–945, 1967.

Walkowicz, ML, Hallet, JW, and Buch, H: Morphological diagnosis of uveitis — Fact or fancy. *Ann. Ophthalmol.* 1: 334–336, 1969/1970.

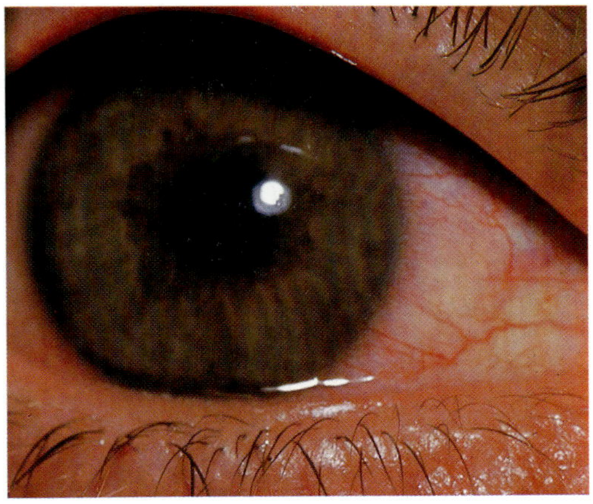

9–1 Iritis in Reiter's syndrome, showing circumcorneal injection and a muddy-appearing iris. One of the major characteristics of an acute iritis is circumcorneal injection with congestion of the iris, which imparts a muddy appearance to the substance of the iris. In this patient with Reiter's syndrome, the injection of the globe and the congestion of the iris are intense.

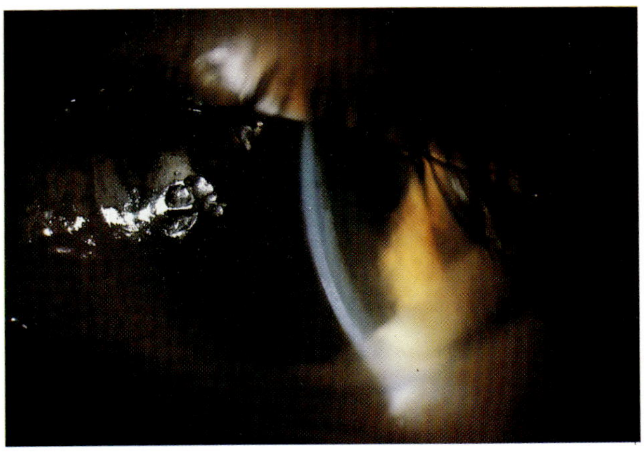

9–2 Hypopyon iritis with plasmoid aqueous. In severe iritis, the aqueous humor may become plasmoid as a result of leakage of protein from the inflamed vessels of the iris and ciliary body. In addition, a hypopyon may develop following diapedesis of white cells from the vessels. In this patient with a severe iridocyclitis, a hypopyon and clot of aqueous are evident.

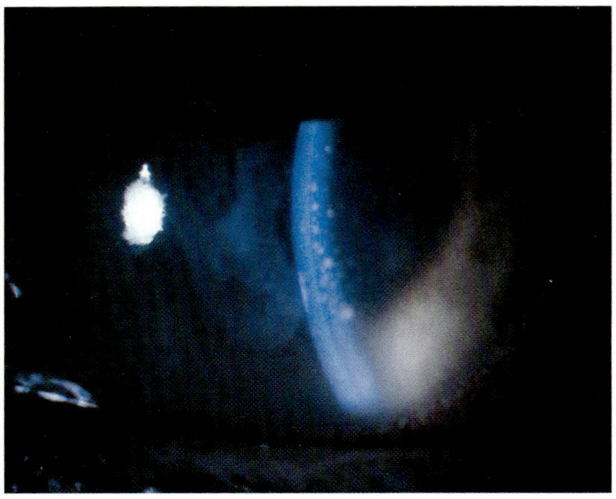

9–3 Slit lamp photograph of medium-sized, white keratic precipitates. Medium-sized, white KPs deposited on the posterior surface of the cornea are readily visible in this slit lamp photograph of a patient with acute iridocyclitis.

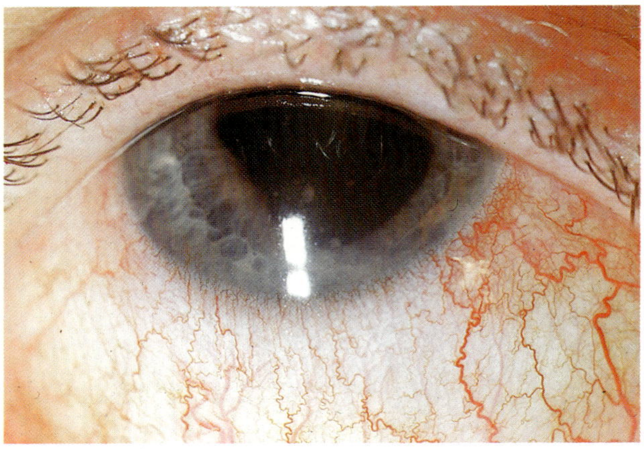

9–4 Large pigmented keratic precipitates, mild circumcorneal injection, and posterior synechiae. Keratic precipitates represent cellular and pigmentary deposits on the posterior surface of the cornea. In most instances they are deposited in a triangular pattern with the base of the triangle directed inferiorly. Pigmented KPs are often old deposits, but in some cases they merely reflect the amount of circulating pigment within the anterior chamber which is easily phagocytized by the inflammatory cells. Posterior synechiae represent adhesions between the posterior surface of the iris and the anterior surface of the lens. In this patient, a broad synechia (adhesion) is visible at the 7:00 to 9:00 region.

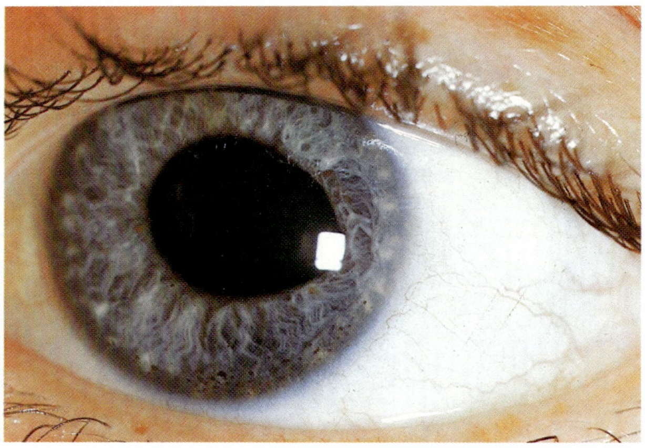

9–5 Pigmented keratic precipitates and iris atrophy. In this patient, small pigmented KPs are evident near the lower border of the pupil, and large clumps of pigmented KPs are evident in the area of the inferior angle. Iris atrophy has also occurred. In this case, both the pigmented corneal precipitates and the iris atrophy are the aftermath of a herpetic keratoiritis.

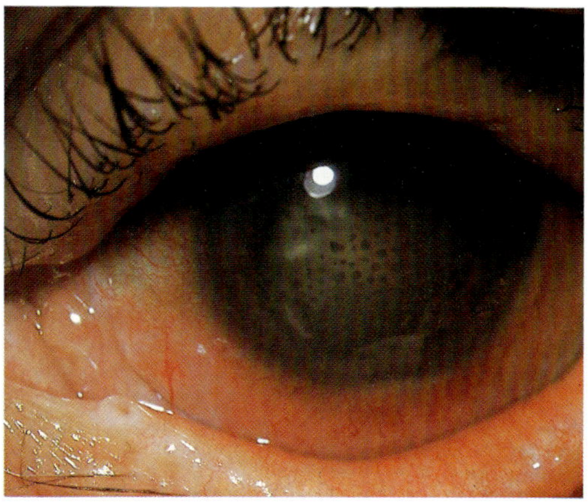

9–6 Mutton-fat keratic precipitates, hypopyon, and hypermature cataract. Mutton-fat KPs appear greasy and are usually quite large. In this patient with a severe iritis resulting from a hypermature lens, multiple, large, greasy-appearing (mutton-fat) keratic precipitates are evident. The hypopyon and iritis formed as a reaction to the lens products that have escaped from the lens capsule in this hypermature lens.

9–7 Pigmented keratic precipitates in herpes simplex keratoiritis. In this 28-year-old female, a disciform keratitis with superficial neovascularization of the cornea superiorly and multiple medium-sized pigmented KPs resulted from a prolonged herpes simplex keratoiritis.

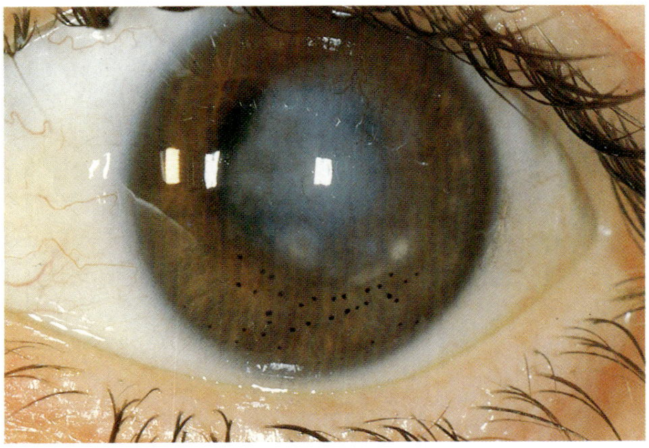

9–8 Posterior synechiae in sarcoid. Posterior synechiae (adhesion of the posterior surface of the iris to the anterior surface of the lens) frequently occurs in iritis or iridocyclitis unless treatment is prompt and adequate. The synechiae often occur at the sites of Koeppe nodules, but may occur wherever the iris is markedly inflamed and approximated to the anterior lens capsule. In this patient with sarcoid uveitis, synechiae developed for almost 360 degrees. A laser iridotomy was performed to prevent occlusion of the pupil.

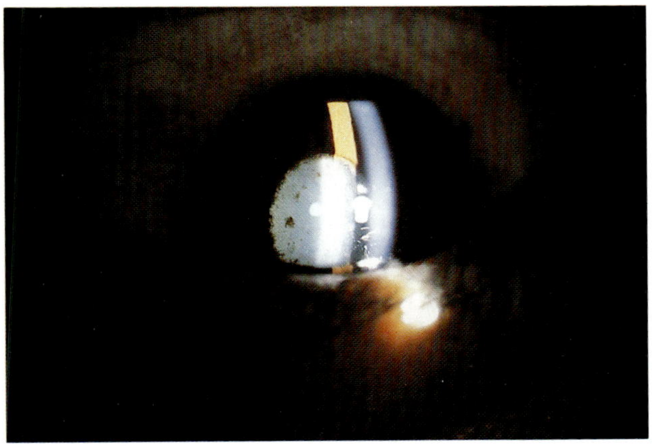

9–9A Herpes simplex focal iritis, keratic precipitates, and corneal scarring. A focal iritis may be seen in herpes simplex keratoiritis, and probably represents actual infection of the iris with the herpes virus. The iritis is usually associated with glaucoma and is often difficult to treat. In this patient with herpes simplex focal iritis, marked circumcorneal injection is evident together with a corneal scar, keratic precipitates, and neovascularization of the iris, especially at the 2:00 position.

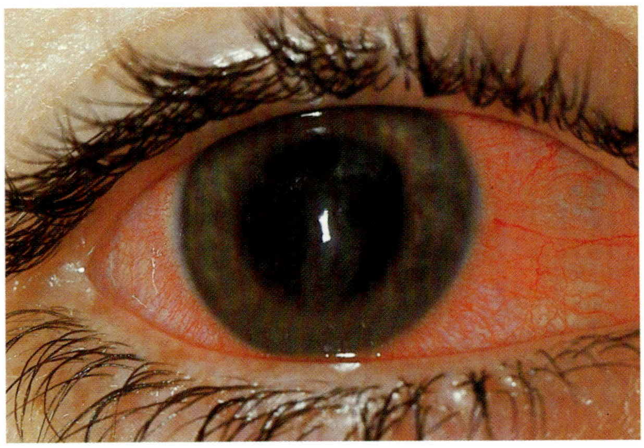

9–9B Focal iris atrophy after subsidence of herpes simplex focal iritis. This is a photograph of the patient in Fig. 9–9A, taken five months later. Iris atrophy is evident at the 2:00 area of the iris, which has caused distortion of the pupil.

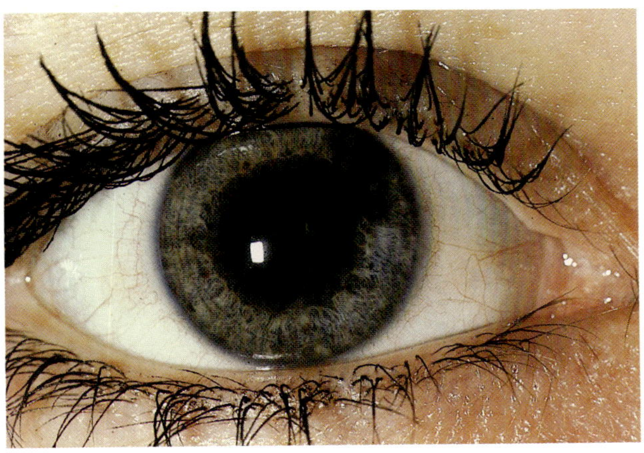

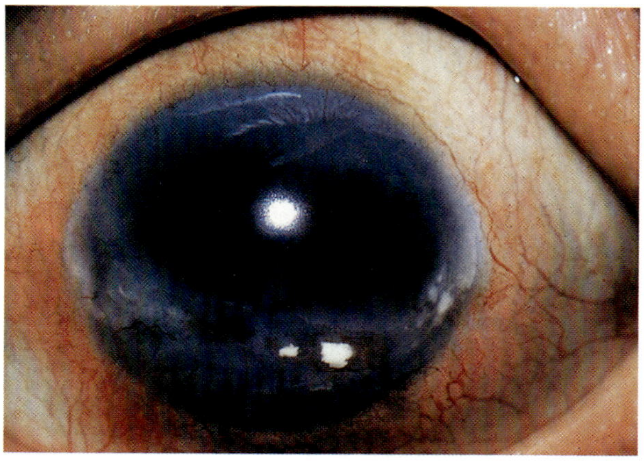

9–10 Iris pearls and iritis in Hansen's disease. Iris pearls are pathognomonic for Hansen's disease. They represent small lepromata that have "worked their way through" the interstices of the iris to reach the iris surface, or are often deposited in the inferior angle of the anterior chamber. The iris pearls resemble small grains of sand lying on the surface of the iris. In this patient, the iris pearls can be seen on the nasal side near the pupil at the 9:00 and 10:00 positions, and on the temporal side midway between the pupil and the limbus at 3:30. The severe inferior scarring of the cornea has resulted from prolonged corneal exposure.

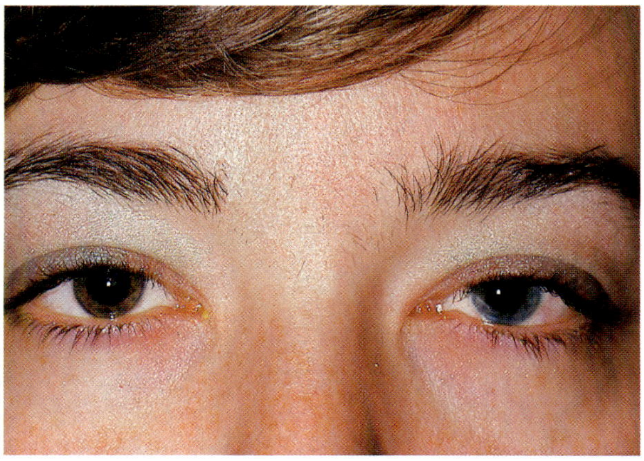

9–11 Fuchs' heterochromia. Fuchs' heterochromia is a mild form of chronic iridocyclitis that persists for many years with minimal sequelae, except for the occasional formation of posterior synechiae (where Koeppe nodules are present) and cataracts. In most instances Fuchs' heterochromia is unilateral, although bilateral cases are occasionally recognized. It is characterized by a mild inflammation of long duration, depigmentation of the iris, and a poor response to anti-inflammatory agents. Note the difference in color of the patient's two irises.

Index

Numbers refer to text pages